URVISH SHAH, M.D.

ERCP
Diagnostic and Therapeutic Applications

CURRENT TOPICS IN GASTROENTEROLOGY

Series Editor
David Zakim, MD

Vincent Astor Professor of Medicine
Cornell University Medical College
Director, Division of Digestive Diseases
The New York Hospital–Cornell Medical Center
New York

Transplantation of the Liver
Willis C. Maddrey, MD

ERCP: Diagnostic and Therapeutic Applications
Ira M. Jacobson, MD

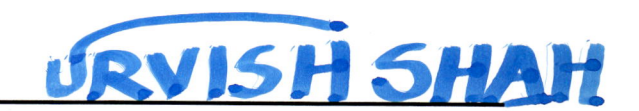

ERCP
Diagnostic and
Therapeutic Applications

Edited by

Ira M. Jacobson, MD
Assistant Professor of Medicine
Department of Medicine
The New York Hospital–Cornell Medical Center
New York

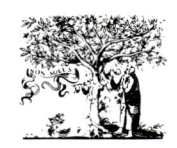

Elsevier
New York • Amsterdam • London

No responsibility is assumed by the publisher for any injury and/or damage to persons or property as a matter of products liability, negligence or otherwise, or from any use or operation of any methods, products, instructions, or ideas contained herein. No suggested test or procedure should be carried out unless, in the reader's judgment, its risk is justified. Because of rapid advances in the medical sciences, we recommend that independent verification of diagnoses and drug dosages should be made. Discussions, views, and recommendations as to medical procedures, choice of drugs, and drug dosages are the responsibility of the authors.

Elsevier Science Publishing Co., Inc.
655 Avenue of the Americas
New York, New York 10010

Sole distributors outside the United States and Canada:

Elsevier Science Publishers B.V.
P.O. Box 211, 1000 AE Amsterdam, The Netherlands

© 1989 by Elsevier Science Publishing Co., Inc.

This book has been registered with the Copyright Clearance Center, Inc.
For further information please contact the Copyright Clearance Center, Inc.,
Salem, Massachusetts.

This book is printed on acid-free paper.

Library of Congress Cataloging-in-Publication Data

ERCP : diagnostic and therapeutic applications / edited by Ira M. Jacobson.
    p. cm.—(Current topics in gastroenterology)
  Includes index.
  ISBN 0-444-01483-7 (alk. paper)
  1. Endoscopic retrograde cholangiopancreatography.   I. Jacobson, Ira M.   II. Series.
    [DNLM: 1. Cholangiopancreatography, Endoscopic Retrograde. WI 750 E65]
RC847.5.E53E73   1989
616.3'6—dc20
DNLM/DLC
for Library of Congress   89-7668
                                                                                                CIP

Current printing (last digit):
10 9 8 7 6 5 4 3 2

Manufactured in the United States of America

Contents

Foreword to the Series by David Zakim, MD / **vii**
Preface / **ix**
Contributors / **xi**

Chapter **1**
Introduction / **1**
Ira M. Jacobson, MD

Chapter **2**
ERCP in the Diagnosis of Pancreatic and Biliary Disease / **9**
Robert H. Schapiro, MD

Chapter **3**
Technique of Endoscopic Sphincterotomy / **41**
Jack A. Vennes, MD

Chapter **4**
Complications of Endoscopic Sphincterotomy / **61**
James W. Ostroff, MD, and Howard A. Shapiro, MD

Chapter **5**
Management of Bile Duct Stones Retained after Sphincterotomy / **75**
Stephen E. Silvis, MD

Chapter **6**
ERCP in Acute Cholangitis and Pancreatitis / **91**
John P. Neoptolemos, MA, MB, BChir (Cantab), MD (Leics), FRCS (Eng), and
David L. Carr-Locke, MA, MB, BChir (Cantab), MRCP (UK)

Chapter **7**
Endoscopic Sphincterotomy in Patients with Intact Gallbladders / **127**
Ira M. Jacobson, MD

Chapter 8
Function and Dysfunction of the Sphincter of Oddi / 139
James A. Gregg, MD

Chapter 9
Endoscopic Management of Benign Biliary Stricture, Biliary Tract Fistulae, and Sclerosing Cholangitis / 171
Jerome H. Siegel, MD

Chapter 10
Endoscopic Treatment in Nonmalignant Pancreatic Disease / 189
Justin H. McCarthy, MD, Joseph E. Geenen, MD, and Walter J. Hogan, MD

Chapter 11
Endoscopic Stents for Biliary Obstruction Due to Malignancy / 203
Anthony G. Speer, BE, MBBS, FRACP, and Peter B. Cotton, MD, FRCP

Chapter 12
Preoperative Biliary Decompression / 225
Robert C. Kurtz, MD

Chapter 13
Iridium-192 Irradiation of Biliary Tract Malignancy / 239
B. H. Laurence, MB, BS, BMed Sci(Hons), FRACP

Chapter 14
Direct Cholangiopancreatoscopy / 251
Richard A. Kozarek, MD

Index / 263

Foreword to the Series

The fund of knowledge and technology that is the basis for practicing gastroenterology has increased rapidly in the recent past. And, as for other medical specialties, there is good reason to believe that the rate of this increase is accelerating. Thus, advances in science and engineering are illuminating new ways to think about, to investigate, and to interdict the pathophysiology of digestive diseases. This kind of maturation of a field leads naturally to fragmentation of the knowledge-base and its diffusion through an ever-expanding literature.

While these developments pose problems for gastroenterologists, they are not to be lamented. They attest to the strong scientific base and intellectual vitality of our speciality. On the other hand, the problem of keeping current with a rapidly expanding discipline needs to be addressed, which is the purpose of the series *Current Topics in Gastroenterology*. Each volume in this series will be a critical and definitive synthesis of the knowledge-base in a selected topic. Each volume will be organized around a set of closely related clinical problems of broad concern to gastroenterologists and will provide up-to-date discussions of clinical issues as well as the scientific background needed to interpret clinical data in the context of current concepts of pathophysiology. Because of their organization, the volumes in the series will provide more penetrating analyses of problems than are usually available in textbooks; yet each volume will be "user friendly" because of its size and readability. The series approach to publishing an extended treatise on gastroenterology also acknowledges that different aspects of the field are likely to advance at different rates. Our hope is that *Current Topics in Gastroenterology* will help to define the field of gastroenterology as it expands and that it will provide practicing gastroenterologists, academicians, and investigators alike with an exciting set of books for keeping current with the expanding frontiers of our specialty.

David Zakim, MD

Preface

The introduction of ERCP as a diagnostic procedure was followed by its adaptation as a powerful therapeutic tool. Each application of ERCP has required critical evaluation of its indications, efficacy, limitations, and complications. With each innovation it has been necessary to formulate strategies to address still unsettled problems, such as unextractable common duct stones and clogging of stents, to name just two examples.

Predictably, a wealth of literature addressing all the facets of this complex procedure has appeared. Many of the major contributions to the field have been made, and continue to be made, by pioneers of ERCP with vast experience in this procedure. Even among internationally known authorities, diverse approaches to the same problem may exist. Increasing numbers of endoscopists are performing the procedure, and changes in the volume of cases are inevitable at many centers. As ERCP becomes more widely available, critical assessment of its applications becomes ever more important.

The goal of this volume is to provide, under one cover, a comprehensive, critical review of the present status of ERCP and its evolving applications. As such it is intended not only for those who perform these procedures, but for all physicians and surgeons who care for patients with pancreatic and biliary disease. Experienced authorities have contributed reviews of specific areas in which they have worked extensively and, in many cases, have played a major developmental role. Where appropriate, their personal experience has been integrated into a more general discussion. The major themes of the book include the basis for our present applications of ERCP, questions about ERCP that still need to be answered, including areas of controversy, and the techniques in an early phase of development that promise to make this an exciting, dynamic field for many years to come.

Contributors

David L. Carr-Locke, MA, MB, BChir (Cantab), FRCP (UK)
Consultant Physician in Gastroenterology, Department of Gastroenterology, Leicester Royal Infirmary, Leicester, England

Peter B. Cotton, MD, FRCP
Professor of Medicine, Department of Medicine and Gastroenterology, Duke University, Durham, North Carolina

Joseph E. Geenen, MD
Clinical Professor of Medicine, Medical College of Wisconsin; Director, Digestive Disease Center, St. Luke's Hospital, Racine, Wisconsin

James A. Gregg, MD
Assistant Clinical Professor of Medicine, Harvard Medical School; Gastroenterologist, New England Deaconess Hospital, New England Baptist Hospital, Boston, Massachusetts

Walter J. Hogan, MD
Professor of Medicine, and Chief, Gastrointestinal Diagnostic Section, Medical College of Wisconsin, Milwaukee

Ira M. Jacobson, MD
Assistant Professor of Medicine, Department of Medicine, The New York Hospital-Cornell Medical Center, New York

Richard A. Kozarek, MD
Associate Clinical Professor of Medicine, University of Washington, Section of Therapeutic Endoscopy, Virginia Mason Clinic, Seattle, Washington

Robert C. Kurtz, MD
Associate Attending Physician, Gastroenterology Service, Department of Medicine, Memorial Sloan-Kettering Cancer Center, New York

B. H. Laurence, MB, BS, BMed Sci (Hons), FRACP
Gastroenterologist, Gastroenterology/Liver Unit, Sir Charles Gairdner Hospital, Western Australia, Australia

Justin H. McCarthy, BSC (Med), PhD, FRACP, MBBS
Assistant Professor of Medicine, University of Texas, Southwestern Medical School; Director of Therapeutic Endoscopy, Parkland Memorial Hospital, Dallas, Texas

John P. Neoptolemos, MA, MB, BChir (Cantab), MD (Leics), FRCS (Eng)
Senior Lecturer, Department of Surgery, University of Birmingham Honorary Consultant Surgeon, Dudley Road Hospital, Birmingham, England; Hunterian Professor of Surgery, Royal College of Surgeons of England

James W. Ostroff, MD
Clinical Assistant Professor of Medicine, Department of Medicine, University of California at San Francisco

Robert H. Schapiro, MD
Associate Clinical Professor of Medicine, Harvard Medical School; Physician and Director, Gastrointestinal Endoscopy, Massachusetts General Hospital, Boston, Massachusetts

Howard A. Shapiro, MD
Clinical Professor of Medicine, Department of Medicine, University of California at San Francisco

Jerome H. Siegel, MD, FACP
Assistant Clinical Professor of Medicine, Mount Sinai School of Medicine, City University of New York (CUNY); Chief, Gastroenterology, Doctors Hospital, New York

Stephen E. Silvis, MD
Staff Physician, Minneapolis Veterans Administration Medical Center; Professor of Medicine, University of Minnesota, Minneapolis

Anthony G. Speer, BE, MBBS, FRACP
Gastroenterologist, Department of Gastroenterology, The Royal Melbourne Hospital, Parkville, Victoria, Australia

Jack A. Vennes, MD
Professor of Medicine, University of Minnesota, Minneapolis Veterans Administration Medical Center, Minneapolis

Chapter 1

Introduction

Ira M. Jacobson, M.D.

It is just two decades since pioneering endoscopists began to cannulate the papilla of Vater under direct vision with fiberoptic endoscopes.[1-6] The first endoscopic sphincterotomies were reported about 5 years later.[7-10] By the early 1980s, with the accumulation of experience with nasobiliary tubes[11,12] and, shortly thereafter, endoprostheses,[13-15] the basic tools in the therapeutic biliary endoscopist's armamentarium were in place.

During the years since these early developments, endoscopic retrograde cholangiopancreatography (ERCP) has profoundly altered the diagnostic and therapeutic approach to patients with pancreatic and biliary disease, to a degree that rivals the changes wrought by revolutionary technological advances in other branches of gastroenterology and medicine. The modern trainee in gastroenterology would do well to read the early reports in this field to grasp a sense of the excitement and challenge experienced by those who crossed the frontier into this previously inaccessible area.

Paralleling the evolution of ERCP was the development of percutaneous transhepatic cholangiography, which was given particular impetus by the introduction of the Chiba thin-needle technique.[16,17] Percutaneous transhepatic biliary drainage preceded endoscopic biliary drainage by a very short time.[18-21] Similarly, extraction of common bile duct stones through the tract of a T tube with a Dormia basket and steerable catheter was introduced slightly before endoscopic sphincterotomy.[22] In many places the development of percutaneous and endoscopic techniques proceeded simultaneously.[23]

In the early phases of their evolution, percutaneous and endoscopic biliary techniques were often viewed as competitive and tended to be developed independently, with little collaboration between radiologists and endoscopists. Some groups did, however, perform comparative trials.[24,25] Particularly gratifying in recent years have been collaborative efforts between radiologists and endoscopists in the performance of difficult sphincterotomies and in the placement of biliary stents.[26-32] Implicit in this trend is a growing, if not universal, consensus that for the diagnosis and nonsurgical treatment of obstructive jaundice, ERCP is the preferred initial modality, except, arguably, for patients with obstruction of the proximal biliary tree. Endoscopists, on the other hand, are prepared to defer to interventional radiologists for certain problems, such as retained bile duct stones in patients with T tubes.[33]

The cornerstone of therapeutic ERCP, endoscopic sphincterotomy, emerged relatively rapidly as the preferred treatment for common duct stones in patients who have had a cholecystectomy. Rates of success at performing sphincterotomy were over 90–95% in experienced hands[34–41] and for clearance of duct stones about 85–90%.[37–39,41] The efficacy of the procedure, combined with the avoidance of general anesthesia and an abdominal incision, and the decrease in cost and hospitalization time, were so appealing that surgery was relegated to a subsidiary role in many centers. In retrospect it is striking, and a tribute to the success of the technique's early pioneers, that this development occurred in the absence of any controlled trials comparing endoscopic sphincterotomy with surgery. In this respect the evolution of sphincterotomy was somewhat analogous to that of colonoscopic polypectomy. It is not obvious that this should have been so given the greater risk in sphincterotomy than in polypectomy, the fact that it alters a physiologic function, and the concern about late stenosis—factors that were the basis for serious reservations about sphincterotomy in some parts of the medical and especially surgical communities. Nevertheless, the mortality rate of 0.5–1.2% for sphincterotomy[34–39] compared favorably with figures such as 2.1%[42] for choledochotomy and 2.9%[43] for elective cholecystectomy and choledocholithotomy. Even if mortality rates are comparable in young patients, it should be realized that mortality rates for biliary surgery rise with age,[42,44] and that published figures for endoscopic sphincterotomy were derived in large part from experience with high-risk patients.[39]

The complication rate of 6–10%[34–39] for sphincterotomy, on the other hand, clearly separates it, along with the low but real mortality, from virtually all other endoscopic procedures in terms of degree of risk. Biliary endoscopists must convey a healthy respect for this procedure to their trainees and other colleagues. Such considerations and the intrinsic complexity of the procedure have led to attempts to establish guidelines for eligibility to perform sphincterotomy, along with the caveat that most gastroenterological trainees should not expect to master this procedure during their fellowships.[45] The additional concerns about long-term complications related to loss of sphincter of Oddi function or stenosis led no less an authority than Classen to write as recently as 1986 that he reserves sphincterotomy for patients over 50.[46] However, such concerns appear to be abating with the appearance of long-term reports demonstrating relatively low rates of restenosis or stone recurrence, and few if any problems related to bactobilia.[47–48]

Even as sphincterotomy continues to be offered as the treatment of choice to most patients with choledocholithiasis following cholecystectomy, we must critically evaluate its expanding applications to other groups. Only careful long-term studies[49–51] are assuring us that the increasingly popular practice of performing sphincterotomy in patients with intact gallbladders is appropriate for elderly or sick patients. These results cannot be extrapolated to other patients. As another example, in patients with acute biliary pancreatitis it is useful to show that urgent sphicterotomy is no more hazardous than routine sphincterotomy and that it appears to abort the illness.[52,53] But even better, albeit quite difficult to perform, are randomized controlled trials such as the recent one from the Leicester group[54] defining which patients appear to benefit from early endoscopic intervention.

The suitability of endoscopic placement of stents for malignant biliary strictures has been subjected to controlled trials,[55,56] but here too the relative simplicity and conceptual appeal of the procedure, along with high published success rates,[57,58] were more instrumental in leading to its widespread adoption. Some surgical protagonists continue to argue that since the stents eventually clog, and duodenal obstruction may develop, the extent to which they reduce hospitalization time over the course of the patient's lifetime requires further assessment. One study of transhepatic stents versus surgery did not, in fact, demonstrate a difference in total hospitalization time,[59] while in at least one study of endoscopic stents versus surgery stents did emerge favorably.[55]

There are other areas in which the application of presently available technology requires further evaluation. For example, we still need to know if preoperative biliary drainage by the endoscopic route will fare better in prospective, randomized trials than did percutaneous drainage.[60–62] It is still unclear if and when biliary endoscopists must perform sphincter of Oddi manometry—as suggested by the meticulous studies of Geenen, Hogan, and co-workers[63] without universal agreement[64]—in order to identify optimally those patients with suspected "papillary stenosis" or "biliary dyskinesia" who are likely to benefit from ablation of the sphincter of Oddi. We need more data on the significance of various manometric abnormalities and their response to treatment. In patients with benign biliary strictures[65] and sclerosing cholangitis,[66] questions remain about patient selection and optimal nonsurgical techniques, and longer term follow-up of patients who have been treated endoscopically will be required.

Many applications in early phases of development are being explored with great interest. A major remaining frontier is the pancreas. Endoscopic therapy of pancreatic disease has recently come under critical evaluation.[67] Cholangioscopes, which can be passed through the channel of standard large-channel duodenoscopes, have intriguing diagnostic and therapeutic potential. Such forms of therapy as electrohydraulic lithotripsy or laser therapy may, for example, be applicable through such instruments.[68] Extracorporeal shock wave lithotripsy seems likely to influence our management of some large bile duct stones.[69] The implantation of radiotherapeutic agents through endoscopes may add to our ability to treat the usually refractory malignancies that affect the bile duct.[70,71] Whether or not we are able to affect the growth of tumors by endoscopic techniques, our management of patients with biliary strictures might be improved by the introduction of nonclogging stents as we learn more about the mechanisms of clogging.[72,73]

The rate of progress in the field of ERCP leaves little doubt that techniques now in an early phase of development will emerge as standard approaches to pancreaticobiliary problems in the next 10 years, just as has happened during the last decade. Inevitably, the number of patients with biliary and pancreatic disease who can be treated nonsurgically by endoscopic or other methods will increase still further, and refinements can be expected in areas where patients already are being treated nonsurgically. Even as this occurs, collaboration with surgical and radiologic colleagues remains essential; and endoscopists must continue to critically evaluate and report the successes, limitations, and complications of their techniques, including comparisons with other modalities, if ERCP is to completely fulfill its enormous potential.

References

1. Watson WC: Direct vision of the ampulla of Vater with the gastroduodenal fiberscope. *Lancet* 1966;1:902–903.

2. McCune WS, Short PE, and Moscovitz H: Endoscopic cannulation of the ampulla of Vater. *Ann Surg* 1968;167:752–756.
3. Oi I, Takemoto T, and Kondo T: Fiberduodenoscope: Direct observation of the papilla of Vater. *Endoscopy* 1970;17:59–62.
4. Takagi K, Ikeda S, Nakagawa Y, Sakaguchi N, Takahashi T, Kumakura K, Maruyama M, Someya N, Nakano H, Takeda T, Takekoshi T, and Kim T: Retrograde pancreatography and cholangiography by fiberduodenoscope. *Gastroenterology* 1970; 59:445–452.
5. Cotton PB, Salmon PR, Beales JSM, and Burwood RJ: Endoscopic trans-papillary radiographs of pancreatic and bile ducts. *Gastrointest Endosc* 1972;19:60–62.
6. Kawai K, Akasaka Y, Murakami K, et al: Endoscopic sphincterotomy of the ampulla of Vater. *Gastrointest Endosc* 1974;20:148–151.
7. Classen M, and Demling L: Endoskopische Sphinkterotomie der papilla Vateri and Steinextraktion aus dem Ductus choledochus. *Dtsch Med Wochenschr* 1974;496–497.
8. Classen M, and Safrany L: Endoscopic papillotomy and removal of gallstones. *Br Med J*: 1975;4:371–374.
9. Zimmon DS, Falkenstein DB, and Kessler RE: Endoscopic papillotomy for choledocholithiasis. *N Engl J Med* 1975;293:1181–1182.
10. Cotton PB, Chapman M, Whiteside CG, and LeQuesne LP: Duodenoscopic papillotomy and gallstone removal. *Br J Surg* 1976;63:709–714.
11. Wurbs D, Classen M: Transpapillary long-standing tube for hepatobiliary drainage. *Endoscopy* 1977;9:192–193.
12. Cotton PB, Burney PG, and Mason RR: Transnasal bile duct catheterization after endoscopic sphincterotomy: Method for biliary drainage, perfusion and sequential cholangiography. *Gut* 1979;20:285–287.
13. Sohendra N, and Reijnders-Frederix V: Palliative bile duct drainage. A new endoscopic method of introducing a transpapillary drain. *Endoscopy* 1980;12:8–11.
14. Laurence BH, and Cotton PB: Decompression of malignant biliary obstruction by duodenoscopic intubation of bile duct. *Br Med J* 1980;280:522–523.
15. Huibregtse K, and Tytgat GN: Palliative treatment of obstructive jaundice by transpapillary introduction of large bore bile duct endoprostheses: Experience in 45 patients. *Gut* 1982;23:371–375.
16. Tsuchiya Y: A new safer method of percutaneous transhepatic cholangiography. *Jpn J Gastroenterol* 1969;66:438–452.
17. Okuda K, Tanikawa K, Emura T, Kuratomi S, Jinnouchi S, Urabe K, Sumikoshi T, Kanda Y, Fukuyama Y, Musha H, Mori H, Shimokawa Y, Yakushija F, and Matsuura Y: Nonsurgical percutaneous transhepatic cholangiography: Diagnostic significance in medical problems of the liver. *Am J Dig Dis* 1974;19:21–36.
18. Kaude JV, Weidenheimer CH, and Agee OF: Decompression of bile ducts with the percutaneous transhepatic technic. *Radiology* 1969;93:69–71.
19. Nakayama T, Ikeda A, and Okuda K: Percutaneous transhepatic drainage of the biliary tract: technique and results in 104 cases. *Gastroenterology* 1978;74:554–59.
20. Ring EJ, Oleaga JA, Freiman DB, Husted JW, and Lunderquist A: Therapeutic applications of catheter cholangiography. *Radiology* 1978;128:333–338.
21. Hoevels J, Lunderquist A, and Ihse I: Percutaneous transhepatic intubation of bile ducts for combined internal-external drainage in preoperative and palliative treatment of obstructive jaundice. *Gastrointest Radiol* 1978;3:23–31.
22. Burhenne HJ: The technique of biliary duct stone extraction. *Radiology* 1974;113:567–572.
23. Mason RR: Percutaneous extraction of retained gallstones. *Clinics in Gastroenterology* 1985;14:403–419.
24. Matzen P, Malchow-Moller A, Lejerstofte J, Stoge P, and Juhl E: Endoscopic retrograde cholangiopancreatography and transhepatic cholangiography in patients with suspected obstructive jaundice. A randomized study. *Scand J Gastroenterol* 1982;17:731–735.

25. Speer AG, Cotton PB, Russell RCG, Mason RR, Hatfield ARW, Leung JWC: Randomized trial of endoscopic versus percutaneous stent insertion in malignant obstructive jaundice. *Lancet* 1987;2:57–62.
26. Long WB, Schwarz W, and Ring EJ: Endoscopic sphincterotomy assisted by catheterization antegrade. *Gastrointest Endosc* 1984;30:36–39.
27. Shorvon PJ, Cotton PB, Mason RR, Siegel JH, and Hatfield AR: Percutaneous transhepatic assistance for duodenoscopic sphincterotomy. *Gut* 1985;26:1373–1376.
28. Tanaka M, Matsumoto S, Ikeda S, Miyazaki K, and Yamauchi S: Endoscopic sphincterotomy in patients with difficult cannulation: use of an antegrade guide. *Endoscopy* 1986;18:87–89.
29. Tsang T-K, Crampton AR, Bernstein JR, Ramos SR, and Wieland JM: Percutaneous-endoscopic biliary stent placement: a preliminary report. *Ann Intern Med* 106:389–392.
30. Robertson DAF, Ayres R, Hacking CN, Shepherd H, Birch S, and Wright R: Experience with a combined percutaneous and endoscopic approach to stent insertion in malignant obstructive jaundice. *Lancet* 1987;2:1449–1452.
31. Brambs HJ, Billman P, Pausch J, Holstege A, and Salm R: Non-surgical biliary drainage: Endoscopic conversion of percutaneous transhepatic into endoprosthetic drainage. *Endoscopy* 1986;18:52–54.
32. Kerr RM, and Gilliam JH III: The team approach to biliary tract intervention: current status of combined percutaneous-endoscopic techniques. *Gastrointest Endosc* 1988;432–434.
33. Lambert ME, Martin DF, and Tweedle DEF: Endoscopic removal of retained stones after biliary surgery. *Br J Surg* 1988;75:896–898.
34. Safrany L: Duodenoscopic sphincterotomy and gallstone removal. *Gastroenterology* 1977;72;338–343.
35. Nakajima M, Kizu M, Akasaka Y, and Kawai K: Five years experience of endoscopic sphincterotomy in Japan: a collective study from 25 centers. *Endoscopy* 1979;11:138–141.
36. Seifert E, Endoscopic papillotomy and removal of gallstones. *Am J Gastroenterol* 1978;69:154–159.
37. Geenen JE, Vennes JA, and Silvis SE: Resume of a seminar on endoscopic retrograde sphincterotomy (ERS). *Gastrointest Endosc* 1981;27:31–38.
38. Leese T, Neoptolemos JP, and Carr-Locke DL: Successes, failures, early complications and their management following endoscopic sphincterotomy: Results in 394 consecutive patients from a single centre. *Br J Surg* 1985;72:215–219.
39. Cotton PB: Endoscopic management of bile duct stones; (apples and oranges). *Gut* 1984;25:587–597.
40. Siegel JH: Endoscopic papillotomy in the treatment of biliary tract disease: 258 procedures and results. *Dig Dis Sci* 1981;26:1057–1064.
41. Haagenmuller F, and Classen M: Therapeutic endoscopic and percutaneous procedures for biliary disorders. In: Popper, H., Schaffner, F., eds.: *Progress in Liver Disease*, New York, Grune and Stratton, 1982, pp. 299–318.
42. McSherry CK, and Glenn F: The incidence and causes of death following surgery for nonmalignant biliary tract disease. *Ann Surg* 1980;191:271–275.
43. Martin JK, Jr, and van Heerden JA: Surgery of the liver, biliary tract, and pancreas. *Mayo Clin Proc* 1980;55:333–337.
44. Doyle PJ, Ward-McQuaid JN, and McEwen-Smith A: The value of routine pre-operative cholangiography: A report of 4000 cholecystectomies. *Br J Surg* 1982;69:617–619.
45. Cohen S, Sachar DB, Eitan A, Lee W, Sorrell MF, and Duane W: Training and third-tier certification in gastroenterology. *Gastroenterology* 1988;94:1083–1086.
46. Classen M: Endoscopic papillotomy. In: Sivak, M.V., Jr.: *Gastroenterologic Endoscopy*. Philadelphia, W.B. Saunders, 1987, pp. 631–651.
47. Hawes R, Vallon AG, Holton JM, and Cotton PB: Long term follow-up after duoden-

oscopic sphincterotomy (DS) for choledocholithiasis in patients with prior cholecystectomy. *Gastrointest Endosc* 1987;33:157 (Abstract).
48. Riemann JF, Lux G, Forster P, and Altendorf A: Long-term results after endoscopic papillotomy, *Endoscopy* 1983;15:165–68.
49. Rosseland AR, and Solhaug JH: Primary endoscopic papillotomy (EPT) in patients with stones in the common bile duct and the gallbladder in situ: A 5–8 year follow-up study. *World J Surg* 1988;12:111–116.
50. Davidson BR, Neoptolemos JP, and Carr-Locke DL: Endoscopic sphincterotomy for common bile duct calculi in patients with gallbladder in situ considered unfit for surgery. *Gut* 1988;29:114–120.
51. Cotton PB: 2–9 year followup after sphincterotomy for stones in patients with gallbladders. *Gastrointest Endosc* 1986;32:157 (Abstract).
52. Safrany L, and Cotton PB: A preliminary report: Urgent duodenoscopic sphincterotomy for acute gallstone pancreatitis. *Surgery* 1981;89:424–428.
53. Escourrou J, Liguory C, Boyer J, and Sahel J: Emergency endoscopic sphincterotomy in acute biliary pancreatitis: Results of a multicenter study. *Gastrointest Endosc* 1987;33:187 (Abstract).
54. Neoptolemos JP, Carr-Locke DL, London NJ, Bailey IA, James D, and Fossard DP: Controlled trial of urgent endoscopic retrograde cholangiopancreatography and endoscopic sphincterotomy versus conservative treatment for acute pancreatitis due to gallstones. *Lancet* 1988;2:979–983.
55. Shepherd HA, Royle G, Ross APR, Diba A, Arthur M, and Colin-Jones D: Endoscopic biliary endoprosthesis in the palliation of malignant obstruction of the distal common bile duct: a randomized trial. *Br J Surg* 1988;75:1166–1168.
56. Dowsett JF, Russell RCG, Hatfield ARW, et al: Malignant obstructive, jaundice: A prospective randomized trial of by-pass surgery versus endoscopic stenting. *Gastroenterology* 1989;96:A128.
57. Huibregtse K, Katon RM, Coene PP, and Tytgat GNJ: Endoscopic palliative treatment in pancreatic cancer. *Gastrointest Endosc* 1986;32:334.
58. Siegel JH, and Snady H: The significance of endoscopically placed prostheses in the management of biliary obstruction due to carcinoma of the pancreas: Results of nonoperative decompression in 277 patients. *Am J Gastroenterol* 1986;81:634.
59. Bornman PC, Harries-Jones EP, Tobias R, Van Steigmann G, Terblanche J: Prospective controlled trial of transhepatic biliary endoprostheses versus bypass surgery for incurable carcinoma of head of pancreas. *Lancet* 1986;1:69–71.
60. Hatfield ARW, Tobias R, Terblanche J, Girdwood AH, Fataar S, Harries-Jones R, Kernoff L, and Marks IN: Preoperative external drainage in obstructive jaundice: A prospective controlled clinical trial. *Lancet* 1982;2:896–899.
61. McPherson GAD, Benjamin IS, Hodgson HJF, Bowley NB, Allison DJ, and Blumgart LH: Preoperative percutaneous biliary drainage: the results of a controlled trial. *Br J Surg* 1984;71:371–375.
62. Pitt HA, Gomes AS, Lois JF, Monn LL, Deutsch LS, and Longmire WP: Does preoperative percutaneous biliary drainage reduce operative risk or increase hospital cost? *Ann Surg* 1985;201:545–553.
63. Geenen JE, Hogan WJ, Dodds WJ, Toouli J, Venu RP: The efficacy of endoscopic sphincterotomy after cholecystectomy in patients with sphincter-of-Oddi dysfunction. *N Engl J Med* 1989;320:82–87.
64. Thatcher BS, Sivak MV, Jr, Tedesco FJ, Vennes JA, Hutton SW, and Achkar EA: Endoscopic sphincterotomy for suspected dysfunction of the sphincter of Oddi. *Gastrointest Endosc* 1987;33:91–95.
65. Huibregtse K, Katon RM, and Tytgat GN: Endoscopic treatment of benign biliary strictures. *Endoscopy* 1986;18:133–137.
66. Johnson GK, Geenen JE, Venu RP, and Hogan WJ: Endoscopic treatment of biliary duct strictures in sclerosing cholangitis: Follow-up assessment of a new therapeutic approach. *Gastrointest Endosc* 1987;33:9–12.

67. Geenen JE: A/S/G/E Distinguished Lecture: Endoscopic therapy of pancreatic disease: A new horizon. *Gastrointest Endosc* 1988;34:386–389.
68. Kozarek RA, Low DE, Ball TJ: Tunable dye laser lithotripsy: In vitro studies and in vivo treatment of choledocholithiasis. *Gastrointest Endosc* 1988;34:418–420.
69. Sauerbruch T, Stern M, and the Study Group for Shock-Wave Lithotripsy of Bile Duct Stones: Fragmentation of bile duct stones by extracorporeal shock waves: a new approach to biliary calculi after failure of routine endoscopic measures. *Gastroenterology* 1989;96:146–152.
70. Siegel JH, Pullano W, Ramsey WH, Rosenbaum A, Halpern G, Nonkin R, Jacob H, Lichenstein J: Endotherapy: Iridium implantation and drainage. One step therapy for malignant biliary obstruction. *Gastrointest Endosc* 1987:33:177–78.
71. Levitt MD, Laurence BH, Cameron F, and Klemp PF: Transpapillary iridium-192 wire in the treatment of malignant biliary tract obstruction. *Gut* 1988;29:149–52.
72. Groen AK, Out T, Huibregtse K, Delzenne B, Hoek FJ, Tytgat GNJ: Characterization of the content of occluded biliary endoprostheses. *Endoscopy* 1987;19:57–59.
73. Speer AG, Cotton PB, Rode J, Seddon AM, Neal CR, Holton J, and Costerton JW: Biliary stent blockage with bacterial biofilm. A light and electron microscopic study. *Ann Intern Med* 1988;108:546–553.

Chapter 2

ERCP in the Diagnosis of Pancreatic and Biliary Disease

Robert H. Schapiro, M.D.

Introduction

Over the last decade and a half, the diagnostic landscape available for the evaluation of pancreatic and biliary disorders has been transformed from a desert to a jungle. A surfeit of new technologies competes for the clinician's attention. These include imaging techniques such as ultrasound (US), computerized body tomography (CBT), magnetic resonance imaging (MRI), and nuclear medicine scans (HIDA), as well as direct cholangiographic and pancreatographic techniques using percutaneous (PTC) or endoscopic (ERCP) approaches. Furthermore, these new techniques provide a platform for additional diagnostic and therapeutic manipulations including biopsy, aspiration, stone removal, and placement of stents and drains. The task of the clinician is to select the proper test or sequence of tests for safe, accurate, and efficient diagnosis and therapy.

With the current climate of cost control, it is no longer acceptable to fire both barrels of the shotgun at a clinical problem. However, the least expensive test is not necessarily the most cost-effective if it is imprecise or delays resolution of the problem. What may be acceptable in the unhurried investigation of intermittent abdominal pain in an outpatient setting may not be appropriate for the ill, hospitalized patient with a high probability of organic disease. If cost accounting is to be realistic, an inexpensive study that prolongs a hospital stay by even 1 day becomes an expensive study.

I believe that the development of new therapeutic endoscopic techniques, as well as the need for efficient diagnosis, has increased the importance of ERCP in the approach to pancreatic and biliary disease.

Initial Resistance to ERCP

In the past, ERCP suffered under the burdens of being thought too difficult, too invasive, and too costly. As experience has expanded, both in number of procedures and in number of practitioners, it has become clear that the first two of these objections are overstated while the third one may be largely artificial. As an advanced endoscopic technique, ERCP requires prior mastery of conventional esophagogastroduodenoscopy, an apprenticeship in which the peculiar "tricks of the trade" of cannulation are learned and practiced, and continued exposure to maintain expertise. Not every gastrointestinal trainee will want to invest the time and effort necessary to acquire this skill, nor in a given medical center will the demand for this skill be sufficient for every gastrointestinal endoscopist to be effective at ampullary cannulation.

Nevertheless, the numerous GI training programs and the widespread geographic dissemination of capable practitioners has assured that someone will be available in most sizable urban and suburban areas who can provide this service. Reasonable skill at ERCP means the ability to cannulate the duct of choice at least 85%, and preferably 95%, of the time,[1] and in most cases to be able to perform the procedure in substantially less than a half hour. The degree of discomfort experienced by the patient should be akin to that of conventional upper endoscopy, and the patient certainly should not remember the experience as an ordeal. Cannulation of the ampulla of Vater in patients who have had a previous partial gastrectomy with Billroth I anastamosis should be equally facile. A Billroth II anastamosis will reduce the success rate to about 50%.[2] After partial gastrectomy with Roux-en-Y gastrojejunostomy, success is very rare.

Although the "invasive" nature of ERCP has been stressed, in truth the complication rate associated with the procedure is quite modest. In 1975, Takemoto reported that the total Japanese experience to that date included an overall complication rate of 1.19%, with a fatality rate of 0.12%.[3] In the interim, similar figures have been reported from widely separate areas, with the most recent report[4] quoting 0.8% complications with one death in 1,930 cases (0.05%). Serious complications can be roughly divided, in order of frequency, into those due to pancreatitis, sepsis, and mechanical perforation. While striking (4–30) postprocedure serum elevations of a variety of pancreas-derived enzymes (amylase, isoamylase, lipase, trypsin, elastase) are very common,[5,6] symptomatic pancreatitis requiring hospitalization is said to occur in less than 1% of diagnostic studies. This complication may tend to be underestimated, however, as the occurence of pancreatitis in various series has ranged from 1% to as high as 7%.[4] Clearly, the frequency with which pancreatitis occurs may reflect the vigor with which pancreatic duct injection is pursued. Repeated injections into the pancreatic duct[7] and overfilling with acinarization, or more importantly, urographic visualization,[8] have been implicated as increasing the likelihood of pancreatitis.

The complication of fever after ERCP occurs primarily in the setting of an obstructed duct, especially when there has been recent septicemia. Prophylactic broad-spectrum systemic antibiotics are indicated if such obstruction is anticipated, although biliary excretion is variable and evidence that these antibiotics penetrate into the pancreatic ductal system to any sizable degree is lacking.[9,10] The addition of antibiotics, such as gentamicin, to the contrast agent has not been documented to be of value.[11] The most effective method to avoid sepsis in the biliary system is to guarantee effective drainage during the procedure, either by removal of an obstructing stone or through placement of an internal stent or nasobiliary drain. Attention to the sterile cleaning of the endoscope channels, regular cleaning of the water bottles, and use of sterile irrigating fluids can help prevent nosocomial infections.[12]

The costliness of ERCP compared to other procedures is of concern in the efficient use of medical resources, although in general rapid diagnosis is usually the least costly. In this institution, the combined professional and technical costs of biliary ultrasound, CBT, PTC, and ERCP are in the ratio of 1:3:3:7.5. This discrepancy may in part reflect academic, political, and socioeconomic factors rather than represent a fair measure of the comparative consumption of resources. When comparing PTC to ERCP, the expenditure of physician time, the need for ancillary personnel, and the use of the radiology suite may not be much different.

Keeping in mind these comments on the traditional objections to ERCP, let us try to reevaluate the role of this procedure in a variety of situations encountered in gastrointestinal practice. After briefly reviewing the advantages of the endoscopic component of the examination, the following sections will consider specific clinical problems: the patient presenting with jaundice, the nonjaundiced patient with symptoms suspicious of pancreatic carcinoma, the patient with recurrent pain and documented pancreatitis, and, finally, the vexing problem of pancreobiliary-type pain in the absence of documented disease.

Endoscopic Contributions to Diagnosis

A major advantage of ERCP is that it affords the opportunity to perform an endoscopic examination en route to obtaining a radiologic image of the bile or pancreatic duct. An adequate view can be obtained of the entire stomach, duodenal loop, and beyond, and, with some effort, of the lower esophagus and duodenal cap. Systematic viewing of these areas is time consuming and, by prolonging the procedure, may restrict the ability to obtain appropriate radiographs. Nevertheless, in appropriate situations, one should seize the opportunity to obtain useful information, and a careful endoscopy should be planned prior to attempted cannulation. The unexpected discovery of ulcer disease or tumors may clarify occult pain syndromes. Rigidity, nodularity, or narrowing of the duodenal angle or loop may indicate carcinoma, and pancreatic cysts may be identified as smooth masses protruding into the lumen.

More importantly, the cause of the patient's symptoms may be evident on visualization of the ampulla of Vater itself (Figure 2-1, **Plate 1**). Ampullary enlargement may be due to benign or malignant tumors, impacted stones, or, occasionally, to a normal variant. Frequently, an impacted biliary stone may cause the ampullary orifice to gape slightly, and cannulation may actually be facilitated. Alternately, the ampullary face may be normal but the infundibulum above may bulge, producing an appearance reminiscent of the "snake that ate the pig."

Ampullary tumors represent a special type of problem. They may appear obviously malignant or suggest a benign villous adenoma.[13-17] Biopsies may prove diagnostic but should be treated with some skepticism when the pathologic interpretation is of a villous adenoma with or without dysplasia, since frank carcinoma may lurk deeper in the mass. As a rule of thumb, when a patient

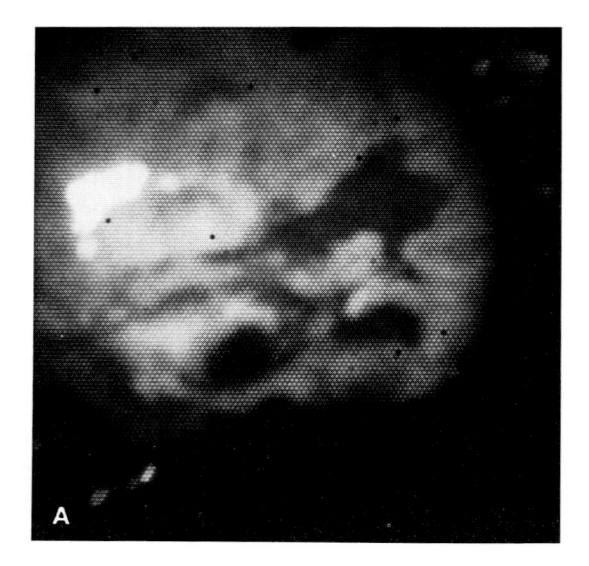

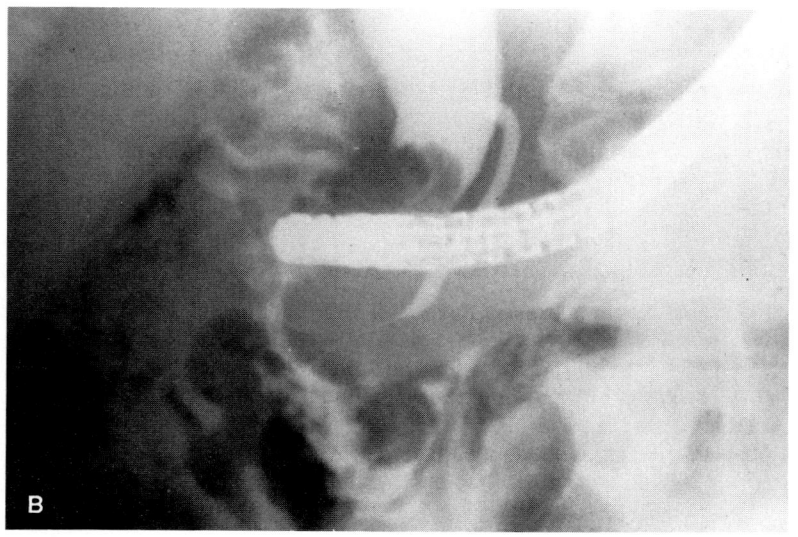

Figure 2-1 (A) (Plate 1) Endoscopic view of ampullary carcinoma and **(B)** radiographic view of ampullary carcinoma. Note the smooth-filling defect in both the pancreatic and bile ducts in the patient in **B**.

presents with obstructive jaundice, any ampullary tumor should be assumed to be malignant.[14,17] In an operable candidate, local resection should be eschewed and consideration given to a potentially curative Whipple procedure. The yield from endoscopic biopsies may be improved by prior papillotomy, with the biopsies taken on the inside surface of the ampulla. Since ampullary tumors are often soft and villous in appearance, the normal orifice may be obscured. In this situation, duct opacification can often still be obtained by poking the cannula through the mass in an appropriate plane of cannulation. Finally, it should be remembered that the Gardner's variant of familial polyposis is associated with a very high incidence of benign and malignant ampullary tumors.[18] In one series of 14 such patients undergoing surveillance, 5 patients had ampullary adenomas at the time of diagnosis and 7 additional patients developed them within a mean of 2.5 years.

ERCP in the Diagnosis of the Jaundiced Patient

The conventional approach to diagnosis of the jaundiced patient involves an initial evaluation by an imaging procedure, usually ultrasound. Are imaging procedures sufficient? Are they ever superfluous? Clearly, ultrasound fulfills the requirements for a rapidly available, totally safe, and relatively inexpensive diagnostic procedure. However, when used in this clinical setting, it is not a precise technique. Ultrasonography generally visualizes the common hepatic duct rather than the common bile duct. The latter and the general area of the head of the pancreas are often obscured by gas. Stones that present in the lower portions of the bile duct can easily be overlooked. When common duct stones are reported on ultrasound, the finding is highly specific[18] but at best stones can be detected in only a bare majority of cases where they are present. Table 2-1 summarizes a number of studies in which US has been prospectively assessed in the diagnosis of common duct stones.[18-22] The sensitivity of this technique has ranged from 19 to 55%.[18-27] Even the accuracy of US as the putative gold standard in the diagnosis of cholelithiasis must be viewed with healthy clinical skepticism. Using ERCP, Venu et al demonstrated a very high percentage of missed gallbladder stones in symptomatic patients with transient abnormalities of liver function tests but normal gallbladder ultrasound and oral cholecystograms.[28]

In most situations, the effectiveness of ultrasound is primarily related to its ability to identify dilated bile ducts as a marker for mechanical obstruction,

Table 2-1 Sensitivity of Ultrasound in Choledocholithiasis

Author	Study population	% Diagnosed	% Nondilated bile ducts
Gross (19) 1983	PTC + ERCP confirmed stones	25	24
Cronan (20) 1983	All stones	13	36
Laing (21) 1983	All stones	29	30
O'Connor (18) 1986	Postcholecystectomy	45	14
Cronan (22) 1986	All stones	55	33

Note: Table shows representative experience with the use of ultrasound in the diagnosis of patients found to have common duct stones. Diagnostic accuracy has improved in recent series. Substantial percentages of patients have normal-size ducts by ultrasonic measurement.

Table 2-2 Etiology of Biliary Obstruction in a University Hospital

Diagnosis	% Total cases
Common duct stones	24
Pancreatic cancer	24
Bile duct cancer	20
Benign stricture of bile duct	19
Chronic pancreatitis	13
Other lesions	6

Source: Reported by Thomas, Pelligrini, Way.[24]

recognizing that this may not distinguish between specific causes of obstruction. Even then, "falsely negative" undilated ducts may be found in 24–36% of patients with common duct stones (28) and 16–45% of patients ultimately shown to have jaundice on an obstructive basis.[23,24,29] This error rate seems unacceptable in a situation where mechanical relief is essential for the patient's recovery. Table 2-2 illustrates the spectrum of conditions found to cause biliary obstruction at one university hospital.[24] Common duct stones represent only one-quarter of the cases, and the range of possibilities is broad. The therapeutic approaches to such a disparate group of conditions are varied. Not only is more reliable proof of mechanical obstruction needed; more precise identification of the cause is needed as well.

In practice, the diameter of the common duct demonstrated by ultrasound does not correlate well with the diameter as measured on ERCP.[30] The differences in size do not necessarily reflect some fixed ratio dependent on the technical aspects of the measurements. Freise *et al* showed in 20% of patients that the diameter of the common bile duct determined by ERCP was twice that of the value determined by sonography.[31] They ascribed the differences to the use of anticholinergic drugs and high injection pressures at ERCP and considered the sonographic findings to be "physiologic." Experienced endoscopists argue that no matter how forceful the injection, a bile duct will not dilate so dramatically unless it was previously stretched to that size.

Computerized body tomography has been advanced as a suitable substitute for US and a remedy for some of ultrasound's deficiencies. Sensitivities as high as 90% have been reported in the diagnosis of common duct stones[24] by using a variety of CBT imaging criteria. Recent evidence suggested that these figures are unduly optimistic.[32] Baron performed a retrospective review of CBT in a highly selected and optimal subgroup of patients who had subsequently undergone cholangiography for suspected biliary obstruction. Even eliminating the 20% of patients with a normal-size bile duct, a specific diagnosis of common duct stones could be made in only 76% of those patients ultimately documented to have them. The criterion used was the demonstration of a "target sign" or calcified stone. Other CBT criteria could not reliably differentiate between stone, carcinoma, or normal duct. Although sensitivity is certainly improved, the increased cost and decreased availability of CBT on an emergency basis added to the still substantial number of imprecise diagnoses has limited the use of CBT as the sole basis for deciding therapeutic strategy in the jaundiced patient. In discussing such high-technology imaging procedures, one should not overlook or denigrate the skills of the experienced physician. Although a positive finding by CBT or ultrasound may be highly predictive, overall clinical judgment based on history, physical, and routine liver chemistries has an excellent record for differentiating between hepatocellular and obstructive jaundice.[23]

Formal decision analysis modeling has been used to test the cost effectiveness of various strategies in suspected obstructed jaundice. Richter et al[33] concluded that when the clinical suspicion of obstructive jaundice was 20% or less, the confirmation of nondilated ducts by imaging techniques was sufficiently accurate to justify a strategy of observation. Percutaneous liver biopsy could be done if there was a need for a specific diagnosis as to the variety of hepatocellular disease. However, if the clinical suspicion of obstruction was greater than 20%, then direct cholangiography with PTC or ERCP became appropriate, even in the face of nondilated bile ducts, because of the unacceptable consequences of overlooking a correctable mechanical problem.

If a specific diagnosis of choledocholithiasis can be made by imaging techniques in a good-risk patient with gallbladder in place, this may be considered evidence enough to proceed to surgery. However, when the cause of obstruction is not so clearly defined, or when the patient is postcholecystectomy, more specific information is often desirable. Although it may be more a matter of style than of substance, most surgeons would prefer a road map rather than a vote of confidence. The management of the mass lesion in the head of the pancreas, dilated bile ducts in the postcholecystectomy patient, or constricting lesions in the porta hepatis may all be optimized by postponing surgery until there is a clearer view of the nature and extent of the problem. The cholangiogram that is available in the operating room is a poor substitute for the quality studies that can be obtained preoperatively. Limited by the absence of fluoroscopy and by a single plane of viewing, operative cholangiography is of only limited benefit in stone disease, and of little or no benefit when the cause of biliary obstruction is more complicated. Where the diagnosis is uncertain, cholangiography prior to surgery is a wise and appropriate first step. Options such as endoscopic or percutaneous drainage may allow debilitated patients or those with limited life expectancy to be better treated by nonoperative means. If there is benign obstruction from a stone, surgery is often avoidable (Figures 2-2 and 2-3).

A substantial amount of heat has been generated among radiologists and endoscopists over which cholangiographic technique is most appropriate. Both agree that intravenous cholangiography has long since been relegated to the medical museums, since the bile duct rarely visualizes in the jaundiced patient. Even in the nonjaundiced patient, stones are missed fully 50% of the time.[34] Numerous comparisons have been made between percutaneous transhepatic cholangiography and endoscopic retrograde cholangiopancreatography. In general, these have shown the two techniques to be more or less equal in terms of their technical success in a broad series of jaundiced patients, their complication rate, and the frequency of nondiagnostic information (7%).[24,35]

Personal observation suggests also that there is no appreciable difference in patient acceptance of the two procedures. In some specific clinical situations one technique or the other may have some advantage. PTC is more frequently successful in patients with dilated bile ducts and more accurate in assessing the details when there is disease of the porta hepatis. In general, it is less costly. In the presence of a bleeding diathesis or ascites, however, it may be unduly

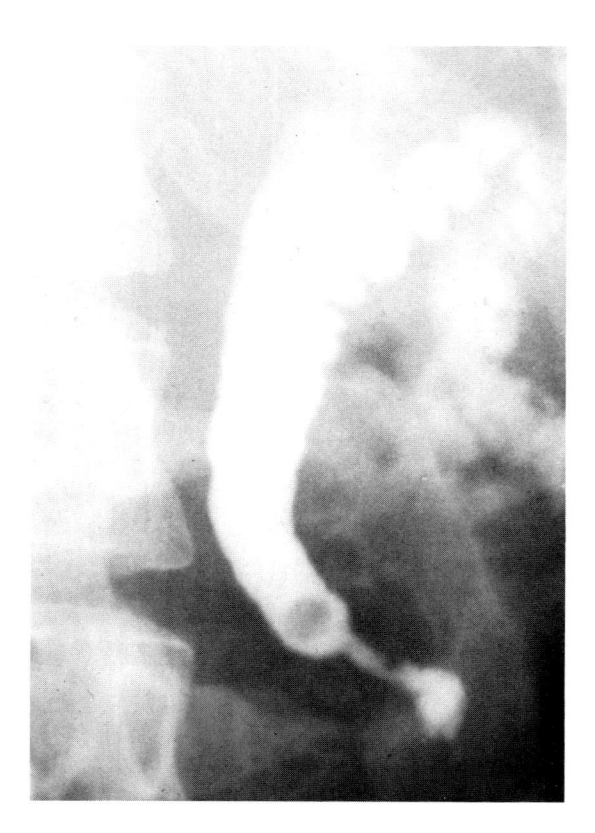

Figure 2-2 A solitary rounded stone at the bottom of a dilated bile duct. The cystic duct remnant is also dilated.

hazardous. ERCP is more often successful in patients with nondilated bile ducts, more accurate in assessing disease of the lower bile ducts and ampulla, and provides a pancreatogram. Jaundice due to chronic pancreatitis, pancreatic cancer, and choledochal cysts (aberrant bile duct takeoff) involves significant pancreatic duct changes.[36] On the other hand, gastric outlet obstruction or a Roux-en-Y anastomosis makes ERCP impossible, and a Billroth II gastrojejunostomy may require a technical tour de force.

In the current era, it is unusual for a sizable hospital not to have a physician available who is skilled in each of these techniques. To my mind, the era of interventional endoscopy, discussed elsewhere in this book, has shifted the balance toward the use of ERCP as the preferred means of direct cholangiography in most clinical situations. Reference to Table 2-3 indicates that most of the common causes of clinical jaundice are preferentially diagnosed and/or treated by this means. The biliary stone can be removed through an endoscopic papillotomy, the pancreatic or ampullary cancer stented, the stricture dilated. Only with cholangiocarcinoma does transhepatic cholangiography have a competitive clinical advantage. It has greater success in defining both right and left hepatic duct systems for possible surgical anastomosis and can be reliably anticipated to accomplish at least external biliary drainage.

Stents and drains can be placed both percutaneously and endoscopically. The percutaneous route is usually associated with considerable initial discomfort. This is a consequence of both bile leakage into the peritoneum from vio-

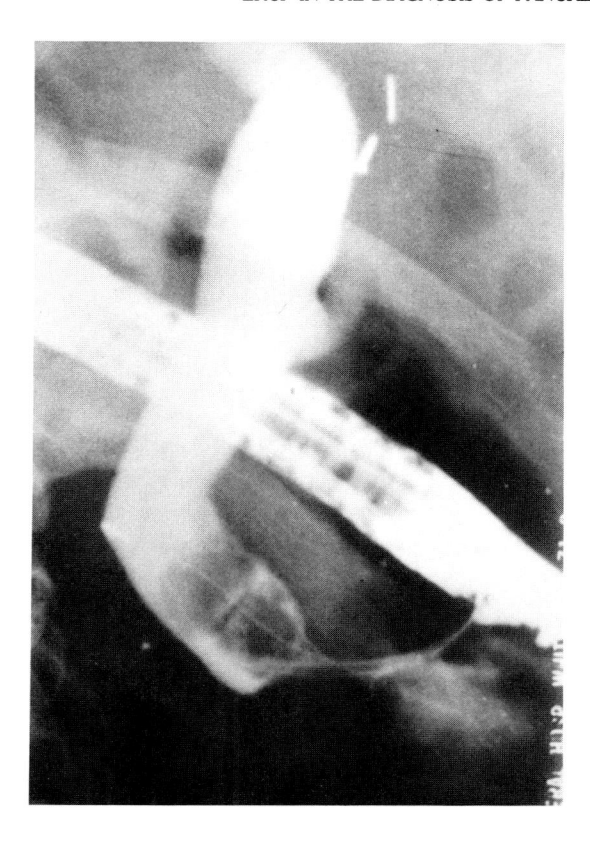

Figure 2-3 Two common duct stones within a basket following endoscopic sphincterotomy.

lation of the liver capsule and the presence of a foreign body extending between the rib cage and the mobile liver. Placement of a large-caliber internal drain usually has to be deferred for at least several days until the path through the liver has become sufficiently enlarged.

In contrast, large endoscopic stents can usually be placed with the initial attempt. Thus logic favors the primary use of ERCP in diagnosis and therapy, with a backup of PTC if that should be unsuccessful. A recent randomized trial

Table 2-3 Choice of Cholangiography in the Jaundiced Patient

Etiology	Preferred approach	Advantages
Hepatocellular disease	ERCP	Higher success rate
Common duct stones	ERCP	Endoscopic papillotomy
Pancreatic CA	ERCP	Pancreatogram, definitive stent placement
Cholangio CA	PTC	Certain drainage, better views
Chronic pancreatitis	ERCP	Diagnostic pancreatogram
Ampullary CA	ERCP	Biopsy, definitive stent placement
Biliary stricture	ERCP	Dilate stricture
Sclerosing cholangitis	ERCP	Greater success rate

Source: Table shows the author's preferred cholangiographic technique in various clinical situations. Although special circumstances may affect the balance, only in suspected cholangiocarcinoma is an initial approach by PTC preferable.

supports this approach.[37] Only in the patient with evidence suggestive of cholangiocarcinoma, ie, ultrasonographic evidence of a normal bile duct and dilated intrahepatic ducts, does the reverse order make sense. Even then, recent reports[38,39] suggested that a combination of the two procedures can solve most technical failures encountered at endoscopy and allow for the reliable placement of large-bore endoprostheses at an initial "sitting."

One of the most important aspects of the diagnosis of obstructive jaundice is the stipulation that it be done efficiently and rapidly. Ideally, direct cholangiography should be performed within 24 hr of admission, or as soon as it is evident from the history and routine laboratory studies that there is a reasonable likelihood of mechanical obstruction. Ultrasound may define the occasional patient who can be routed directly to surgery, but it is in many cases superfluous. It does not substitute for the definitive diagnostic and therapeutic potential of direct cholangiography and it is not essential that it be done beforehand. In some areas of the country clinical availability of PTC or ERCP may be limited and may, therefore, affect the route for bile duct visualization. However, where expertise exists in both techniques, the diagnostic and therapeutic potential of ERCP makes it my procedure of choice.

Diagnostic Strategies in Suspected Pancreatic Carcinoma

The ability of any diagnostic strategy to detect pancreatic carcinoma at a curable stage is extremely limited. For this reason, ERCP, as well as radiologic imaging techniques, has been largely relegated to the function of closing the barn door after the horse has been stolen. The diagnostic revolution that occurred in the 1970s in regard to pancreatic and biliary disease has not appreciably shortened diagnostic delay nor improved survival in pancreatic cancer.[40] Early diagnosis remains elusive. In one study, at least 70% of patients discovered to have pancreatic carcinoma had been hospitalized in the previous year without the establishment of the correct diagnosis.[41] Even should it prove feasible to diagnose pancreatic cancer when still limited in size, the overall survival may not prove much more satisfactory. In a cooperative Japanese study, only 2.1% of a collected series of pancreatic cancers were 2 cm or less in size at discovery, and of this very select group, only 44% were stage 1 (without regional nodes, capsular invasion, retroperitoneal spread, or vascular invasion). The overall 5-year survival for the group was 30.3% and for stage 1 tumors only 37%.[42] At best, less than 1% of pancreatic cancers were curable. Nevertheless, other series[43,44] have suggested that sizable percentages (22–30%) of carcinomas located in the head of the pancreas may be at least surgically resectable by the Whipple procedure or total pancreatoduodenectomy, with modern operative mortalities that are less than 10% and probably closer to 4%.[42] Such an aggressive approach is justified by the finding that one-third of such resected specimens were potentially curable. As would be anticipated, resected patients have a more prolonged survival than nonresectable patients.[43] Whether this advantage only reflects resection of earlier and less aggressive tumors or whether there is also a palliative value to removal of the primary tumor has not been established.

The identification of serologic assays capable of early detection of pancreatic carcinoma has been a Holy Grail for pancreatic researchers for some

Table 2-4 Comparison of Techniques in Diagnosis of Pancreatic Carcinoma

		% Correct diagnosis		
Study		US	CBT	ERCP
Anacker[46] 1981		—	77	90
Frederic[47] 1983		75	—	94
Ariyama[48] 1983		91	84	94
Nix[43] 1984		54	58	92
Van Dyke[49] 1985		78	92	94
Yankaskas[50] 1985	(nonjuandiced)	40	65	53
		63	85	63
Tsuchiya[42] 1986	(low cutoff)	78	72	94
	(high cutoff)	83	79	100
Gilinsky[51] 1980		54	63	80

Note: Wide variations in sensitivity appear to reflect differing criteria for abnormality.

years. Candidate assays have included carcino embryonic antigen (CEA), galactasyltransferase II, leukocyte adherence inhibition assay, pancreatic oncofetal antigen, and serum ribonuclease. All of these determinations have suffered from problems of insufficient sensitivity and specificity. These limitations have precluded their effectiveness in screening populations with minimal or no symptoms, especially as no specific "population at risk" has been defined. The newest and apparently most promising of these assays is the CA 19-9,[45] a carbohydrate antigenic determinant defined by a monoclonal antibody. This has been reported to be highly sensitive for pancreatic cancer (86–90%). Abnormal values increase with increasing size of the tumor, but resectable cancers have also been reported to have a sizable detection rate in the range of 78–93%. The limitations of the assay include a false positive rate of about 10% in benign pancreatic diseases and benign causes of jaundice, as well as occasionally in other disorders. False negative tests occur, especially in patients who lack the structurally related Lewis blood group. The usefulness of this test has not yet withstood the test of time. At best, it may flag as highly suspicious the patients with suggestive but nonspecific symptoms. The significant overlap with benign disease will require the addition of some more definitive diagnostic studies.

The standard diagnostic studies currently used in the diagnosis of pancreatic cancer include ultrasound, computerized body tomography, and ERCP. As yet, MRI has not been shown to have any supplemental value in this condition. Angiography has been relegated to the role of helping to judge resectability in equivocal cases because of its cost, potential complications, and the unusual skill required. The diagnostic accuracy of the three primary techniques has been compared in innumerable studies. Some of the more recent reports are summarized in Table 2-4.[42,43,46–51] Precise comparisons are impossible due to case selection, differences in physician commitment and expertise, and variations in the threshold for declaring the presence of an abnormality by imaging procedures. As an example, the sensitivity of ultrasound varies between 54 and 91%. Although the 91% figure is impressive, the positive predictive value of an abnormal scan was only 14%. The vast majority of the abnormalities being identified were not due to cancer.[48] Most clinicians are in general agreement about the relative value of the techniques. Computer body tomography is considered more sensitive than ultrasound, and ERCP is thought to be more sensitive than either.

Ultrasound is often technically unsatisfactory due to obesity, bowel gas, surgical dressings, ostomies, and so forth. Although the percentage of such unsatisfactory exams may be as low as 14% in some centers with acknowledged expertise, the proportion of CBT exams that are unsatisfactory is usually less than 2%.[49] One study found that CBT was thought to be the sole necessary imaging modality in 75% of cases.[52] As seen in Table 2-4, ultrasound may rival CBT in diagnostic sensitivity, but in other studies it may prove considerably inferior.

In contrast, in most studies ERCP equals and usually exceeds CBT in diagnostic sensitivity (Table 2-4) and commonly provides diagnostic information when the results on CT scan are abnormal but indeterminate. Eight carcinomas were diagnosed in 18 such indeterminate cases in one study[53] and 6 in 26 cases in another.[54] Only one subsequently proven cancer was missed by ERCP in each study.

The diagnostic confusion arises because some findings on computerized scans lack specificity. Subacute and chronic pancreatitis may present as focal mass-like enlargements on CT scan, while pancreatic cancer can appear as a generalized enlargement suggestive of pancreatitis. Even detection of a dilated duct on CBT will not necessarily differentiate between the two entities. To add to the problem, normal congenital variations in ductal anatomy such as pancreas divisum or duplications of the main pancreatic duct may appear as focal enlargements of the head or tail of the gland on CBT.[55]

Nevertheless, CBT has an enviable record in diagnosis of pancreatic cancer with a reported sensitivity ranging from 58 to 92% (Table 2-4). The advantage of CBT over ERCP as a primary diagnostic modality lies in its ease of performance, lower cost, and its ability to provide information in regard to tumor resectability. The detection of retroperitoneal invasion, arterial thickening, or hepatic metastases can, *a priori*, indicate unresectability.[56–58] In addition, CBT-guided fine-needle percutaneous aspiration biopsy (actually cytology) can establish a tissue diagnosis and resolve the nature of indeterminate masses. The complications of such biopsies are surprisingly infrequent,[59] although the report of a malignant implant along the needle tract may cause some concern if resection for cure is a realistic alternative.

Recently a new procedure, endoscopic ultrasound (EUS), has been suggested as a potentially important technique for the diagnosis of pancreatic cancer. In a recent report on 50 patients, of whom 42 had cancer of the pancreas and 8 has "pseudotumorous pancreatitis," EUS was found to be superior to all conventional imaging modalities, including ERCP, in the detection of tumors under 30 mm in size, though its ability to distinguish benignity from malignancy declined with tumors under 20 mm. In addition to its sensitivity in the detection of small lesions, EUS appeared to be valuable in the detection of vascular invasion by pancreatic cancers.[60] Because of its sensitivity, EUS, especially as the technology is refined and experience accrues, may assume an increasingly important role in the diagnosis of pancreatic cancer. Whether it is substantially less "invasive" than ERCP is unclear.

Nonetheless, a role clearly remains for ERCP in the investigation of suspected pancreatic carcinoma if CBT is abnormal but equivocal, if guided biopsy is nondiagnostic as it is in 20–30% of lesions,[59] or if CBT facilities are inadequate or unresponsive to clinical needs. ERCP is useful when resection of pancreatic carcinoma is contemplated and may define possible biliary encroachment as well as the extent of pancreatic ductal involvement. Most importantly, ERCP is appropriate for the patient with a normal CBT where sufficient clinical suspicion of cancer is present. Just what level of diagnostic suspicion is sufficient is an arguable point. It should be appreciated that with cancers of the head of the pancreas, for example, the early complaints are often nonspecific: unexplained wieght loss, change in bowel habits, tiredness and malaise, sudden onset of diabetes mellitus, and nonspecific upper abdominal discomfort.[43] Jaundice and classic abdominal pain patterns are usually late symptoms. Perhaps it is to this population that the newer serologic studies may make the greatest difference by defining a group where diagnosis should be vigorously pursued.

The ERCP diagnosis of pancreatic cancer may be made on the basis of the duodenoscopic findings, the pancreatogram, or the cholangiogram.[53] Diagnostic radiographic findings (Figure 2-4) include abrupt lancet-shaped or rat-tailed cutoff of the main pancreatic duct (2-4A), irregularity of the duct with absence of secondary ducts in that region (2-4B), ductal disorganization (2-4C), and long strictures with dilated ducts behind (2-4D). The double-duct sign (Figure 2-5), ie, abnormalities of both the bile and pancreatic ducts, has been frequently and appropriately touted as an indicator of pancreatic carcinoma (2-5A). It must be understood, however, that benign pancreatic disease may also cause secondary stricture or displacement of the bile duct (2-5B).[61] The specific characteristics that point toward malignancy are total bile duct obstruction, close proximity of the bile ductal lesion to a pancreatic lesion, a short stenotic segment of the common bile duct removed from the papilla, and an abrupt irregular transition from normal to stenotic or obstructed duct.[62]

As with any diagnostic test, infallibility is rarely achieved. Although accepted as the most specific diagnostic study, a recent series of ERCPs still reported a 5% false-positive and 7.7% false-negative rate in the diagnosis of pancreatic cancer (compared with 37% false-negative rate for CBT in the same patients).[51] Several techniques have been suggested to enhance ERCP precision. Lavelle[63] suggested combining digital subtraction techniques with more forceful endoscopic injection in order to provide parenchymal detail and more clearly define defects due to neoplasm. The increased filling of the secondary ducts may, however, carry a higher risk of producing pancreatitis. Pancreatic ductal cytology may also allow definitive assessment at ERCP[64] and has been reported to provide very few false positive diagnoses. However, even in centers with a tradition of cytologic excellence, this can only serve as an adjunct to diagnosis and not as a substitute for cholangiopancreatography.

Thus, the diagnostic strategy to be employed[65] in suspected pancreatic cancer depends on the presenting complaint. When the presenting complaint is one of jaundice (7–30% of cases),[44] prompt cholangiography can provide an opportunity not only for diagnosis but also for therapeutic relief of biliary obstruction, and may even permit an attempt at curative resection. When the problem is one of weight loss, pain, or more nonspecific symptoms, then an initial imaging exam complemented by percutaneous fine-needle aspiration biopsy may provide diagnostic evidence of pancreatic carcinoma and spare the patient the further misfortune of an unnecessary and unhelpful laparotomy. Although ultrasound

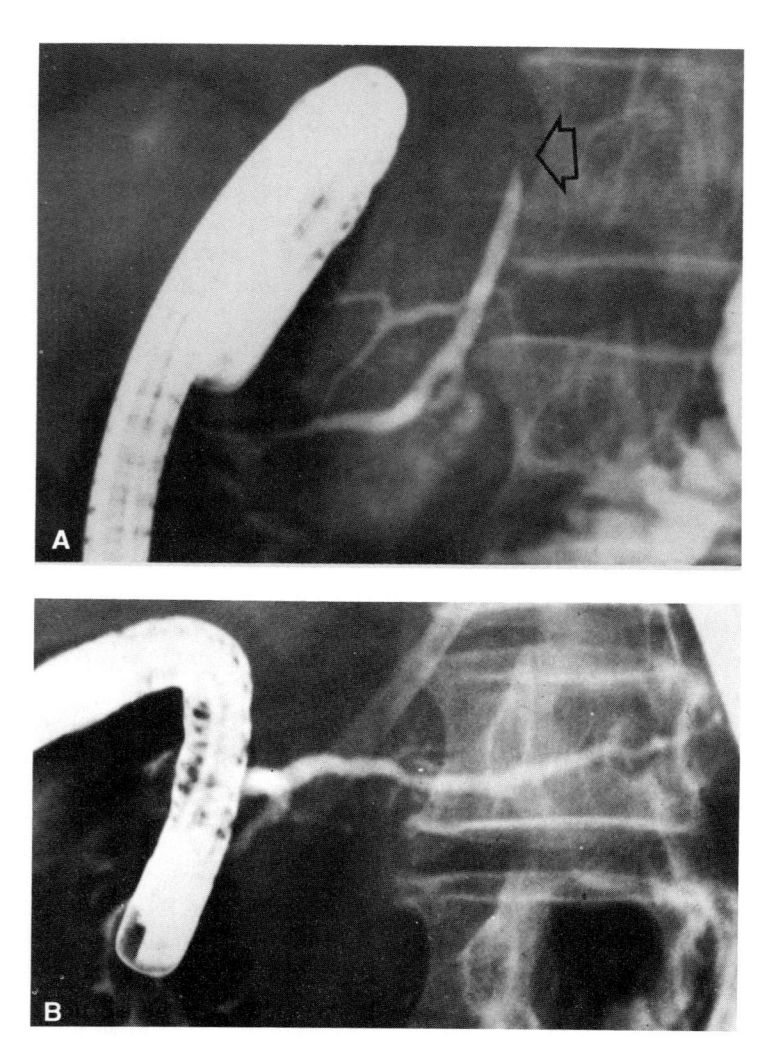

Figure 2-4 A & B

and ultrasound-guided needle biopsy may be sufficient to detect some pancreatic carcinomas, the use of CBT as the initial diagnostic test may actually represent a more cost-effective use of resources in a hospitalized patient with a high probability of disease. If CBT is abnormal but nondiagnostic, ERCP is indicated. If CBT is normal, ERCP should be done whenever the diagnostic suspicion is appreciable.

The Value of ERCP in Pancreatitis

ERCP is of special value in patients with inflammatory lesions of the pancreas and may contribute at a variety of levels to diagnosis and to the planning of appropriate therapy. This section will discuss its use in patients in whom a diagnosis of pancreatitis has been established. The appropriateness of ERCP in patients with unexplained and recurrent pain suggestive of pancreobiliary origin will be considered later.

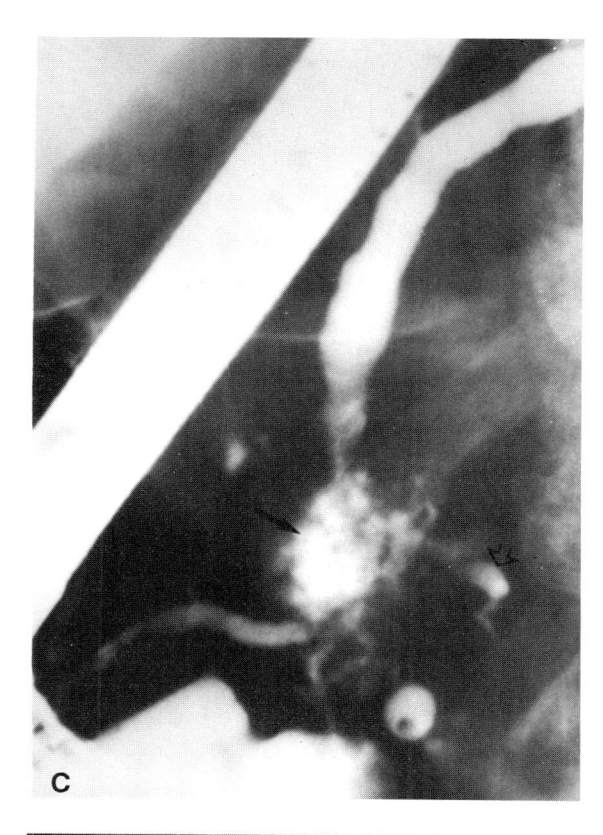

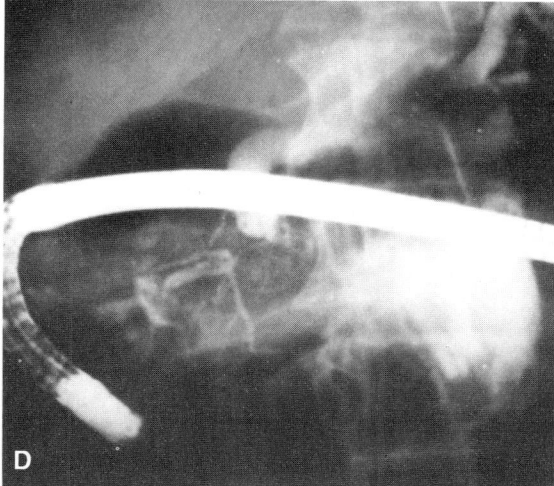

Figure 2-4 Characteristic ERCP appearance in pancreatic cancer. **(A)** Pancreatogram in a 70-year-old woman presenting with nonspecific mid- and lower abdominal pain and 20-lb weight loss. An abrupt cutoff of the main pancreatic duct is present in the body of the gland. Arrow indicates a sharp margin at the point of obstruction. If obstruction were due to a stone, a meniscus effect would be anticipated. **(B)** A 55-year-old alcoholic female with weight loss and back pain. Diffuse enlargement of the pancreas on ultrasound and computed body tomography were interpreted as due to pancreatitis. Although the diffuse irregularity of the duct is nonspecific, the absence of secondary ducts suggested carcinoma. The diagnosis was ultimately confirmed at laparotomy. **(C)** A 45-year-old man with abdominal pain and diarrhea and a mass in the head of the pancreas on CBT. Black arrow indicates an area of disorganization in the head of the gland with parenchymal infiltration of contrast and dilated secondary ducts (white arrow). These patchy collections of contrast can be distinguished from the confluent extravasations that might be seen in a benign pseudocyst. **(D)** A 60-year-old man who presented with jaundice. CBT was interpreted as normal. Endoscopic cholangiogram was unsuccessful. Pancreatography showed a 1-cm area of narrowing in the head with dilatation proximally. The carcinoma was surgically resectable but recurred 3 years later.

Although the greatest contributions of this technique are in patients with chronic or recurrent pancreatitis, it can occasionally be helpful in patients presenting with acute disease. The pancreatographic findings in acute pancreatitis are nonspecific. When pancreatography is done in the acute setting, the findings consist either of normal ducts or minimal change pancreatitis, with the occa-

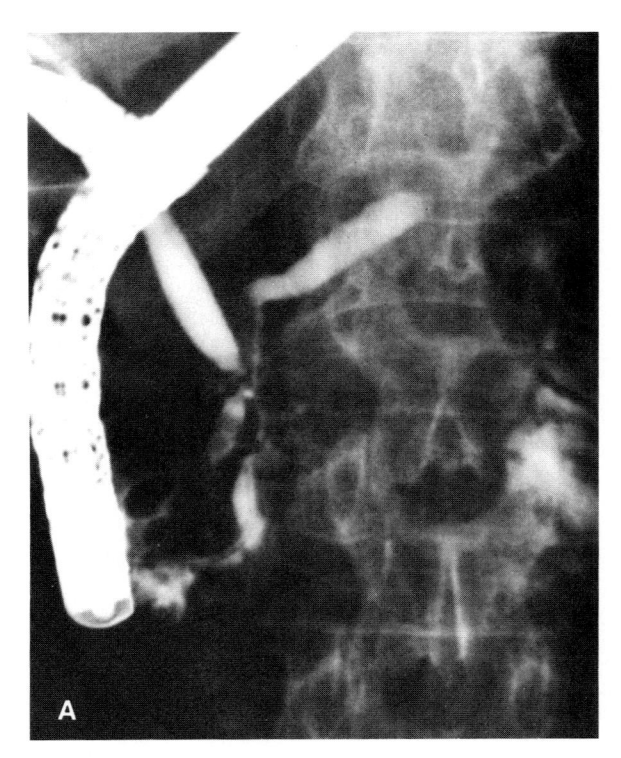

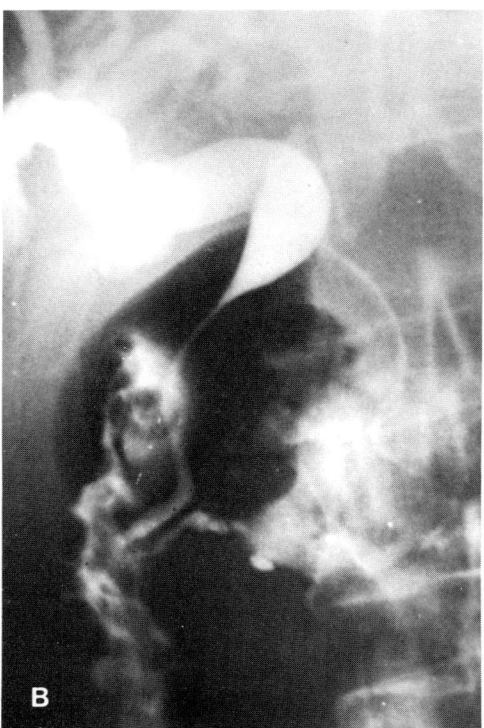

Figure 2-5 Appearance of malignant and benign bile duct strictures in pancreatic disease. **(A)** Malignant stricture: classic "double-duct" sign of pancreatic cancer. Pancreatic and bile duct obstruction are geographically adjacent. There is abrupt transition to a totally obstructed bile duct at a distance removed from the ampulla. **(B)** Stricture associated with chronic pancreatitis. There is smooth, narrowing of the bile duct, often asymmetrically deviated involving the extent of the intrapancreatic bile duct. Characteristically, a short segment immediately adjacent to the ampulla may return to normal caliber.

sional discovery of unsuspected chronic pancreatitis. ERCP is *not* recommended as a technique for monitoring the course of patients presenting with fulminant attacks of acute hemorrhagic pancreatitis. In such patients pain and fever may persist, or recrudesce, 2 or 3 weeks into the course. The critical decision to be made in these patients is whether surgical debridement or drainage of a pancreatic phlegmon or abscess is needed. This decision is best made with the aid of computerized body tomography, abetted by plain abdominal films and occasionally by ultrasound. Only on the rare occasions when the attack of pancreatitis has dragged on in a subacute fashion for a month or months is it helpful to define the ductal anatomy before surgical intervention.

In nonalcoholic patients with acute pancreatitis, choledocholithiasis may be suspected as the cause on the basis of the ultrasonographic demonstration of either stones in the gallbladder or a dilated common duct. Here, emergent ERCP may play a role. The early endoscopic removal of impacted common duct stones in gallstone pancreatitis is a controversial subject discussed elsewhere in this volume. Although the therapeutic advantage of such an aggressive approach has not yet been unequivocally validated, early studies have suggested that ERCP can be safely performed in the acute stages of gallstone pancreatitis. Both Rosseland and Solhaus[66] and Neoptolemos *et al*[67] reported no complications attributable to this procedure in their studies.

On the other end of the spectrum, ERCP may be helpful in defining the etiology of unexplained acute pancreatitis after the attack has subsided. Depending on the population studied, cholelithiasis is usually listed as the first or second most common cause of pancreatitis. Abdominal ultrasound and oral cholecystogram are thought to be the two most sensitive studies for the detection of cholelithiasis. Nevertheless, one group investigating idiopathic pancreatitis determined that gallstones were missed by these tests in 13% of the cases. Of these, 11% were subsequently diagnosed by ERCP.[68] In another study,[69] 23 of 73 patients with unexplained pancreatitis were found on ERCP to have potentially curable lesions, 9 due to gallstones and 5 due to pancreatic duct abnormalities. Standing views of the gallbladder should be done following ERCP in all unexplained cases.

In chronic pancreatitis, ductal morphology as determined by ERCP has proved the most sensitive measure of chronic pancreatic injury, whether compared to a pancreatic function test like the secretin pancreozymin test (PFT),[70] the Bentiromide test and PFT,[71] or CBT.[72] Ductal changes usually consist of obstruction or dilation of the main pancreatic duct, dilation with clublike terminations of the secondary ducts, or irregularities in the main pancreatic duct with focal fibrosis, extravasations, or chain-of-lakes appearance. Interestingly, although pancreatic calcifications seen on plain film are indicative of chronic pancreatitic damage and calcifications greater than 5 mm almost always indicate obstruction of the duct,[73] there are some gross discrepancies between the amount of calcification and the actual degree of functional impairment. Clearly, one can have pancreatic calcifications without actual enzyme insufficiency and insufficiency without calcifications.[74] Finally, even in the absence of symptoms of pancreatitis, a population at high risk, such as chronic alcoholics, may have an almost 50% incidence of ductal changes ranging from mild to advanced.[74]

The technical ability to visualize the pancreatic duct by means of endoscopy is not synonymous with the need to perform this procedure. If a diagnosis of alcoholic or hereditary pancreatitis has been established clinically, the detailed

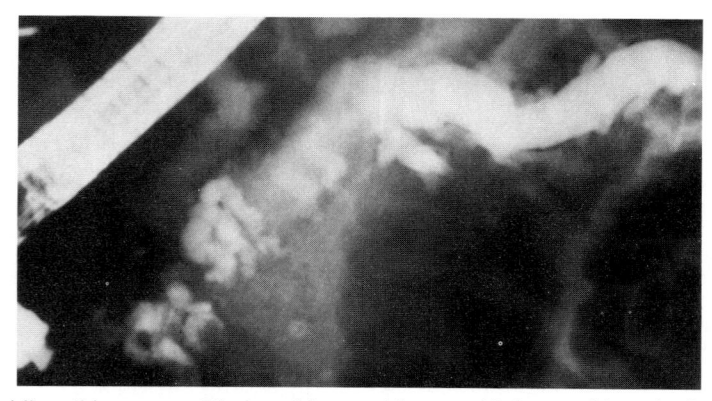

Figure 2-6 Idiopathic pancreatitis in a 24-year-old man with intractable pain despite abstinence. A Roux-en-Y lateral pancreatojejunostomy afforded relief.

anatomy of the pancreatic ductal system is only of value when surgical therapy is contemplated. If the frequency of pancreatitis or severity of chronic pain is not sufficient to justify the risks of surgery, ERCP should be deferred. Some authors have questioned the wisdom of any operative approaches to the pain associated with chronic pancreatitis.[75] They contend that with time pancreatic inflammation will "burn out" and pain subside, and that no ductal pattern correlates with intractable pain.[76] Nevertheless, this author feels that there are certain patterns amenable to limited surgery and that such surgery can be performed with the reasonable expectation of pain relief.[77] In general, about one-half of the patients studied will be found to have lesions amenable to operative intervention short of subtotal or total pancreatectomy.[78,79]

Examples of such favorable lesions are illustrated in the pancreatograms in Figures 2-6 to 2-9. Figure 2-6 depicts the pancreatic ductogram of a 24-year-old

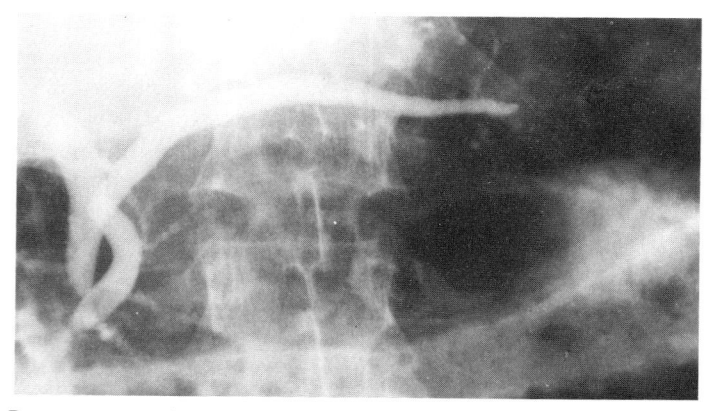

Figure 2-7 Pancreatogram in a patient who had presented 10 years before with pancreatic insufficiency. He was noted to have a dilated duct and an atrophic gland on ERCP and CBT. Only in the 3 years prior to this examination did pain become a problem. Repeat ERCP showed a dilated, truncated duct with pancreatic calcification extending well beyond the end of the duct (white arrow).

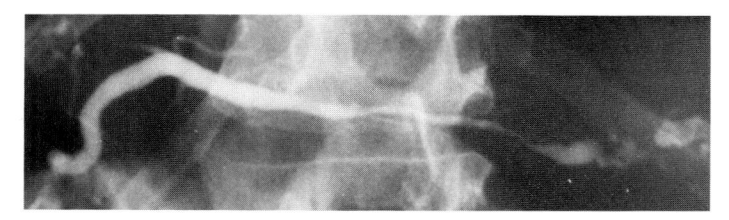

Figure 2-8 Recurrent pancreatic pain over 20 years with recent crescendo symptoms. Visible abnormalities when confined to the tail of the pancreas and were treated by distal pancreatectomy with preservation of the spleen.

man with a 5-year history of idiopathic pancreatitis and recurrent pancreatic pain. This massively dilated pancreatic duct was ideally suited for a Roux-en-Y lateral pancreatojejunostomy (modified Puestow procedure) which was done with relief of his pain. Figure 2-7 shows the pancreatogram of a man who presented at the age of 65 with weight loss and diarrhea. Pancreatic insufficiency was diagnosed and the patient responded to replacement therapy. Only after several years did he begin to experience disabling abdominal pain. In the figure, the pancreatic duct is dilated and total ductal obstruction is noted at the junction of the body and tail of the pancreas. Pancreatic calcifications clearly are evident in the nonvisualized area of the tail (white arrow). This patient was successfully treated by amputation of the tail of the pancreas in addition to a Puestow procedure. This illustrates the complex procedures that may be necessary in a given case. Figure 2-8 illustrates the ductogram of a patient with many years of recurrent attacks of pain. Despite the absence of dilated ducts, she developed ductal irregularity and extravasation of contrast exclusively in the tail of the gland. A distal pancreatectomy was done with preservation of the spleen. Figure 2-9 shows the pancreatogram of a patient with familial pancreatitis and incidental pancreas divisum. Gross destruction of the duct of Wirsung is present in

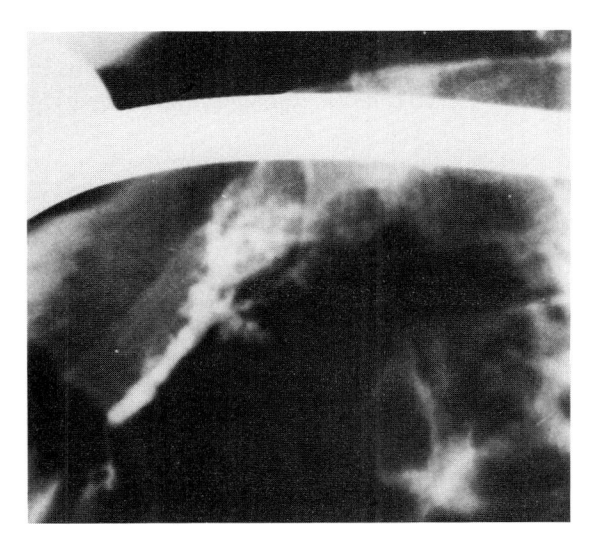

Figure 2-9 Pancreatogram taken through the ampulla of Vater in a patient with pancreas divisum and recurrent pancreatitis. Diffuse abnormality was present involving the duct of Wirsung. A separate injection through the lesser ampulla revealed a normal main pancreatic duct.

the head of the gland while the duct of Santorini, filled through the minor ampulla, showed a normal anatomy. A pylorus-sparing Whipple pancreatoduodenectomy was done. This case demonstrates that the type of ductal change may not be consistent despite closely related types of pancreatitis. Affected members of families with hereditary pancreatitis may have vastly different patterns on pancreatography.[80] None of the other affected members of this particular kinship had pancreas divisum.

Obviously, there is no assurance that the presence of a ductal anatomy amenable to limited surgical intervention will guarantee relief of symptoms of pain after surgery. Patients suffering from pancreatic pain are complex. Long-term use of narcotics runs the risk of resultant narcotic dependency, especially in alcoholics or other addictive personalities. In addition, pancreatitis may persist in the parts of the gland without overt ductal changes. The presence of a dilated duct is not equatable with mechanical obstruction. It may simply reflect shrinkage and atrophy of the gland. Often no obstructing stone is present, and the value of a diverting procedure in that context is rightly suspect.

Few good, long-term follow-up studies are available. One study reported good or excellent relief of pain in 70% of cases after Puestow procedures, although there was no decrease in the subsequent development of either pancreatic insufficiency or diabetes mellitus.[77] In contrast, a recent report[81] suggested that up to 20% of patients with exocrine pancreatic failure may have early ductal obstruction of the gland with the potential for renewed function. These patients may have exocrine recovery after diverting surgery or after abstinence from alcohol. Such patients may be identified by the presence of high serum trypsin levels in the face of low urinary para-aminobenzoic acid (PABA) excretion. Despite this report, surgery in general is only appropriate for the relief of pain.

In addition to pancreatic ductal anatomy, it is equally important to assess bile duct anatomy when surgery is considered. Bile duct strictures secondary to chronic pancreatitis can present as cholangitis, jaundice, pain, or a secondary biliary cirrhosis-type picture.[61] These may occur even in the absence of obvious pancreatitis. On the other hand, without a high index of suspicion biliary strictures may be overlooked when surgery is done for chronic pancreatitis, with the potential for severe postoperative problems.[82] An elevated alkaline phosphatase is the best indicator of bile duct abnormalities and is an absolute indication for preoperative endoscopic or percutaneous transhepatic cholangiography.[83]

A special problem occurs in patients who present with pancreatic pseudocysts that require drainage, either because of great chronicity or as a means to relieve associated symptoms of pain, obstruction, and the like. Concern that the performance of ERCP in this setting will result in clinical infection of the pseudocysts seems unfounded.[84,85] Less than 5% incidence of sepsis is reported if surgery is done within 24 hours and even if surgery is delayed beyond that time there are rarely untoward results. Antibiotics should be given prophylactically and the procedure scheduled as close to the operative date as possible. At ERCP, most pseudocysts will fill off the pancreatic duct, and additional pseudocysts missed on ultrasound may be detected.[85] The choice of operative procedure is affected in about half of patients.[84] Unless the operative possibilities are limited by the poor condition of the patient or the huge size of the cyst, it is inadvisable to proceed to definitive surgery without first obtaining endoscopic directions.

A similar caveat applies to patients with pancreatic ascites and pancreatic fistula. Pancreatic ascites usually presents as insidiously progressive abdominal distension with high concentrations of amylase in the ascitic fluid. Abdominal pain may be minimal. Almost always this syndrome reflects intra-abdominal rupture of a pseudocyst or intra-abdominal drainage of ductal fluid following inflammatory pancreatic disease. Although conservative treatment over several weeks may occasionally lead to resolution, definitive surgery after precise definition of the ductal anatomy by ERCP is the most effective route. Limited pancreatic resection including the site of leakage is usually necessary.[85-87] In any condition that disrupts the pancreatic duct and leads to fistula, rational surgery is also best planned by identifying the site of leak. Such problems can occur after resective surgery, attempted local removal of islet cell adenomas, and traumatic pancreatic disruption such as may result from steering wheel impact in motor vehicle accidents.

In summary, ERCP has little use in acute pancreatitis as a diagnostic procedure alone, except occasionally to define a cause in patients whose attacks remain unexplained after the usual imaging procedures. However, when operative intervention is contemplated for chronic pancreatitis, the surgeon will be able to reach his destination best with the aid of an endoscopic road map.

Unexplained Pain of Suspected Pancreatic or Biliary Origin

Many patients consult their physicians because of recurrent episodes of upper abdominal pain, reminiscent in location and character of the pain associated with pancreatitis or biliary tract disease. The pain is usually episodic and postprandial, but it may be constant. It is often associated with abdominal tenderness, and discomfort may persist after an acute attack for hours or days. Epigastric or costal margin location of pain may radiate through to the back. A common pattern is one of intermittent attacks, initially spaced weeks or months apart and gradually increasing in frequency, occasionally progressing to daily or constant pain. Some of these patients will prove to have occult cholelithiasis, others to have peptic ulcer disease[88,89] that may not be appreciated until ERCP. In patients at a high risk for pancreatitis, such as chronic alcoholics, ERCP may reveal a surprisingly high incidence of pancreatic disease even in the absence of clinical elevations of pancreatic enzymes.[89] In older patients, or when symptoms of weight loss and anorexia are prominent, pancreatic carcinoma must be suspected. A preceding section has already dealt with an appropriate workup in that situation. However, in most cases, neither weight loss nor systemic symptoms are present. Often the patients are young or middle-aged, and most frequently they are women.

When such symptoms occur following a cholecystectomy, they are labeled with the umbrella diagnosis "postcholecystectomy syndrome." Often the symptoms experienced are identical to those that preceded the cholecystectomy. Such renewed symptoms after cholecystectomy may be attributable to a variety of causes. These include retained or recurrent common duct stones, operative trauma, long intramural cystic duct stump, secondary pancreatitis, or erroneous initial diagnosis. A number of authors[90-93] suggested that ampullary dysfunction and spasm with functional obstruction of bile flow may underlie the symptom complex in a sizable proportion of these patients. If the patient's pain is accompanied by episodic elevations of transaminase and alkaline phosphatase, the bile duct is dilated to greater than 15 mm on ERCP, and remains full of contrast for 45 minutes after the procedure, the diagnosis is clinically easy and extensive studies would be superfluous.

However, the vast majority of cases are not so accommodating. A number of techniques have been suggested for identifying those patients who might in a similar way benefit from a surgical or endoscopic sphincterotomy. These have ranged from provocative tests,[94] biliary scintigraphy,[95] and ultrasonic monitoring of duct size[96] to, most recently, endoscopic manometry of the ampullary sphincter.[90,97,98] This subject is discussed in great detail in the succeeding chapter and will not be treated further here. The concept of functional ampullary stenosis is not reserved exclusively for the postcholecystectomy patient and may be applied to patients with either pancreatic or biliary pain. Again, this concept is discussed in the next chapter.

There is one controversial area requiring further consideration here: the relationship between recurrent attacks of pancreatitis or pancreatic pain, and the developmental anomaly of the pancreatic ductal system known as pancreas divisum. In this group of patients, pancreatic pain has putatively been ascribed to an ampullary stenosis-type mechanism involving the accessory papilla. The term *pancreas divisum* describes a congenital anatomic variant of pancreatic development in which there is failure of fusion between the duct systems of the embryologic dorsal and ventral pancreatic anlages. In this situation, the ventral pancreas drains through a foreshortened duct of Wirsung at the papilla of Vater, while the bulk of the pancreatic drainage escapes through the duct of Santorini at the lesser papilla. Extensive clinical and autopsy studies[99,100] showed an overall incidence of this anomaly in about 9% of the general population. However, the frequency of this condition is often underestimated at routine ERCP. In 4–5% of patients, no ductal drainage occurs through the ampulla of Vater and the duct of Wirsung is entirely absent. Failure to visualize the pancreatic duct in this situation may be ascribed to the patient's disease or to a technical failure of endoscopy. A true estimate of the incidence of pancreas divisum requires an attempt to cannulate the dorsal pancreatic duct at the lesser ampulla whenever a duct of Wirsung of appropriate length cannot be demonstrated through the ampulla of Vater.

The lesser ampulla, if it exists, is always located proximal[101,102] to the main ampulla. Usually, it is 2–3 cm proximal and about 1 cm anterior to the major papilla on the medial duodenal wall. It may be flat or present as a small nipple, 1–1.5 mm in diameter, or may on other occasions be so prominent as to be mistaken for the main ampulla. In these situations, it can usually be differentiated from the ampulla of Vater by the absence of a longitudinal fold above the lesser ampulla and confluent arrowlike folds converging on its inferior border. Technically, the successful cannulation of the lesser ampulla in the majority of patients requires the use of a variant of the new, fine, metal-tipped catheters such as the Cremer catheter. The lesser ampulla can best be lined up on direct introduction of the endoscope into the second portion of the duodenum without the use of a pull-back maneuver. The Belgian group[99] reports a success rate of 90% in their recent experience and our own success rate is approximately 80%.

22. Cronin JJ: US diagnosis of choledocholithiasis: A reappraisal. *Radiology* 1986;161: 133–134.
23. O'Connor KW, Snodgrass PJ, Swonder JE, Mahoney S, Burt R, Cockerill EM, and Lumeng L: A blinded prospective study comparing four current noninvasive approaches in the differential diagnosis of medical versus surgical jaundice. *Gastroenterology* 1983;84:1498–1504.
24. Thomas MJ, Pellegrini CA, and Way LW: Usefulness of diagnostic tests for biliary obstruction. *Am J Surg* 1982;144:102–108.
25. Myllyla V, Paivansalo M, Pyhtinen J, Kairaluoma MI, and Niemela S: Sensitivity of ultrasonography in the demonstration of common bile duct stones and its ranking in comparison with intravenous cholangiography and endoscopic retrograde cholangiopancreatography. *ROFO* 1984;141:192–194.
26. Cooper D, Tarrant J, Whelan G, Styles CB, Cook M, and Desmond PV: Ultrasound in the diagnosis of jaundice: A review. *Med J Aust* 1985;143:381–385.
27. Honickman SP, Mueller PR, Wittenberg J, Simeone JF, Ferrucci JT Jr, Cronan JJ, and vanSonnenberg E: Ultrasound in obstructive jaundice: Prospective evaluation of site and cause. *Radiology* 1983;147:511–515.
28. Venu RP, Geenan JE, Toouli J, Stewart E, and Hogan WJ: Endoscopic retrograde cholangiopancreatography: Diagnosis of cholelithiasis in patients with normal gallbladder x-ray and ultrasound studies. *J Am Med Assoc* 1983;249:758–761.
29. Raval R, Lamki N, and Bandali K: Radiologic investigation of suspected extrahepatic biliary obstruction. *Can Med Assoc J* 1982;127:1191–1194.
30. Niederau C, Sonnenberg A, and Mueller J: Comparison of the extrahepatic bile duct size measured by ultrasound and by different radiographic methods. *Gastroenterology* 1984;87:615–621.
31. Freise J, Kleine P, and Gebel M: Lumenweite des ductus hepatocholedochus: sonographie im vergleich zur ERCP. *Rontgenblatter* 1985;38:241–243.
32. Baron RL: Common bile duct stones: Reassessment of criteria for CT diagnosis. *Radiology* 1987;162:419–424.
33. Richter JM, Silverstein MD, and Schapiro RH: Suspected obstructive jaundice: A decision analysis of diagnostic strategies. *Ann Intern Med* 1983;99:46–51.
34. Goodman MW, Ansel HJ, Vennes JA, Lasser RB, Silvis SE: Is intravenous cholangiography still useful? *Gastroenterology* 1980;79:642–645.
35. Matzen P, Haubek A, Holst-Christensen J, Lejerstofte J, and Juhl E: Accuracy of direct cholangiography by endoscopic or transhepatic route in jaundice: A prospective study. *Gastroenterology* 1981;81:237–241.
36. Rattner DW, Schapiro RH, and Warshaw AL: Abnormalities of the pancreatic and biliary ducts in adult patients with choledochal cysts. *Arch Surg* 1983;118:1068–1073.
37. Speer AG, Cotton PB, Russell RCG, et al: Randomized trial of endoscopic versus percutaneous stent insertion in malignant obstructive jaundice. *Lancet* 1987;2:57–62.
38. Long W, Schwartz W, Ring E. Endoscopic sphincterotomy assisted by catheterization antegrade. *Gastroint Endosc* 1984;30:36–39.
39. Tsang T, Crampton AR, Bernstein JR, Ramos SR, and Wieland JM: Percutaneous-endoscopic biliary stent placement: A preliminary report. *Ann Intern Med* 1987; 106:389–382.
40. Kairaluoma MI, Myllyla V, Partio E, Stahlberg M, Laitinen S, Juvonen T, and Suramo I: Impact of new imaging techniques on survival in cancer of the head of the pancreas and the periampullary region. *Acta Chir Scand* 1985;151:69–72.
41. Moosa AR, and Levin B: Collaborative studies in diagnosis of pancreatic cancer. *Cancer* 1981;47:1988–1697.
42. Tsuchiya R, Noda T, Harada N, Miyamoto T, Tomioka T, Yamamoto K, Yamaguchi T, Izawa K, Tsunoda T, Yoshino R, and Eto T: Collective review of small carcinomas of the pancreas. *Ann Surg* 1986;203:77–81.

43. Nix GA, Schmitz PI, Wilson JH, Van Blankenstein M, Groeneveld CF, and Hofwijk R: Carcinoma of the head of the pancreas. Therapeutic implications of endoscopic retrograde cholangiopancreatography findings. *Gastroenterology* 1984;87:37–43.
44. Moosa AR: Pancreatic Cancer: approach to diagnosis, selection for surgery and choice of operation. *Cancer* 1982;50:2689–2698.
45. Steinberg WM, Gelfand R, Anderson KK, Glenn J, Kurtzman SH, Sindelar WF, and Toskes PP. Comparison of the sensitivity and specificity of the CA 19-9 and carcinoembryonic antigen assays in detecting cancer of the pancreas. *Gastroenterology* 1986;90:343–934.
46. Anacker H, Lamarque JL, and Pistolesi GF: Editorial-Efficiency of different radiodiagnostic techniques in pancreatic disorders. *Eur J Radiol* 1981;1:79–84.
47. Frederic N, Deltenre M, d'Hondt M, deRueck M, Hermanus A, and Potvliege R: Comparative study of ultrasound and ERCP in the diagnosis of hepatic, biliary, and pancreatic diseases: A prospective study based on a continuous series of 424 patients. *Eur J Radiol* 1983;3:208–211.
48. Ariyama J, Sumida M, Shimaguchi S, and Shirakabe H: Integrated approach to the diagnosis of pancreatic carcinoma. *Rad Med* 1983;1:46–51.
49. Van Dyke JA, Stanley RJ, and Berland LL: Pancreatic imaging. *Ann Intern Med* 1985;102:212–217.
50. Yankaskas BC, Staab EV, Rudnick SA, and Fletcher RH: The radiologic diagnosis of pancreatic cancer. *Invest Radiol* 1985;20:73–78.
51. Gilinsky NH, Bornman PC, Girdwood AH, and Marks IN: Diagnostic yield of endoscopic retrograde cholangiopancreatography in carcinoma of the pancreas. *Br J Surg* 1986;73:539–543.
52. Freeny PC, Marks W, and Ball TJ: Impact of high-resolution computed tomography of the pancreas on utilization of endoscopic retrograde cholangiopancreatography and angiography. *Radiology* 1982;142:35–39.
53. Freeny PC, and Ball TJ: Endoscopic retrograde cholangiopancreatography (ERCP) and percutaneous transhepatic cholangiography (PTC) in the evaluation of suspected pancreatic carcinoma: Diagnostic limitations and contemporary roles. *Cancer* 1981;47:1666–1678.
54. Frick MP, Feinberg SB, and Goodale RL: The value of endoscopic retrograde cholangiopancreatography in patients with suspected carcinoma of the pancreas and indeterminant computed tomographic results. *Surg Gynecol Obstet* 1982;155:177–182.
55. Siegel JH, Yatto RP, and Vander RJ: Anomalous pancreatic ducts causing "Pseudomass" of the pancreas. *J Clin Gastroenterol* 1983;5:33–36.
56. Itai Y, Araki T, Tasaka A, and Maruyama M: Computed tomographic appearance of resectable pancreatic carcinoma. *Radiology* 1982;143:719–726.
57. Megibow AJ, Bosniak MA, Ambos MA, and Beranbaum ER: Thickening of celiac axis and/or superior mesenteric artery: a sign of pancreatic carcinoma on computed tomography. *Radiology* 1981;141:449–453.
58. Jafri SZH, Aisen AM, Glazer GM, and Weiss CA: Comparison of CT and angiography in assessing resectability of pancreatic carcinoma. *Am J Radiol* 1984;142:535–529.
59. Wittenberg J, Mueller PR, Ferrucci JT Jr, Simeone JF, vanSonneberg E, Neff CC, Palermo RA, and Isler RJ: Percutaneous core biopsy of abdominal tumors using 22 gauge needles: Further observations. *Am J Radiol* 1982;139:75–80.
60. Yasuda K, Mukai H, Fujimoto S, et al: The diagnosis of pancreatic cancer by endoscopic ultrasonography. *Gastrointest Endosc* 1988;34:1–8.
61. Warshaw AL, Schapiro RH, Ferrucci JT Jr, and Galdabini JJ: Persistent obstructive jaundice, cholangitis, and biliary cirrhosis due to common bile duct stenosis in chronic pancreatitis. *Gastroenterology* 1976;70:562–567.
62. Plumley TF, Rohrmann CA, Freeny PC, Silverstein FE, and Ball TJ: Double duct sign: reassessed significance in ERCP. *Am J Radiol* 1982;138:31–35.

63. Lavelle MI, Tait NP, Walsh T, Alderson D, and Record CO: Demonstration of pancreatic parenchyma by cholangiopancreatography. *Clin Radiol* 1985;36:405–407.
64. Hunt DR, and Blumgart LH: Preoperative differentiation between carcinoma of the pancreas and chronic pancreatitis: The contribution of cytology. *Endoscopy* 1982;14:171–173.
65. Silverstein MD, Richter JM, Podolsky DK, and Warshaw AL: Suspected pancreatic cancer presenting as pain or weight loss: Analysis of diagnostic strategies. *World J Surg* 1984;8:839–845.
66. Rosseland AR, and Solhaus JH: Early or delayed endoscopic papillotomy (EPT) in gallstone pancreatitis. *Ann Surg* 1984;199:165–167.
67. Neoptolemos JP, London N, Slater ND, Carr-Locke DL, Fossard DP, and Moosa AR: A prospective study of ERCP and endoscopic sphincterotomy in the diagnosis and treatment of gallstone acute pancreatitis. Arch Surg 1986;121:697–702.
68. Goodman AJ, Neoptolemos JP, Carr-Locke DL, Finlay DB, and Fossard DP: Detection of gall stones after acute pancreatitis. *Gut* 1985;26:125–132.
69. Feller ER: Endoscopic retrograde cholangiopancreatography in the diagnosis of unexplained pancreatitis. *Arch Intern Med* 1984;144:1797–1799.
70. Girdwood AH, Hatfield AR, Bornman PC, Denyer ME, Kottler RE, and Marks IN: Structure and function in non-calcific pancreatitis. *Dig Dis Sci* 1984;29:721–726.
71. Mee AS, Girdwood AH, Walker E, Gilinsky NH, Kottler RE, and Marks IN: Comparison of the oral (PABA) pancreatic function test, the secretin-pancreozymin test and endoscopic retrograde pancreatography in chronic alcohol-induced pancreatitis. *Gut* 1985;26:1257–1262.
72. Malfertheiner P, Buchler M, Stanescu A, and Ditschuneit H: Exocrine pancreatic function in correlation to ductal and parenchymal morphology in chronic pancreatitis. *Hepatogastroenterology* 1986;33:110–114.
73. Gilinsky NH, Leung JW, Heron C, and Cotton PB: Calcific pancreatitis: Calcification patterns and pancreatogram correlations. *Clin Radiol* 1984;35:401–404.
74. Testoni PA, Masci E, Passaretti S, Guslandi M, and Tittobello A. Early detection of pancreatic lesions in chronic alcoholism: Diagnostic accuracy of ERP. *J Clin Gastroenterol* 1984;6:519–523.
75. Amman RW, Akovbiantz A, Largiader F, and Schueler G: Course and outcome of chronic pancreatitis: Longitudinal study of a mixed medical-surgical series of 245 patients. *Gastroenterology* 1984;86:820–828.
76. Norup-Lauridsen K, Raahede J, Kruse A, Thommesen P. ERP in chronic pancreatitis—ductal morphology, relation to exocrine function and pain—clinical value. *Roetgenblatter* 1985;38:258–260.
77. Warshaw AL, Popp JW Jr, and Schapiro RH: Long-term patency, pancreatic function, and pain relief after lateral pancreaticojejunostomy for chronic pancreatitis. *Gastroenterology* 1980;79:289–293.
78. Mullens JE: Endoscopic retrograde cholangiopancreatography (ERCP) in the diagnosis of chronic pancreatitis. *Surgery* 1978;84:308–312.
79. Katon RM, Bilbao MK, Eidemiller LR, and Benson JA, Jr, Endoscopic retrograde cholangiopancreatography in the diagnosis and management of non-alcoholic pancreatitis. *Surg Gynecol Obstet* 1978;147:333–338.
80. Makela P, and Aarimaa, M: Pancreatography in a family with hereditary pancreatitis. *Acta Radiol* 1985;26:63–66.
81. Garcia-puges AM, Navarro S, Ros E, Elena M, Ballesta A, Aused R, and Vilar-Bonet J: Reversibility of exocrine pancreatic failure in chronic pancreatitis. *Gastroenterology* 1986;91:17–24.
82. Gregg JA, Carr-Locke DL, and Gallagher MM: Importance of common bile duct stricture associated with chronic pancreatitis. Diagnosis by endoscopic retrograde cholangiopancreatography. Am J Surg 1981;141:199–203.
83. Eckhauser FE, Knol JA, Strodel WE, Achem S, and Nostrant T: Common bile duct strictures associated with chronic pancreatitis. *Am Surg* 1983;49:350–358.

84. O'Connor M, Kolars J, Ansel H, Silvis S, and Vennes J: Preoperative endoscopic retrograde cholangiopancreatography in the surgical management of pancreatic pseudocysts. *Am J Surg* 1986;151:18–24.
85. Levine JB, Warshaw AL, Falchuck KR, and Schapiro RH. The value of endoscopic retrograde pancreatography in the management of pancreatic ascites. *Surgery* 1977;81:360–362.
86. Weaver DW, Walt AJ, Sugawa C, and Bouwman DL: A continuing appraisal of pancreatic ascites. *Surg Gyynecol Obstet* 1982;154:845–848.
87. Stone LD: Pancreatic ascites. *Br J Hosp Med* 1986;35:252–253.
88. Lee MJ, Choi TK, Lai EC, Wong KP, Ngan H, and Wong J: Endoscopic retrograde cholangiopancreatography after acute pancreatitis. *Surg Gynecol Obstet* 1986;163:354–358.
89. Ruddell WSJ, Lintott DJ, and Axon ATR: The diagnostic yield of ERCP in the investigation of unexplained abdominal pain. *Br J Surg* 1983;70:74–75.
90. BarMeir S, Geenen JE, Hogan WJ, et al: Biliary and pancreatic duct pressures measured by ERCP manometry in patients with suspected papillary stenosis. *Dig Dis Sci* 1979;24:209–213.
91. Venu RP, and Geenen JE: Diagnosis and treatment of diseases of the papilla. *J Clin Gastroenterology* 1986;15:439–456.
92. Guelrud M, Mendoza S, Vicent S, et al: Pressures in the sphincter of Oddi in patients with gallstones, common duct stones, and recurrent pancreatitis. *J Clin Gastroenterology* 1983;5:37–41.
93. Tanaka M, Ikeda S, Matsumoto S, et al: Manometric diagnosis of sphincter of Oddi spasm as a cause of postcholecystectomy pain and the treatment by endoscopic sphincterotomy. *Ann Surg* 1985;202:712–719.
94. Nardi GL, Michelassi F, and Zannini P: Transduodenal sphincteroplasty. *Ann Surg* 1983;198:453–461.
95. Zeman RK, Burrell MI, Dobbins J, Jaffe MH, and Choyke PL: Postcholecystectomy syndrome: Evaluation using biliary scintigraphy and endoscopic retrograde cholangiopancreatography. *Radiology* 1985;156:787–792.
96. Warshaw AL, Simeone J, Schapiro RH, et al: Objective evaluation of ampullary stenosis with ultrasonography and pancreatic stimulation. *Am J Surg* 1985;149:65–72.
97. Geenen JE, Hogan WJ, Dodds WJ, et al: Intraluminal pressure recordings from human sphincter of Oddi. *Gastroenterology* 1980;78:317–324.
98. Toouli J, Roberts-Thomson IC, Dent J, et al: Manometric disorders in patients with suspected sphincter of Oddi dysfunction. *Gastroenterology* 1985;88:1243–1250.
99. Delhaye M, Engelholm L, and Cremer M: Pancreas divisum: Congenital anatomic variant or anomaly? *Gastroenterology* 1985;89:951–958.
100. Sugawa C, Walt AJ, Nunez DC, and Masuyama H: Pancreas divisum: Is it a normal anatomic variant? *Am J Surg* 1987;153:62–7.93.
101. Grant JCB. *An Atlas of Anatomy*, 4th ed. Baltimore, Williams and Wilkins, 1956, p. 140.
102. Sisfusson BF, Wehlin L, and Lindstrom CG: Variants of pancreatic duct system of importance in endoscopic retrograde cholangiopancreatography. Observations on autopsy specimens. *Acta Radiol (Diag)* 1983;24:113–128.
103. Warshaw AL, and Cambria RP: False pancreas divisum. Acquired pancreatic duct obstruction simulating the congenital anomaly. *Ann Surg* 1984;200:595–595.
104. Warshaw AL, Richter JM, and Schapiro RH: The cause and treatment of pancreatitis associated with pancreas divisum. *Ann Surg* 1983;198:443–452.
105. Cotton PB: Pancreas divisum—curiosity or culprit? *Gastroenterology* 1985;89:1431–1435.
106. Madura JA, Fiore AC, O'Connor KW, Lehman GA, and McCammon RL: Pancreas divisum. Detection and management. *Am Surg* 1985;51:353–537.

107. Steer ML: More doubts about the clinical significance of pancreas divisum. *Gastroenterology* 1987;93:206–207.
108. Warshaw AL, and Schapiro RH: Pancreas divisum and pancreatitis. *Surg Annual*, to be published.
109. Warshaw AL: Reply to selected summary: More doubts about the clinical significance of pancreas divisum. *Gastroenterology* 1987;93:1140–1041.

Chapter **3**

Technique of Endoscopic Sphincterotomy

Jack A. Vennes, M.D.

Introduction

Endoscopic retrograde sphincterotomy (ERS) is a very gratifying procedure which frequently offers patients permanent relief from pain, sepsis, and pruritis. The parent procedure, endoscopic retrograde cholangiopancreatography (ERCP), ushered in new diagnostic possibilities requiring new skills. ERS is a valuable therapeutic descendant also involving new skills, risks, benefits, anatomic precision, and technical detail.[1-7] The aspects of ERS are the primary focus of this chapter (Table 3-1).

The indications for endoscopic sphincterotomy (ES) are listed in Table 3-2. Other conditions on which clinical experience is being gathered without clear consensus at present include gallstone pancreatitis, choledocholithiasis in standard-risk patients with gallbladders in situ, recurrent acute pancreatitis, pancreatitis with pancreas divisum, and chronic pancreatitis with chronic pain. Most of these clinical entities are treated in some detail elsewhere in this book. Finally, the sump syndrome[8] and choledochocoele[9] may be successfully managed by ES, but their diagnosis and assessment of clinical significance together with their rarity removes them from the indications list.

Preparation

Preparation of ourselves and the patient for ERS differs from that for ERCP largely in degree and detail. Discussion with the patient is more complete because the clinical consequences of success are frequently more far reaching than those of ERCP, and the risks are the risks of ERS plus those of ERCP. When discussing risks with patient and family, we include the risk of failure, since this prompts a preliminary discussion of what the next options will be in that event. The additive risks of ERCP and sphincterotomy in most hands approximates 10%[4,10] (see Chapter 4).

Preparation includes continuing attention to disinfection of equipment, as using a contaminated endoscope has serious potential consequences for the patient undergoing ERCP or ERS. Patients frequently have an obstructed biliary tree which may or may not already be infected. When ductal obstruction is

Table 3-1 Endoscopic Retrograde Sphincterotomy—Technical Steps

1. Preparation
2. Diagnostic ERCP
3. Free cannulation of bile duct
4. Sphincterotomy
5. Sphincterotomy variations
6. Sphincterotomy alternatives

promptly relieved by endoscopic sphincterotomy, further complications from endogenous or exogenous infection are greatly reduced. However, when ERCP is performed and when subsequent attempts at sphincterotomy are unsuccessful, the risks of an infection from organisms already present or from *Pseudomonas* newly introduced[11] becomes significant. When this occurs we regard it as urgent that ductal drainage be accomplished by one of several measures, including nasobiliary drainage, transhepatic cholangiography, or immediate surgical management. In patients who are already on antibiotics or in whom antibiotic infusion was begun shortly before the ERS attempt, antibiotics are continued. Antibiotics may be chosen on the basis of specific culture data; often the institutional preference is for two antibiotics providing coverage against enteric pathogens.

Dealing more generally with the potential problems of infection due to contaminated endoscopes, we advocate the following:

1. Strict adherence to details of endoscopic disinfection including a final rinse of alcohol and air drying to prevent growth of water-loving organisms[12]
2. Routine monitoring of post-ERCP or post-ERS bile cultures if the patient subsequently comes to laparotomy
3. Periodic monthly cultures of all endoscopes and related equipment
4. Repeating the disinfection and rinsing cycle just prior to ERCP on all instruments which have been hanging for more than 24 hr

Utilizing these measures plus the judicious and early use of appropriate antibiotic coverage has reduced endoscopically related infections to negligible numbers.

It is important that we take all cost-effective measures to preclude bleeding after ES. As a general rule hemostasis is adequate when the prothrombin time is no more than 2 sec outside the normal range and the platelet count is at least 80,000 in a patient with a negative bleeding history. Platelet dysfunction due to

Table 3-2 Indications for Endoscopic Sphincterotomy

1. Choledocholithiasis
    Patient over 50 years of age
    Previous cholecystectomy
    Gallbladder in situ, high surgical risk
    Often with acute cholangitis
2. Papillary stenosis
3. Stent placement across malignant extrahepatic duct strictures

recent therapy with aspirin, nonsteroidal drugs, or newer generation penicillins may be at least additive factors in deciding about platelet transfusions or in timing procedures.

Performing the Diagnostic ERCP

In this discussion we shall assume that before doing the ERCP the need for probable sphincterotomy is recognized and therefore the preparations are for cholangiography to be followed by a sphincterotomy if indicated. This is desirable but not always possible; however, the interval should be brief between the ERCP and referral for sphincterotomy.

A successful and safe sphincterotomy requires that several special observations be made during the diagnostic cholangiography. First of course, the contents and contours of the duct must be accurately detailed. The *number* of calculi when present and the *least diameter* of the largest stone provide important information in making sphincterotomy decisions. Next, the endoscopic view of the visible intramural segment is a critical measurement, since safe cutting limits are thus defined. As an example, if the largest stone is 10 mm in diameter, we need to know that a sphincterotomy can be made within the confines of the intramural duct which is large enough to permit retrieval and passage of a 10-mm calculus. Visualizing all of the calculi in the duct can be a tricky business and requires attention to detail. If the duct is rather large and the contrast column is therefore fairly dense, raising the K_v will improve the contrast image of ductal contents. Many calculi are situated just above the intramural segment and as filling is begun the stones are fluoroscopically seen to float up at the head of the contrast column. We obtain a spot film immediately at this juncture. The presence of a normal-caliber duct is no assurance that stones are absent, as we find that at least a fourth of the time in patients with choledocholithiasis ductal calibers are normal. Coming back to the measurement of the intramural segment for a moment, it is well to get some initial sense of how long it is and make a mental note on viewing it as to what portion of it will be divided. That is, cutting up to a crossing fold or through a crossing fold is a decision that will often come up, but it can be difficult if deferred until part of the sphincterotomy is made and the anatomic details are unclear.

It is incumbent on the endoscopist to obtain a clear radiographic view of the distal intrapancreatic and preampullary common bile duct. Occasionally this area is variably narrowed, enough so that delivery of all stones is impossible. This is important information *prior* to doing the sphincterotomy. When present, the narrowed distal duct is usually fairly firm, although occasionally thin webs can be easily traversed. Such webs are probably pleats of a tortuous curving duct and of no clinical or endoscopic significance. Once traversed with a cannula they may partially straighten.

The prospect of doing an ERS requires more thorough and thoughtful planning ahead than does a diagnostic ERCP. Discussion with a surgical colleague and often with an invasive radiologist should cover not only the possible complications of the procedure, but also a contingency plan for ERS failure, the inability to remove all stones (particularly large ones during the initial procedure), or the presence of unusual anatomy which makes the procedure more difficult, such as the presence of the papilla inside a diverticulum.

If the distal duct is of smaller caliber than the least diameter of the largest calculus, one must pause as routine sphincterotomy may not be possible. There are several options. One may make a sphincterotomy, then pass a balloon to test whether the narrowing will expand, or whether the large stone separates into several smaller ones when "perturbed" by the balloon. Fragmentation of a single large stone may be possible in at least half of attempts with a mechanical or electrohydraulic lithotripter. Dissolution with monooctanoin delivered via a nasobiliary tube left indwelling for 4–7 days is effective in about half of attempts.[13] Dissolution with more effective solvents, disintegration with extracorporeal lithotripsy or with tunable dye laser may all be effective options fairly soon (see Chapter 5). Alternatives as always include referral for surgical management.

No pancreatogram is routinely done during the ERCP when sphincterotomy is planned. Avoidance of pancreatography may reduce the complication rate of pancreatitis in this group of patients. The exception is the patient with possible papillary stenosis in whom careful evaluation of both systems is essential. Papillary stenosis may be due to papillary *fibrosis* of the Vaterian segment with partial obstruction and dilation of both bile and pancreatic ducts. Pain is usually relieved by ES of the biliary duct, and later additional pancreatic ES is rarely necessary.

Free Cannulation Technique with Variations

When doing diagnostic ERCP, free cannulation of the bile duct is desirable but usually not requisite for success. In contrast, successful and safe endoscopic sphincterotomy absolutely requires that free entry be obtained to the interior of the bile duct since the procedure is designed to provide a free access *from* the interior of the duct *to* the duodenum. Free entry to the duct with a regular cannula and usual ERCP maneuvers is usually possible with some attention to detail. The common bile duct pursues a course within the papilla and certainly within the duodenal wall which is virtually immediately a cephalad one. It is important, therefore, to address the papilla from a rather tucked-under position so that the cannula is easily directed into the papillary orifice immediately cephalad, seeming to almost crawl up under the duodenal mucosa. We believe more common duct cannulations are missed by failing to take this usual anatomy into account than by any other means. Moreover, the successful retrograde approach to the common bile duct often takes advantage of the fact that the duct pursues a course within the papilla which is somewhat right-to-left as viewed from the retrograde position (Figure 3-1). Addressing the papillary orifice, then, with a cephalad orientation and initially some right-to-leftness is sometimes helpful.

What to do when the anatomy seems easily identified and is normal, the pancreatic duct is where it ought to be, and the common duct would seem to be taking off cephalad and perhaps a little to the left as viewed endoscopically, but no common duct cannulation occurs? We look for other ways of doing things and the list of variations in Table 3-3 is worthy of attention. Since this is a troublesome cannulation we're attempting, it occurs to us about this time that if we do freely cannulate, perhaps we ought to have a wire secured in place

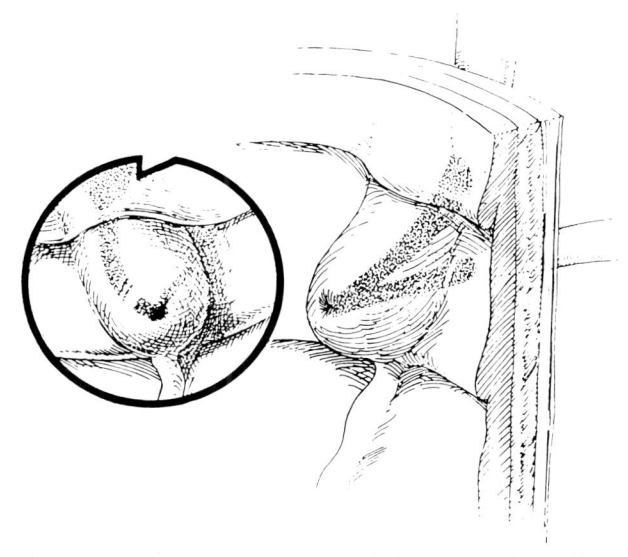

Figure 3-1 Usual course of common bile duct. In its terminal intrapapillary portion the bile duct is commonly submucosal with lateral curving. Therefore in retrograde cannulation it is frequently useful to orient the cannula *immediately* cephalad and in a lateral plane from right to left. This is especially advisable when all roads *seem* to lead to the pancreatic duct.

over which we can pass the sphincterotome, should a sphincterotomy be indicated after cholangiography. It is a vexing circumstance in which after some trial one succeeds in freely cannulating the duct with the regular cannula or a tapered tip cannula, only to fail miserably to ever get a sphincterotome back in the duct after the regular cannula is removed. Therefore the next maneuver we suggest is the use of a regular cannula passed over a 0.035-in. 400-cm wire. The wire may be extruded so that a centimeter or less of its floppy tip is beyond the cannula. One then simply uses the cannula-wire combination in the same maneuvers that have just been unavailing with a regular cannula. As often happens, the common duct was right where we thought it was and is now entered by the tip of the wire with the cannula following to a free duct position. Leaving the cannula well up the duct, the wire can be removed for cholangiography followed by reintroduction of the wire, removal of the cannula, and passage of a two-channel sphincterotome back over the wire. It is quite evident that gentle-

Table 3-3 Free Cannulation of Bile Duct—
Technical Options

1. Regular cannula
2. Tapered tip cannula
3. Regular cannula over 0.035-in. guidewire
4. Sphincterotome as cannula
5. Two-channel sphincterotome over guidewire
6. Precut with wire electrode
7. Choledochoduodenal fistula with needle electrode
8. 3-cm leader on sphincterotome

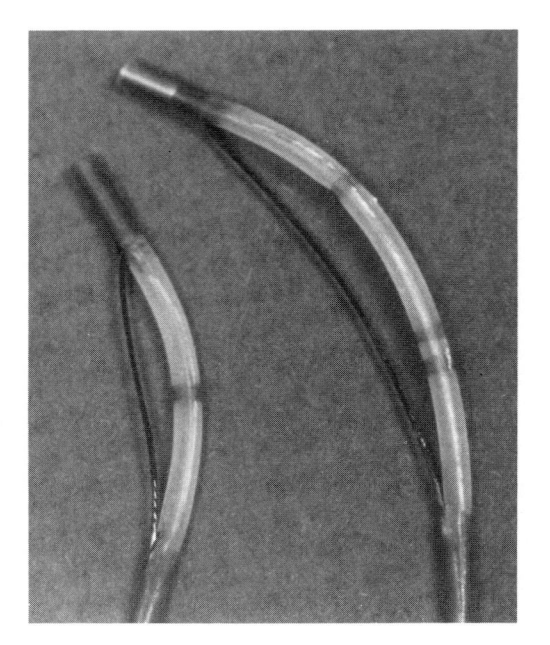

Figure 3-2 Standard sphincterotomes may have 20 or 30 mm of exposed wire in their extended position. Preference for one or the other is usually based on personal familiarity and experience. Both are available with the 5-cm cannula leader out ahead of the wire. This has the advantage of better maintenance of intraductal position during placement of the wire precisely in the desired transpapillary location.

ness is the byword in these wire matters, but with this proviso this is a satisfactory sequencing of steps in a successful free cannulation. The use of the tapered cannula and 0.018- or 0.025-in. wire is less useful because the floppy tip is really too permissive and that system provides no real advantages over the 0.035-in. wire.

The next option which works rather well is to use the sphincterotome as the initial cannulating accessory. This has a distinct advantage in that the tip of the cannula can be oriented in the cephalad direction of the common bile duct by simply having the assistant put a partial flex on the wire. If for some reason a tucked-under and cephalad approach is difficult or impossible, this may work very well, still acknowledging the early cephalad orientation of the common duct within the intramural segment. The trouble with this system is that the sphincterotome must often be in the duct far enough to cover both holes before injecting contrast, or else contrast leaks back through the proximal hole rather than running into the duct. Either 20-mm or 30-mm sphincterotomes work well for this purpose (Figure 3-2). If the sphincterotome is misplaced in the pancreatic duct and further passage is impeded by a turn in the duct, one can usually get enough contrast in to confirm this anatomic location even when the proximal hole leaks contrast into the duodenum. Repeated entry of the sphincterotome into the pancreatic duct should be avoided. Use of the sphincterotome as the cannulating instrument abbreviates the whole procedure, particularly the troublesome cannulation component, since from a free position a careful cholangiogram can be made with the sphincterotome remaining in place anchored by placement of a half or three-quarter flexion on the wire.

Several other technical options for obtaining a free position in the common duct included the use of a precut papillotome in which the wire extends to the tip of the catheter[14]; a wire electrode for precutting[15]; a needle electrode for

TECHNIQUE OF ENDOSCOPIC SPHINCTEROTOMY 47

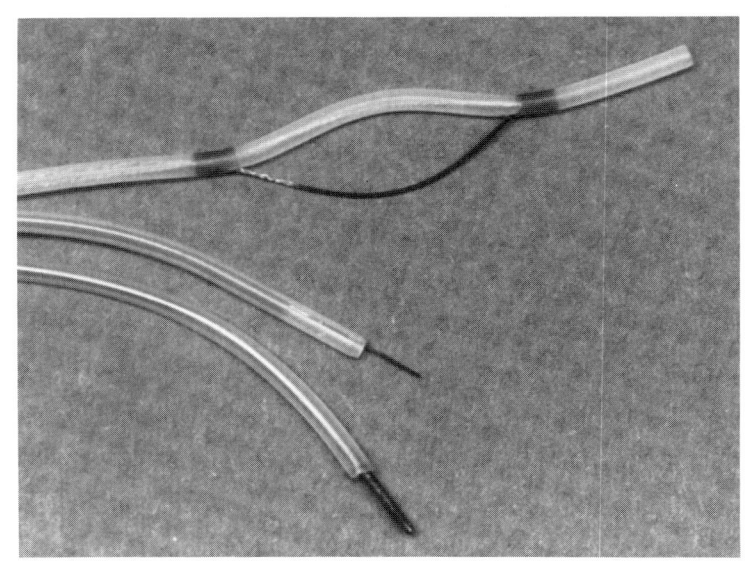

Figure 3-3 Alternative sphincterotomes. The top is one of the several devices produced to successfully do a sphincterotomy in the patient with a Billroth II anastomosis. The instrument at the bottom of the picture is the older needle knife which is useful for the occasional formation of a choledochoduodenostomy in the intramural portion of the duct. In the middle is the small fine-wire electrode which is useful for occasional precutting. Less current is necessary for smooth cutting with this instrument as compared with a standard sphincterotome, since obviously the electrode is much smaller and the current density therefore higher.

making a choledochoduodenal fistula proximal to the papilla orifice[16] (Figure 3-3); and a two-channel sphincterotome which can be passed over a 0.035-in. guidewire (Figure 3-4).[17] The needle electrode or needle knife has been available for years with an extendable blunt tip whose diameter is about that of a 23-gauge needle. The wire electrode has been introduced more recently by Hui-

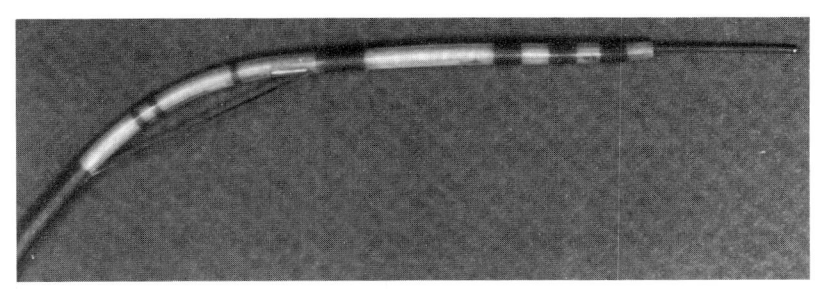

Figure 3-4 A sphincterotome is available with two channels. Having freely cannulated the duct containing stones with a standard cannula, a 0.035-in. wire is passed into the duct and the cannula is removed. The 7 French two-channel sphincterotome is then passed over the wire. The sphincterotome wire is placed in its proper location across the papilla and a sphincterotomy is performed. The two wires are electrically insulated from each other in this model. In the one shown, a 5-cm leader is present. This two-channel variation of the sphincterotomy procedure has the advantage of maintaining a freely cannulated position throughout the procedure once it is obtained, often with some difficulty.

bregtse et al[15] as a flexible wire of even smaller diameter than the "needle." The needle has the purpose of making occasional choledochoduodenal fistulas. The finer wire electrode works well to make a 6-mm precut sphincterotomy. (The fine-wire electrode is sometimes referred to as a "fine needle-knife," creating the possibility of semantic confusion) (Figure 3-3).

Precutting with a precut papillotome or with a thin-wire electrode is usually used in circumstances in which a sphincterotomy is likely going to be indicated, when pancreatic duct position is already demonstrated by pancreatography, and when the ductal orifice is visible. With precut papillotomes one may lose control of the radial direction in which cutting is occurring so that proximity to the pancreatic duct becomes a problem. Accordingly, I have always regarded precut papillotomes with respect and have been so reluctant to use them that we have substituted prolonged patient attempts at free cannulation in their place. When using the thin-wire papillotomes alluded to above, on the other hand, anatomic landmarks remain clear and the radial orientation is readily controlled. Therefore, when all else fails and the free cannulation position is required, we will consider using a fine-wire electrode to make a 6-mm cut in the papilla along the presumed course of the common bile duct (from the central depression up toward 11 o'clock). Entry is thereby gained the majority of the time. This technique has been used extensively in Amsterdam, and their experience is reassuring to the rest of us who are occasionally in need of such options.

When the very distal bile duct is obstructed by impacted stone or by ampullary tumor, and when a well-defined intramural duct impression is seen coursing cephalad to the papilla, free access to the bile duct may be obtained by creating a choledochoduodenal fistula. This is accomplished by use of a wire electrode. The wire is extruded a few millimeters from the cannula, and positioned clearly on the intramural ridge 6–10 mm or so cephalad to the papillary opening. Using less power than used for regular sphincterotomy, with blended current, the tip of the wire is slowly spiraled down through tissue until bile appears and entry to the bile duct is gained. At this point the usual options are open, including the creation of a larger sphincterotomy. This procedure does not appear to have caught on in this country. On the relatively few occasions we have used it, there has been no morbidity, as has also been reported by others. Aabakken and Osnes used this technique as the only decompressing measure for a number of patients with ampullary carcinomas and found that the duct remained open until the demise of the majority of patients.[18]

The Standard Sphincterotomy

There are multiple variations on the basic sphincterotome design, all of which make good sense and work best in the hands of some. I think it comes down to using a design with which one is confident, skilled, and experienced. From personal experience I prefer a 30-mm length of exposed wire largely for these reasons of familiarity. On flexing, the wire comes up smoothly with a symmetric bow in the cannula. Typically, we cut with 10 mm or less of wire in touch with tissue. Added flexion of the cannula as needed provides a smooth means of enlarging a cut, holding wire in touch with tissue. The standard 20-mm sphincterotome is used with equal success and enthusiasm by many (Figure 3-2). Technique is altered with the 20-mm sphincterotome in that flexion results in a minimal arc of the cannula, and necessary cephalad cutting takes place with flexion of the scope tip or vertical lift with the elevator. A 3-cm leader provides some insurance against having the sphincterotome fall back into the duodenum during precise placement, particularly if the ductal channel is firm and tight. The disadvantage is that flexion of the wire does not provide the same degree of control over the tip of the sphincterotome, a property of the standard sphincterotome that is sometimes helpful with cannulation.

Let us assume that a good-quality cholangiogram has been obtained and the indications for sphincterotomy have been thereby defined. Any equipment we may need is readily available. A free cannulation backup has been obtained with the standard cannula. Coagulation parameters are satisfactory. A surgical colleague has been consulted. The appropriate amount of power as blended current is known; anatomic details are clear and not confusing. The indifferent electrode (conducting pad) is applied to the gluteal area. Information learned earlier regarding best endoscope position for free cannulation is now recalled. The sphincterotome is passed into endoscopic view. The wire is noted to be radially oriented in a 12 o'clock to 1 o'clock position. If the wire appears more inclined to a 2 or 3 o'clock position, another sphincterotome is passed. One can frequently force the sphincterotome cannula into a more favorable position by removing it and twisting it forcibly over the thumb. This is practically unnecessary and merely switching accessories usually suffices. Moving up close and in a tucked-under position, the sphincterotome is freely passed into the bile duct. Its position in the biliary tree is verified fluoroscopically now *and with each reentry*. Having assuredly positioned the sphincterotome in the common duct, one now requests the assistant to flex the wire to a "half flex" to secure the free duct position.

From now on, tight, clear, verbal communication between the endoscopist and the assistant is required for safe, successful technique. Verbal orders are repeated back.

About now the necessary length of cut is determined. If, for instance, a 10-mm cut will be sufficient to deliver all known calculi, then a 10-mm point proximal to the papillary opening is estimated as the terminus of the cut. This is frequently in some relationship to a first or second crossing fold. It is well to note whether the intramural impression extends above the predicted necessary length of cut. There are times that a longer cut than predicted is necessary on the duodenal side in order to create an opening large enough on the duct side of the sphincterotomy (Figure 3-5). It is advisable to know before landmarks are disturbed whether one has a length of intramural segment required to do so if necessary.

The sphincterotome is now anchored safely in the duct by maintaining flexion of the wire. The endoscope is positioned for most favorable viewing of the sphincterotomy as cutting will proceed in a few minutes. Whereas the tucked-under position was best for free cannulation, sphincterotomy is best done under viewing in a more enface position, looking more directly at the papilla than obliquely under it. In this position the progress of the sphincterotomy is best monitored. Whereas cannulation was often obtained up very close to the papilla, one may now back away a bit for a more panoramic view of the area. Both of these adjustments, the enface and the more distant view, are generally obtained by merely advancing the endoscope a bit, leaving the controls locked. The other positional change that may require attention at this point is the occasional

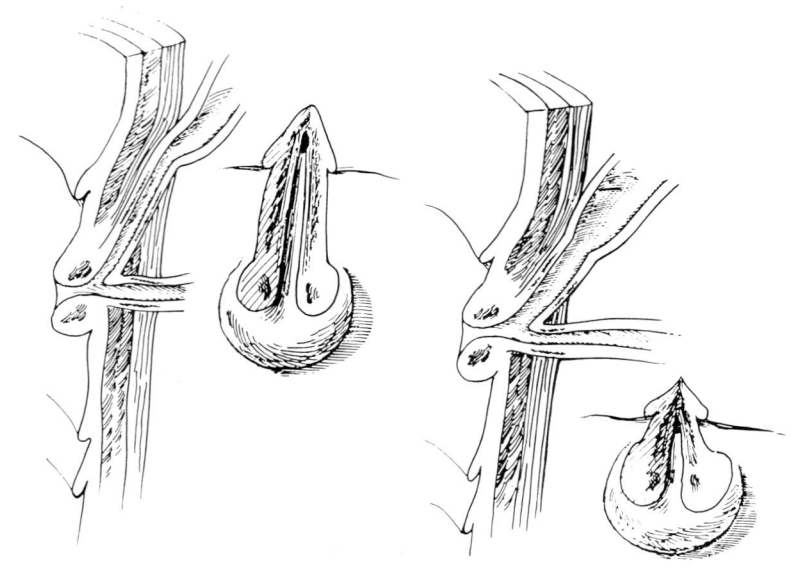

Figure 3-5 Variations in length of intramural segment. The usual length and angulation is schematically shown on the right. An unusually long intramural segment shown on the left may be suspected by the endoscopic view of a long intramural bulge above the papilla. Practically, this means that a cut must be made longer than usual in order to obtain an adequate opening. For example, a 8- to 9-mm opening as judged by retrieval of a 9- to 10-mm balloon may require sequential cutting until a 12- to 14-mm cut is made on the duodenal side.

tendency for the papilla to remain at the far 3 o'clock perimeter of the visual field. Again, with the sphincterotome anchored in the duct, one maneuvers the papilla into the center of view by clockwise rotation of the scope and left lateral flexion.

Our next assignment is to position the sphincterotome wire so that the desired length of wire is in contact with tissue and so that the wire is not pressed firmly but rather is gently flexed to be in touch with the tissue. To accomplish this, the sphincterotome is gently retracted, and if it hangs up then less flexion is called for. The assistant is instructed that "less flexion" at this point means very small decrements of flexion. Now it is a matter of gently repeating these motions until the wire is lying gently across the papilla and intramural duct with 10–15 mm of wire in touch with tissue (Figures 3-6 and 3-7). If undue flexion pressure is placed on the wire, it will merely result in the sphincterotome popping either back up into the duct or into the duodenum. Also, when cutting occurs, the wire which is flexed too tautly into tissue may cut rapidly in an uncontrolled manner.

So now we have the sphincterotome in place with the length of wire inserted being somewhat determined by the length of intramural segment and the length of sphincterotomy planned, but in no case greater than 10–15 mm in length. If one uses a 30-mm sphincterotome, the intraluminal portion of the wire can be kept in visual control so that no inadvertent burning of duodenal folds occurs.

At this point, one calls for "power on." Power settings are at the minimal number of watts considered necessary for the power source being used. With

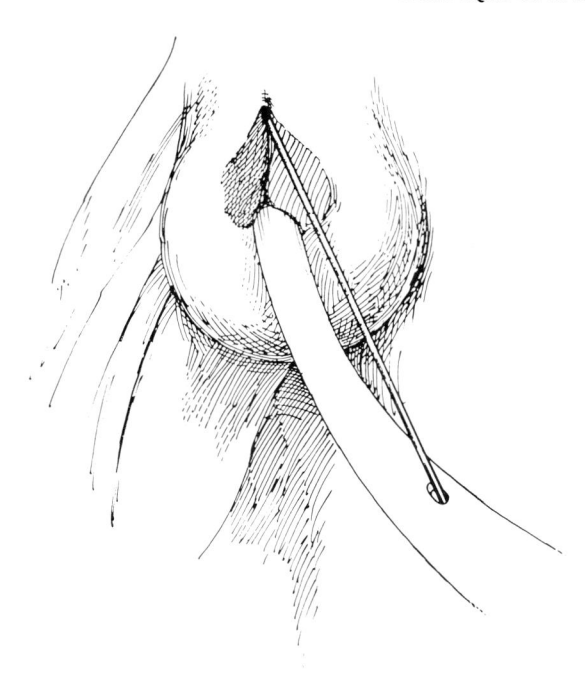

Figure 3-6 Wire position in tissue. Ten millimeters of a 30-mm sphincterotome is in touch with tissue. The entire length of wire was placed free in the duct as fluoroscopically confirmed, then slowly and gently withdrawn with minimal flexion to this position. Cutting proceeds with minimal flexion tension.

everything in place, blended current is applied to the wire for a second or two. Blanching of tissue with or without a little smoke is reassuring evidence that we do indeed have a completed circuit. With the application of another 1- or 2-second burst, cutting begins. The thing to underline in your mind is that at this point, the position of the sphincterotome is maintained or at most is very slightly withdrawn. *Do not* pull the sphincterotome out of the ductal position before cutting has occurred. The ominous possibility exists that tissue coagulation may occur prior to cutting and after the sphincterotome slips out the sphincterotomy reposition may be difficult. If a circuit is complete but cutting is not occurring, we would turn up our power by 10% and continue. Typically, cutting occurs up to 5 or 6 mm at which point the position of the wire with respect to tissue needs adjustment. This is done by calling for more flexion or by elevating the sphincterotome with the left thumb on the elevator. If one had to turn up power to a new power position to initiate cutting, one may frequently turn it back down now to the initial setting in that cutting in the first few millimeters is frequently more difficult, requiring more power than the subsequent completion of cutting (? fibrosis). It will be noted that as cutting continues, the wire length in contact with tissue decreases. This is partly because of the usual position of the sphincterotome and partly because we tend to withdraw the wire in small increments. As cutting then continues smoothly and controllably, a typical gush of bile and contrast signals the arrival of the cut at the ductal end of the intramural length of Vaterian segment, often signaling essentially the completion of the sphincterotomy (Figure 3-8, **Plate 2–5**). A gush of bile is of course dependent on our having filled the duct full enough of contrast that this can happen.

Let's say that the sphincterotomy appears complete but no gush has occurred. At this point one simply passes the sphincterotome back into the duct,

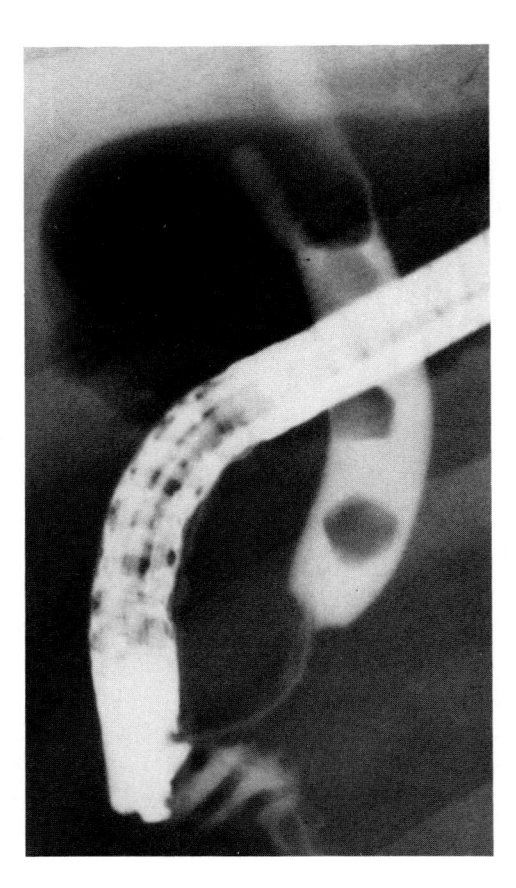

Figure 3-7 Choledocholithiasis. At least four faceted calculi are evident. The duct is only minimally dilated at about 15 mm (the tip of the endoscope is 12 mm in diameter). The sphincterotome wire is poorly visualized, as is the soft-tissue density of the papilla. The wire is minimally flexed and about 12 mm is in touch with tissue. A sphincterotomy of 9–10 mm will be necessary to permit passage of the largest stone, situated proximally in the duct near the cystic duct take-off.

requests full flexion, which for a 30-mm papillotome amounts to about a 9- or 10-mm distance between the wire and flexed cannula, and pulls this gently back into the duodenum. If cutting is complete or nearly complete, the papillotome should pass through unimpeded.

A cautionary note at this point. The optics of modern instruments are such that with wide angles of view, the size of the apparent image drops off quickly as one moves away from it. Therefore, a sphincterotomy made at some distance from the scope may appear rather minimal or inadequate. If this is the case, one should move up close and assess the length, or pass an object through the sphincterotomy of known diameter or radius, i.e., a balloon or a flexed sphincterotome.

Generally at this point, therefore, the papillotome is removed and replaced by a balloon. Standard balloons generally have around 9–14 mm of diameter with 1.5–4.0 cm^3 of air instilled. The balloon is positioned just a short distance up the duct and inflated under fluoroscopic control to a known diameter of 8–10 mm. The balloon can then be pulled through the sphincter area and, as it comes through relatively unimpeded, one has sized the channel and can then determine the success with which existing stones will also pass. The usual maneuver then is to pass the balloon up the duct, inflating it proximal to one or two stones at a time and bringing them down into the duodenum. Stones which are intrahepatic may be induced to come down by using a sucking technique whereby the duct is filled with contrast, and the balloon is distended at the bifurcation and rather quickly pulled down the length of the duct. When successful, the stone will follow the balloon, permitting deflation of the balloon and repositioning proximal to the stone for retrieval (Figure 3-9).

There are a number of anatomic variations on this standard technique. It is disconcerting to find that making a standard sphincterotomy with a directly observable 10- or 12-mm cut on the duodenal side does not always make an opening commensurately large on the duct side. This occurs when the intramural length of duct is unusually long and more directly cephalad in its course than usual (see Figure 3-5). When this occurs, it is required that we go back in and cut a few more millimeters and try again, doing this sequentially and measuring each time with the balloon until the gush of bile or the unimpeded balloon passage signals that we have arrived at the opening of the upper end of a long intramural segment. By this time the duodenal mucosa cut may have been extended to 12 or 14 mm.

The other anatomic variant is the short intramural segment, whereby very little, if any, bulging of the duodenal wall occurs proximal to the papilla. These seem to be more frequent in the case of noncalculous disease, but we're not sure of this. Virtually always in these circumstances, a medium (8–9 mm) sphincterotomy can safely be made without danger of perforation. This is not the kind of circumstance in which to make heroic cuts much greater than this, however.

As a final note in these paragraphs on the standard sphincterotomy technique, it may turn out that the sphincterotomy made is smaller than was anticipated or the stone diameter larger than it initially appeared. In this case recutting is necessary, usually because a stone or balloon has been pulled down into the sphincterotomy area and has failed to pass into the duodenum. It is possible to put fairly large amounts of pressure on these balloons and stones, and they may come gliding through slowly. We suggest slow, steady pulls on the balloon cannula rather than jerky ones. The vector of force for withdrawing a balloon through the cut is made more efficient if downward deflection of the tip of the scope is used. It will be noted that the balloon frequently pulls the whole papilla up against the tip of the scope, obscuring vision. Balloons may come through so suddenly that they are ruptured as they pull back into the elevator of the scope.

If further cutting is indicated, the balloon is deflated; any stone in the distal duct is disimpacted by advancing the sphincterotome. The sphincterotome is repositioned and a cut of usually 2 or 3 mm is made. Stone passage generally occurs with repeat balloon extraction.

Alternatives to balloon stone removal include basket extraction (Table 3-4). Basket configurations vary and both soft braided wire and stiffer, single-strand wire may be used. The unextended basket is passed into the duct, then advanced to open position along or above a stone under fluoroscopic control. The stone is teased into the basket by jiggling motions and captured by partial closure. Basket and stone are firmly retracted through the sphincterotomy opening. The rare but dreaded impaction of the stone-filled basket is prevented by comparatively sizing the stone and sphincterotomy opening by balloons. The use of currently available mechanical lithotripsy baskets for large stones should also prevent this complication.

Alternative methods for dealing with stones left in the bile duct include

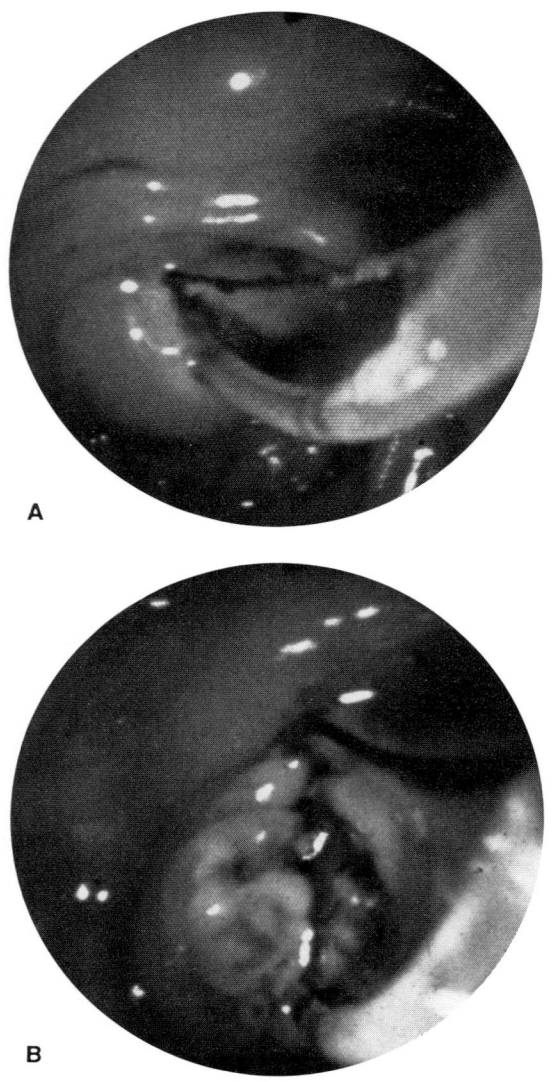

Figure 3-8 (A and B) (Plates 2 and 3) Endoscopic sphincterotomy. The sphincterotome is placed fairly deeply in this instance and cutting is proceeding with at least 10 mm of wire in touch with tissue. Note the pale tan edges of the cut surface. This represents electrical symphysis between common duct epithelium and duodenal mucosa, and results in the equivalent of a surgical sphincteroplasty. It is perhaps for this reason that strictures occur only rarely. In **B** above, sphincterotomy has been completed, as demonstrated by a gush of bile. A sphincterotomy length of 10 mm has remained within the confines of visible intramural duct length. **(C) (Plate 4)** This initial sphincterotomy was inadequate for the release of stones present in the duct, as judged by the fact that the inflated balloon came through the sphincterotomy

only with great difficulty and the stones were approximately the same size as the balloon. Therefore a small, several-millimeter recut was being done as this picture was taken. **(D) (Plate 5)** After sphincterotomy, stone material remaining in the distal duct may be trapped in the sphincterotome and may be released or withdrawn as the sphincterotome is withdrawn, as in this picture. Stones which remain in the very distal or intramural portion of the duct may be a problem during cutting as well, in that stones up against the cutting wire seem to "bleed off" sufficient current that cutting does not occur or occurs only with higher-than-usual settings. This can be discerned at times from the fluoroscopic view of the distal cholangiogram.

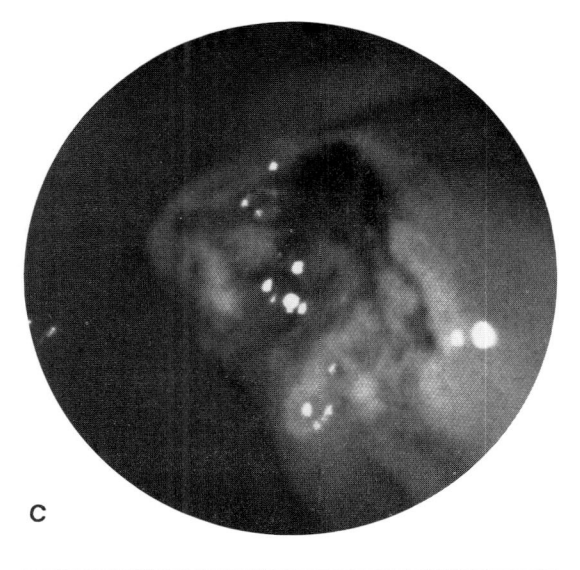

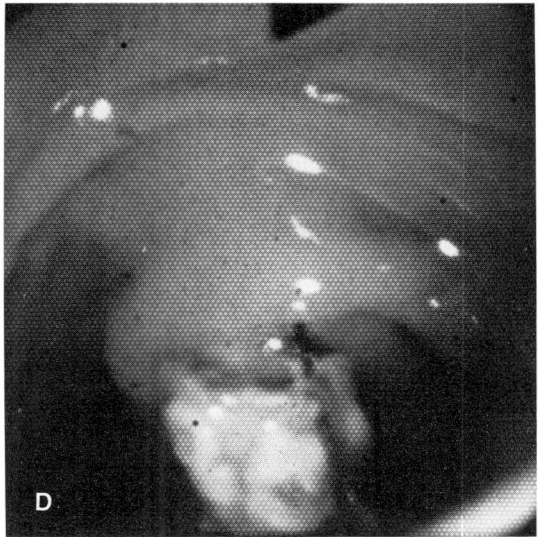

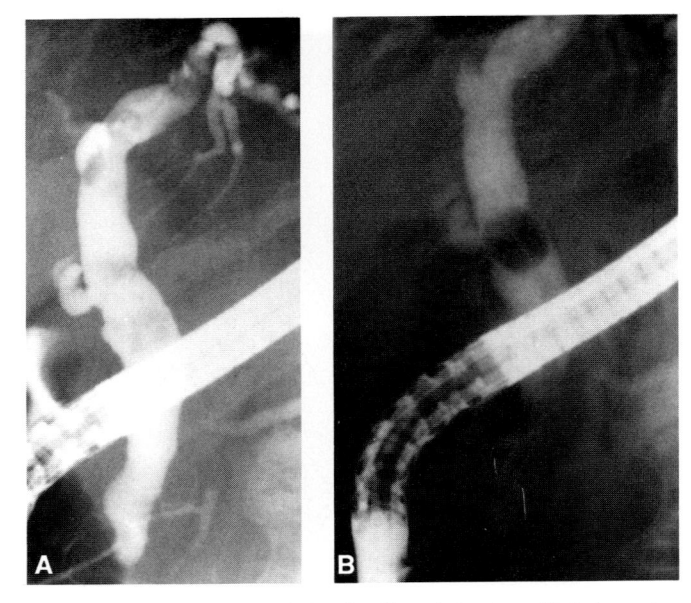

Figure 3-9 Choledocholithiasis. In a minimally dilated duct, multiple lucent areas are seen, appearing irregular in outline **(A)**. After a sphincterotomy, multiple small, soft, pigmented calculi were delivered into the duodenum by serial passage of an 11-mm balloon **(B)**. In this final passage, contrast is injected as the balloon is slowly withdrawn, and the resulting occlusive cholangiogram demonstrates an empty duct. Note that minimal contrast is present in the pancreatic ductal system, introduced during an attempt at cholangiography. A pancreatogram is not a routine part of this procedure.

watchful waiting for several days with a nasobiliary tube in place for decompression in the event of stone reimpaction. Tissues around the sphincterotomy may become soft and pliable in 3–7 days, facilitating subsequent attempts at extraction or even permitting stones to pass, either silently or during a brief painful episode. There are other methods of successfully removing ductal calculi when a sphincterotomy cannot be safely enlarged. These include disintegration by mechanical or electrohydraulic lithotripsy, dissolution with monooctanoin or methyl tert-butyl ether, and, rarely, the permanent installation of a pigtail stent

Table 3-4 Options for Stone Retrieval from Bile Duct

1. Sphincterotomy
2. Balloon extraction
3. Basket extraction
4. Extend sphincterotomy
5. Mechanical lithotripsy
6. Electrohydraulic lithotripsy
7. Nasobiliary drainage
    Wait for spontaneous passage
    Monooctanoin dissolution
8. Pigtail stent placement, leave stones in place

to prevent reimpaction of stone(s) left to reside in the duct. These methodologies are discussed elsewhere in this volume.

Other Sphincterotomy Techniques

We have discussed precut papillotomies and choledochoduodenal fistulotomies in the section on free cannulation techniques because of their role in patients whose bile ducts prove inaccessible to standard approaches. The impression among many experienced biliary endoscopists is that precuts, at least with the older precut papillotomes in which the wire comes down to the tip of the catheter, pose a higher risk of pancreatitis. The use of wire-guided sphincterotomes has become a popular alternative when introduction of a guidewire into the bile duct is possible but deep free cannulation is not.

When a wire-guided sphincterotome is used, we leave the guidewire in place during cutting and find that the two wires are functionally insulated from each other. This is true in our laboratory experiments as well. Leaving the guidewire in place maintains access against the distinct possibility that the sphincterotome may slip out of the already traumatized Vaterian segment, which could be difficult to reenter.

A combined percutaneous transhepatic retrograde endoscopic approach works well and is indicated in several situations: (1) When cholangiography is not possible due to location of the papilla inside a diverticulum; (2) when cholangiography is not possible due to prior Billroth II anastomosis; and (3) when endoscopic stent placement is not possible due to failure to place a guidewire across an extrahepatic duct stricture.

Our procedure consists of transhepatic placement of a 6-Fr catheter into the bile duct. A 400-cm 0.035-inch guidewire is passed through the catheter into the duodenum. The catheter is advanced just across the papilla into the duodenum as well. The wire in the duodenum is picked up by a snare and brought out through the 4.2-mm accessory channel of the endoscope. In the case of stenting a stricture, a small sphincterotomy may have already been made. If not, a two-channel sphincterotome is passed over the wire, and a small sphincterotomy is made. The stent is then passed over the wire and catheter and seated across the stricture. Detailed technical references are available.[19,20]

When a patient with a prior partial gastrectomy and Billroth II anastomosis is a probable candidate for ES, the preprocedure discussion includes the possibility of failure along with other possible complications. A course of action if ES fails is also considered at this point.

Let us assume that successful cholangiography, usually performed by us with a forward-viewing endoscope, confirms the need for ES and stone removal. In our experience, a successful sphincterotomy is possible with the end-viewing endoscope in approximately 20% of attempts. More commonly, a brief trial of sphincterotome placement will induce a longing for the elevator capabilities of a side-viewing scope, so the end-viewing scope is withdrawn, marking the afferent loop opening with a biopsy forceps on the way, and the side-viewing endoscope is inserted. (Some experts begin with a side-viewing endoscope.) We now need to cut from 6–8 o'clock rather than 12 o'clock. If one can easily get the sphincterotome passed up the bile duct, anchoring it there by flexing the distal tip, it is easier to remain in the duct while negotiating a favorable radial position.

If this attempt fails, one of the available Billroth II sphincterotomes is passed, which permits wire extrusion at a nearly 6 o'clock position (Figure 3-3). Typically the endoscopic view is somewhat tangential rather than enface and it is difficult at times to determine the length of wire in contact with tissue. Finally, one may cut down to 6 o'clock from the papillary orifice with a needle electrode. Success rates for sphincterotomy in patients with Billroth II anastomoses have been reported to be as high as 74–92%[21–23] in very experienced hands. In many centers the figures are probably lower.

Juxtaampullary diverticula are seldom responsible for ES failure, as the papilla is typically on the rim of the "tic" or bisects the opening as a ridge moving up the back wall. When the papilla has disappeared into the (usually wide-mouthed) diverticulum and when indications for the procedure are firm, a combined radiologic/endoscopic procedure is indicated, as described elsewhere. It is worth remembering that the diverticular wall consists of a single layer of epithelium which could be perforated by a probing cannula tip.

Conclusion

The technique of endoscopic sphincterotomy continues to evolve with gradual adoption of safer and more successful variations. It is obvious that we have entered a period in which passing cannulas and sphincterotomes over guidewires is a frequent part of sphincterotomy technique along with stent placements. "Above all do no harm" is still an appropriate admonition.

References

1. Koch H, Classen M, Schaffner O, and Demling L: Endoscopic papillotomy: Experimental studies and initial clinical experience. *Scand J Gastroenterol* 1976;10:441–444.
2. Kawai K, Akasaka Y, Murakami K, Tada M, Kohli Y, and Nakajima M: Endoscopic sphincterotomy of the ampulla of Vater. *Gastrointest Endosc* 1974;20:148–151.
3. Cotton PB, Chapman M, Whiteside CG, and LeQuesne LP: Duodenoscopic papillotomy and gallstone removal. *Br J Surg* 1976;63:709–714.
4. Geenen JE, Vennes JA, and Silvis SE: Resume of a seminar on endoscopic retrograde sphincterotomy (ERS). *Gastrointest Endosc* 1981;27:31–38.
5. Cotton PB, and Vallon AG: British experience with duodenoscopic sphincterotomy for removal of bile duct stones. *Br J Surg* 1981;68:373–375.
6. Nakajima M, Kizu M, Akasaka Y, and Kawai K: Five years experience of endoscopic sphincterotomy in Japan: A collective study from 25 centres. *Endoscopy* 1979;11:138–141.
7. Tedesco FJ, Vennes JA, and Dreyer M: Endoscopic sphincterotomy: The USA experience. *Endoscopic Surg* 1984;1:41.
8. Marbet UA, Stalder GA, Faust H, Harder F, and Gyr K: Endoscopic sphincterotomy and surgical approaches in the treatment of the 'sump syndrome'. *Gut* 1987;28:142–145.
9. Venu RP, Geenen JE, Hogan WJ, Dodds WJ, Wilson SW, Stewart ET, and Soergel KH: Role of endoscopic retrograde cholangiopancreatography in the diagnosis and treatment of choledochocele. *Gastroenterology* 1984;87:1144–1149.
10. Leese T, Neoptolemos JP, and Carr-Locke DL: Successes, failures, early complications

and their management following endoscopic sphincterotomy: results in 394 consecutive patients from a single centre. *Br J Surg* 1985;72:215–219.
11. Allen JI, Allen MO, Olson MM, Gerding DN, Shanholtzer CJ, Meier PB, Vennes JA, and Silvis SE: *Pseudomonas* infection of the biliary system resulting from use of a contaminated endoscope. *Gastroenterology* 1987;92:759–763.
12. Gerding D, Peterson L, and Vennes JA: Cleaning and disinfection of fiberoptic endoscopes: Evaluation of glutaraldehyde exposure time and forced-air drying. *Gastroenterology* 1982;83:613–618.
13. Venu RP, Geenen JE, Toouli J, Hogan WJ, Kozlov N, and Stewart ET: Gallstone dissolution using mono-octanoin infusion through an endoscopically placed nasobiliary catheter. *Am J Gastroenterol* 1982;77:227–230.
14. Siegel JH: Precut papillotomy: A method to improve success of ERCP and papillotomy. *Endoscopy* 1981;12:30–33.
15. Huibregtse K, Katon RM, and Tytgat GNJ: Precut papillotomy via fine-needle knife papillotome: a safe and effective technique. *Gastrointest Endosc* 1986;32:403–405.
16. Kozarek RA, and Sanowski RA: Endoscopic choledochoduodenostomy. *Gastrointest Endosc* 1983;29:119–120.
17. Cohen H, and Quinn M: Antegrade assistance for retrograde sphincterotomy using a new sphincterotome. *Gastrointest Endosc* 1986;32:405–407.
18. Aabakken L, and Osnes M: Endoscopic choledochoduodenostomy as palliative treatment of malignant periampullary obstruction of the common duct. *Gastrointest Endosc* 1986;32:41–42.
19. Passi RB, and Rankin RW: The transhepatic approach to a failed endoscopic sphincterotomy. *Gastrointest Endosc* 1986;32:221–225.
20. Shorvon PJ, Cotton PB, Mason RR, Siegel JH, and Hatfield ARW: Percutaneous transhepatic assistance for duodenoscopic sphincterotomy. *Gut* 1985;26:1373–1376.
21. Safrany L, Neuhaus B, Portocarrero G, and Krause S: Endoscopic sphincterotomy in patients with Billroth II gastrectomy. *Endoscopy* 1980;12:16–22.
22. Forbes H, and Cotton PB: ERCP and sphincterotomy after Billroth II gastrectomy. *Gut* 1984;25:971–974.
23. Osnes M, Rosseland AR, and Aabakken L: ERCP and endoscopic papillotomy in patients with a previous Billroth II resection. *Gut* 1986;27:1193–1198.

Chapter 4

Complications of Endoscopic Sphincterotomy

James W. Ostroff, M.D., and Howard A. Shapiro, M.D.

Early Complications

It is often difficult to evaluate complications when different techniques are used to achieve the same end. As a general rule, it appears that for endoscopic sphincterotomy the complication rate of 6–10% holds in most large centers. As with most procedures, there is a definite learning curve. With experience the complication rate decreases.[1]

A mortality of about 1% compares very favorably with figures of 2–3% for surgical choledocholithotomy.[1] Even if the mortality is considered comparable, as in younger, otherwise healthy patients who are good surgical candidates, the endoscopic approach avoids general anesthesia, an abdominal incision, postoperative morbidity,[2] and reduces time spent in the hospital as well as costs. As the popularity of endoscopic sphincterotomy grows, the patients referred to surgeons will not be similar since the greater risk patient will be referred for sphincterotomy.[3]

The total number of sphincterotomies reported in this review includes unsuccessful attempts at sphincterotomy as even these could result in a complication, despite the failure. The probability of going to surgery after a certain complication is undergoing flux because of the emergence of nonsurgical and interventional radiologic techniques, but it remains higher in certain complications than in others.

We will consider each of the major acute complications individually and try to suggest means for prevention and treatment of these complications (see Tables 4-1 and 4-2).

Hemorrhage

A small amount of self-limited bleeding occurs frequently immediately after sphincterotomy, but bleeding is not significant unless it requires transfusions. This complication occurred in 2.5% of the procedures reviewed here. Laporotomy was required in about 18% of the patients who bled and the overall mortality rate for patients with hemorrhage was nearly 10% (Table 4-3).

There are two types of bleeding after sphincterotomy[1]: oozing from mucosal

Table 4-1 Early Complications

Author	No. sphinc.	Compl.	Lap. req.	Death
Mustard[22]	289	39	7	2
Strunk[36]	717	52	15	11
Cotton[37]	679	58	11	7
Tedesco[29]	5790	393	86	22
Geenen[1]	1250	109	23	15
Safrany[2]	243	24	6	3
Escourrou[25]	443	27	7	6
Thatcher[13]	51	8	3	0
Neuhaus[23]	400	27	5	2
Dunham[20]	820	36	5	6
Kawai[30]	496	17	6	2
Leese[8]	394	41	15	3
Total	11572	831 (7.2%)	189 (1.6%)	79 (0.7%)

surfaces or brisk bleeding from a major arterial vessel. In a small percentage of persons the retroduodenal artery is located unusually close to the papilla, within the range of a sphincterotomy incision. Most bleeding occurs immediately or during the first 24 hr following sphincterotomy, but it can also occur up to a week afterward. Potential causes of delayed bleeding include sloughing of a coagulum, the presence of a coagulopathy, the use of nonsteroidal antiinflammatory agents, or the passage of large stones.[1] The risk of bleeding is increased with extension of a prior sphincterotomy, especially if this is performed within a week.[3] This may be due to the increased vascularity of the fresh wound. The longer the sphincterotomy, the greater the predisposition to bleeding.[1,4,5]

Measures to reduce the risk of bleeding after sphincterotomy include the correction of a significant preexistent coagulopathy. In all patients the risk of bleeding may be reduced by exposing less wire to contact with the tissue and reducing the power settings to better control the rate of cutting. Excessive bowing of the wire will impair the degree of control as cutting occurs. Attention to these measures will facilitate the performance of sphincterotomy by incremental electrocoagulation rather than continuous cutting. To address the problem of aberrant retroduodenal arteries, endoscopic Doppler sonography has been proposed as a means of detecting such vessels prior to sphincterotomy, but has not been applied widely.[6]

Table 4-2 Early Complications
11572 Sphincterotomies Attempted

Complication	No.	(%)	Lap. Req.	Death
Hemorrhage	291	(2.5)	50	26
Pancreatitis	232	(2.0)	16	25
Cholangitis	149	(1.3)	51	13
Perforation	130	(1.1)	53	16
Impacted basket	27	(0.2)	18	3

Note: Tables 4-1 and 4-2 include series for which data on all complications, as well as laparotomy and mortality, are included. The succeeding tables contain data from several other series devoted to specific complications.

Table 4-3 Hemorrhage

Author	No.	Lap. req.	Death
Mustard[22]	15	2	1
Grimm[7]	9	0	0
Strunk[36]	18	2	1
Cotton[37]	17	5	1
Tedesco[29]	123	18	11
Geenen[1]	29	5	4
Safrany[2]	7	1	0
Escourrou[25]	18	2	2
Reiertsen[38]	12	1	3
Thatcher[13]	3	0	0
Neuhaus[23]	2	2	0
Dunham[20]	23	3	2
Kawai[30]	5	3	0
Leese[8]	19	6	1
Goodall[39]	14	6	2
Total	314	56 (17.8%)	28 (8.9%)

Some groups[1,7] feel that at the first sign of significant bleeding the application of various combinations of epinephrine (1:10,000) and sclerosant (polidocanol or morrhuate) will result in the immediate cessation of bleeding. In the small number of published cases it is unclear whether the bleeding might not have stopped spontaneously, the others[8] feel it is unlikely that infiltration of the site will be of value. In patients with the most brisk bleeding infiltration would probably be logistically impossible anyway because of the rapidity with which visibility is obscured by blood.

It has been suggested that hemostasis may be achievable by continuing or extending the sphincterotomy, with the rationale being that a completely cut vessel, whose ends can retract, will bleed less briskly than a partially severed one.[8] Whether this actually occurs is unclear, but bleeding does appear to cease sometimes when the sphincterotome is kept within the incision and pure coagulation current is applied. At present there is very little experience with the various modes of coaptive coagulation (Bicap or heater probe) or the noncontact modalities (laser). Tamponade with an inflated balloon inside the sphincterotomy has been suggested.[9]

In some patients with active arterial bleeding it is unlikely that bleeding will stop either spontaneously or with any form of locally applied therapy. Angiographic embolization of the gastroduodenal artery appears to be highly effective[10] and may prove to be the procedure of choice, especially in high-risk patients, when radiologic expertise is available. More reports of this technique are needed. When bleeding is severe or persists and surgery is required, bleeding can be controlled by converting the sphincterotomy to a surgical sphincteroplasty by oversewing the cut edges, extending the sphincterotomy if necessary.[8]

Pancreatitis

In the combined series reported here, pancreatitis occurred in 2.0% of patients. This does not include patients with asymptomatic hyperamylasemia, which is

Table 4-4 Pancreatitis

Author	No.	Lap. req.	Death
Mustard[22]	11	1	0
Strunk[36]	7	1	2
Cotton[37]	20	1	3
Tedesco[29]	122	5	6
Geenen[1]	41	3	6
Safrany[2]	3	0	1
Escourrou[25]	3	2	2
Thatcher[13]	2	0	0
Sarr[12]	6	2	1
Neuhaus[23]	7	2	2
Dunham[20]	5	0	2
Kawai[30]	3	0	0
Leese[8]	8	1	1
Total	238	18 (7.6%)	26 (10.9%)

considerably more common. Most reviews do not differentiate gradations of pancreatitis and are not stratified as to either age or prognostic criteria (see Table 4-4).

There are several potential causes for pancreatitis in the patient who has undergone endoscopic sphincterotomy. During the diagnostic ERCP preceding sphincterotomy, overfilling of the pancreatic duct to the point of acinarization is one such cause. It is also clear, however, that repeated small injections of contrast, even in the absence of acinarization, may precipitate pancreatitis. This usually occurs in the course of repeated attempts to cannulate an elusive common bile duct. Urographic visualization was noted by one group to be strongly associated with post-ERCP pancreatitis.[11] In a patient who has undergone sphincterotomy, damage to the pancratic duct orifice and thermal injury to the pancreas itself are potential causes of pancreatitis.

Patients who develop pancreatitis after ERCP are often asymptomatic immediately after the procedure. Abdominal pain, often accompanied by nausea or vomiting, develops within a few hours but symptoms may not reach their peak intensity until the day after the procedure. In patients who become febrile the temperature usually is elevated by the second or third day. The amylase level in patients with clinically overt post-ERCP pancreatitis is usually markedly elevated during the first 24 hours. The symptoms, physical examination, and laboratory findings usually make the diagnosis clear. Occasionally, however, it may be difficult to distinguish pancreatitis from a retroperitoneal perforation on clinical grounds alone. Sarr et al[12] found CT scanning to be of the greatest discriminatory value.

The treatment of pancreatitis after ERCP with or without sphincterotomy is largely supportive, similar to that of pancreatitis associated with other causes. Patients are fasted and hydrated intravenously. A nasogastric tube should be inserted if the patient is vomiting. Fluid intake and output must be carefully recorded. Particularly in more severe cases, the serum calcium, arterial blood gases, and renal function must be monitored. Antibiotics have not been proven to prevent the development of pancreatic abscesses following pancreatitis of any cause. It is arguable, however, that since post-ERCP pancreatitis follows instrumentation and contrast injection, there may be a role for the use of antibiotics in this setting. Obviously, if there is any suggestion of cholangitis their use is mandatory.

Fortunately, most patients with post-ERCP pancreatitis improve with conservative treatment. However, some patients do develop severe disease and, in addition to parenteral alimentation, may require surgery for drainage and debridement, or drainage of subsequent pseudocysts or abscesses.[8]

Although pancreatitis can occur with the most careful technique, several considerations help to reduce the risk. During the diagnostic phase of the procedure and during placement of the sphincterotome, one should limit the number, volume, and pressure of contrast injections. The position of the sphincterotome and the state of filling of the pancreatic duct must be monitored frequently by flouroscopy.[1,4,13] Forceful, deep cannulation of the pancreatic duct with the sphincterotome should be avoided. The sphincterotomy incision should proceed in the longitudinal axis of the intramural portion of the common bile duct, which is usually at 11 to 12 o'clock in the endoscopist's field of view. One should be cautious in utilizing the precut technique,[5] as it is often considered to be associated with a greater risk than standard sphincterotomy. In situations where deep selective cannulation of the common duct is impossible, needle-knife sphincterotomy or combined transhepatic-endoscopic placement of a sphincterotome over a guidewire may prevent pancreatic injury.

Cholangitis

Cholangitis (Table 4-5) occurs infrequently and is almost totally preventable. Transient bacteremia frequently accompanies instrumentation of an infected system and may be manifested as a single temperature spike to 38.5°C on the evening after the procedure. Significant cholangitis is associated with a more sustained bacteremia and clinical sepsis with positive blood cultures. The risk of cholangitis is higher if the patient presented with it initially.[14]

Because clearance of the bile duct almost always prevents cholangitis in patients with choledocholithiaisis, some authorities reserve antibiotics for patients who still have gallbladders, who have had cholangitis recently, or in whom stones cannot be extracted (which is our approach). In the latter group, anti-

Table 4-5 Cholangitis

Author	No.	Lap. req.	Death
Mustard[22]	5	0	0
Strunk[36]	10	6	4
Cotton[37]	13	2	2
Tedesco[29]	78	26	2
Geenen[1]	25	9	2
Safrany[2]	5	3	2
Reiertsen[38]	4	1	1
Neuhaus[23]	2	0	0
Kawai[30]	4	2	1
Leese[8]	7	3	0
Total	153	52 (34.0%)	14 (9.2%)

biotics are started immediately after the procedure.[5] Others, in contrast, give antibiotics to all patients with biliary obstruction in whom manipulation of the bile duct is planned.[15] In addition to the need for coverage of the usual Gram-negative enteric flora implicated in most biliary infections, special recognition of the role of *Pseudomonas aeruginosa* in post-ERCP cholangitis is necessary. This organism is isolated from bile after ERCP far more commonly than from bile obtained at surgery when ERCP has not been performed[16] and has repeatedly been implicated in patients with biliary sepsis following ERCP. This association is related to the tendency of *P. aeruginosa* to contaminate equipment such as endoscope channels and water bottles. The prevention of infections with this organism warrants meticulous disinfection of equipment used for ERCP and periodic culture surveillance.[17,18]

The most important risk factor for the development of cholangitis after ERCP is the failure to clear the bile duct or, if this is impossible, failure to establish adequate biliary drainage. Following the introduction of nasobiliary drainage for the prophylaxis of stone impaction after endoscopic sphincterotomy, Haagenmuller and Classen[19] noted a decrease in the incidence of cholangitis from 3.3 to 1.0% and a 50% reduction in the overall mortality after sphincterotomy. In patients with malignant strictures of the bile duct, the bile is infected less often than in those with stones but, as in patients with stones, the risk of cholangitis following ERCP is substantial unless drainage is established promptly.

If a large stone is not removable and further attempts are not foreseen, one or two 7F pigtail stents should be placed to prevent impaction of the stone in the distal duct (large-caliber straight stents may also be used; see also Chapter 5). If another attempt is to be made to extract the stone, which may be easier after several days when the edema from sphincterotomy has subsided, or if extracorporeal shock wave lithotripsy is to be used, a nasobiliary catheter is placed deep in the duct for decompression and subsequent transnasal cholangiography. In general, a nasobiliary tube should be placed whenever there is doubt that retained stones will pass spontaneously (Figure 4-1).

Perforation

Perforation is uncommon (Table 4-6) but may require surgery, with an attendant 10% mortality rate. Historically, early surgical treatment was the initial plan of management, but in recent years medical treatment has been advocated with surgery reserved for delayed complications. The diagnosis of a retroperitoneal perforation may be difficult. The initial findings are often subtle and consist of mild pain and low-grade fever without the presence of subcutaneous emphysema or retroperitoneal gas.[4] A review of the symptoms in eight reported perforations exhibits this variability[20]:

Clinical Course	N	Delay in Diagnosis (hr)
Abdominal swelling	8	1–8
Pain	7	0–8
Nausea	4	1–12
Hyperamylasemia	4	12
Fever	3	1–48
Peritonitis	2	48
Septic shock	2	48

COMPLICATIONS OF ENDOSCOPIC SPHINCTEROTOMY 67

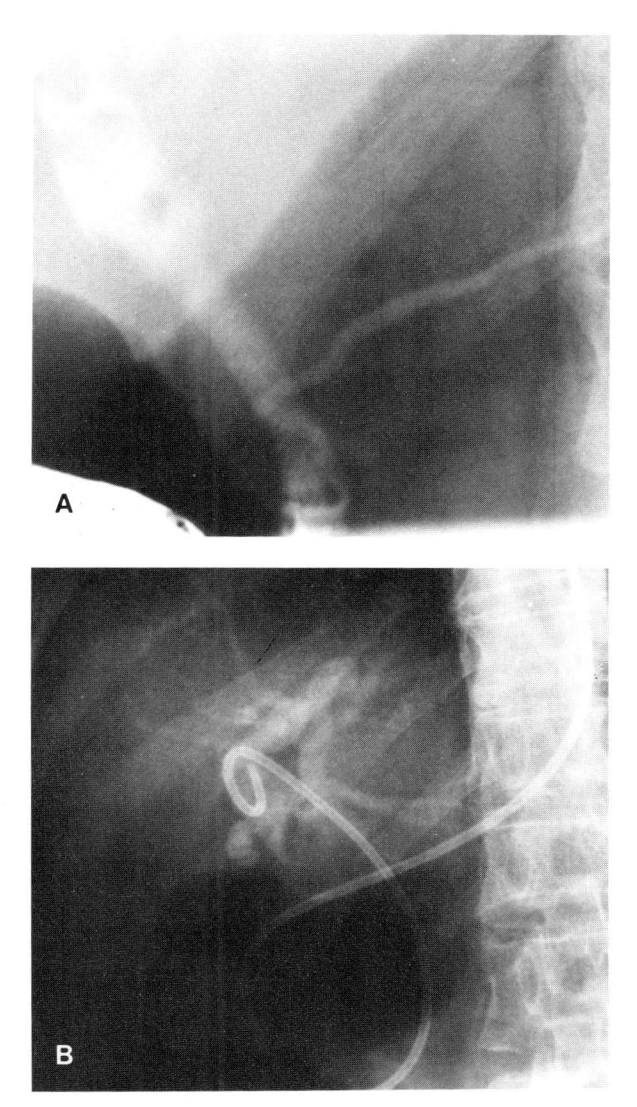

Figure 4-1 **(A)** ERCP revealing at least three stones in the common hepatic duct which could not be extracted immediately after sphincterotomy. **(B)** A nasobiliary tube was inserted proximal to the stones to ensure drainage. The stones were extracted with a balloon and basket 3 days later.

In this series, all patients received conservative therapy, which consisted of fasting, nasogastric suction, and antibiotics. Two required delayed surgical exploration and drainage, and subsequently expired. The diagnosis may be apparent on both a cholangiogram which reveals extravasation of contrast (Figure 4-2) and a CT showing a retroduodenal phlegmon (Figure 4-3). Of four patients with perforation undergoing CT within 5 days reported by Saar,[12] three had a localized periduodenal fluid collection while only two had retroperitoneal air.

Current wisdom suggests treating retroperitoneal perforations conservatively unless sepsis or evidence of abscess formation occurs.[1,4,5,12,21–23] In most

Table 4-6 Perforation

Author	No.	Lap. req.	Death
Mustard[22]	5	3	1
Strunk[36]	14	4	4
Cotton[37]	5	1	1
Tedesco[29]	57	28	1
Geenen[1]	14	6	3
Safrany[2]	8	1	1
Escourrou[25]	6	3	2
Thatcher[13]	4	3	0
Sarr[12]	5	4	0
Neuhaus[23]	3	0	0
Dunham[20]	8	2	2
Kawai[30]	3	0	0
Leese[8]	3	2	1
Byrne[21]	5	1	0
Total	140	58 (41.4%)	16 (11.4%)

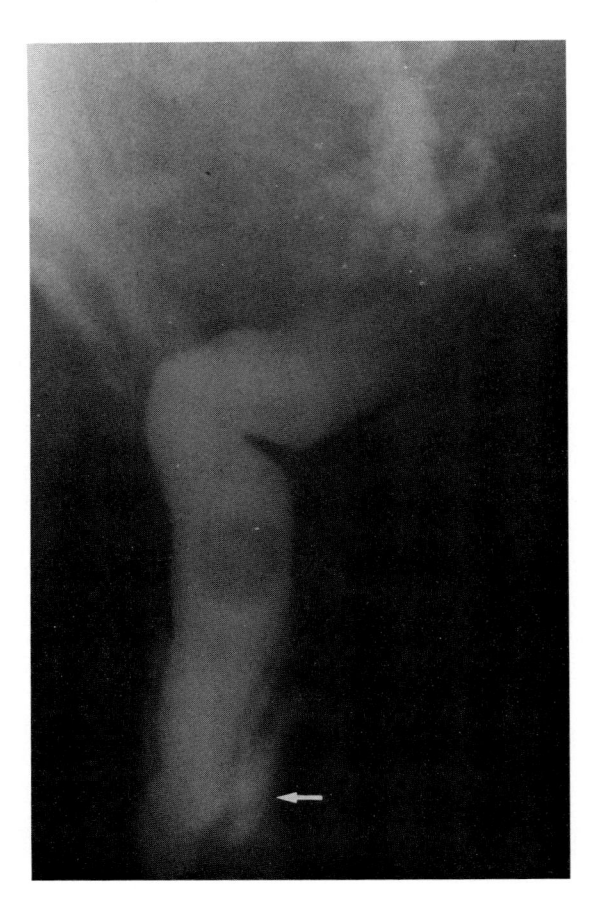

Figure 4-2 Extravasation of contrast after a retroduodenal perforation.

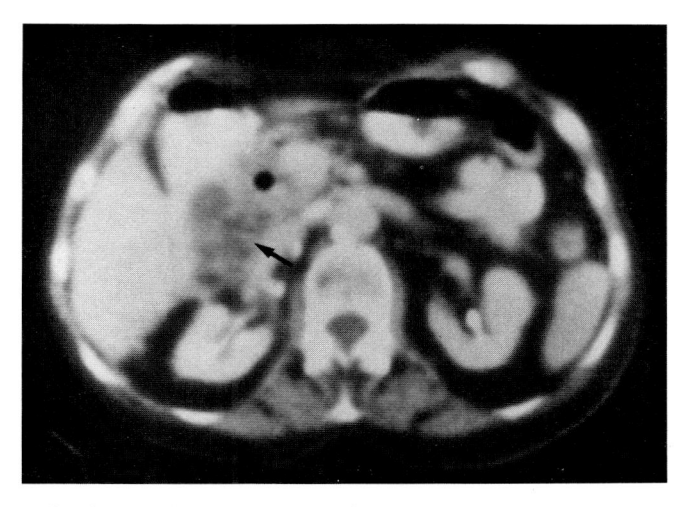

Figure 4-3 Retroduodenal phlegmon resulting from a duodenal perforation.

cases that go to surgery a discrete perforation cannot be located. Some authorities[24] favor early surgery to prevent the excessive mortality that occurs after abscess formation has been established.

The predisposing factors that can lead to a retroperitoneal perforation appear to be long sphincterotomies, a short intramural segment of the distal common bile duct, extraction of very large stones, and possibly the presence of a duodenal diverticulum.[1,12] Retroperitoneal perforation is most feared in instances of uncontrolled incisions ("zipper effect").[23] The more dilated the duct, the longer the cut that may be made,[22] since a large intramural bile duct is visible inpressing the duodenal wall. There is a slightly greater risk in producing a perforation in a patient with a Billroth II gastrojejunostomy because of difficulty in orienting the sphincterotome and controlling the length of the cut. A higher rate of perforation is associated with stenosis of the papilla.[13] The best safeguard against perforation is not to extend the sphincterotomy further than the visible intraduodenal portion of the common bile duct.

Impacted Basket

The incidence of an impacted basket is low (Table 4-7). Very large stones usually cannot be trapped in a basket but if trapped can usually be released. In addition to the problem of unextractable hardware, the hazard of an impacted basket results from obstruction and sepsis secondary to cholangitis that can attend an instrumented closed space.[4] With older baskets the only hope of avoiding surgery resided in cutting off the handle, removing the scope, reinserting it alongside the basket, and extending the sphincterotomy. With the development of mechanical lithotripsy one can cut the handle off the basket and utilize the device to break the basket or fracture the stone. This is accomplished with a metal overtube and a rachet crank which winds the relatively strong wires of the basket until there is either material failure or stone fracture. An alternative approach would be to use extracorporal shock wave lithotripsy to fracture the impacted stone. We have avoided the need to extend the sphincterotomy with the above techniques.

Table 4-7 Impacted Basket

Author	No.	Lap. req.	Death
Mustard[22]	1	1	1
Strunk[36]	3	2	0
Cotton[37]	3	2	0
Tedesco[29]	13	9	2
Safrany[2]	1	1	0
Neuhaus[23]	3	1	0
Leese[8]	3	2	0
Total	27	18 (66.7%)	3 (11.1%)

Cholecystitis

Acute cholecystitis was a feared complication of endoscopic sphincterotomy in patients with their gallbladder in situ. The postulated mechanism related to the observation that most patients who have had barium studies after sphincterotomy are found to have free reflux of barium into the biliary tree,[3] and there is usually an increased bacterial count in the bile. The significance of both these observations in the nonobstructed biliary system in not known. It appears clear that acute cholecystitis is uncommon immediately after sphincterotomy,[25-26] particularly when antibiotics are given prophylactically.[3] Siegel et al,[27] however, reported acute cholecystitis in 8.6% of patients within 10 days after sphincterotomy; a large but unspecified number of these patients had presented with cholangitis. In the same vein, Davidson et al[28] reported empyema of the gallbladder in 5 of 106 patients within 30 days of sphincterotomy and noted that 4 of the 5 had cholangitis on presentation. The subject of sphincterotomy in patients with gallbladders is covered in more detail in Chapter 7.

On some occasions acute cholecystitis may exist concurrently with cholangitis or with choledocholithiasis with no cholangitis. It is important to recognize these situations because sphincterotomy may solve only half the problem and the patient may need either a surgical cholecystectomy or a percutaneous drainage of the gallbladder to completely arrest the sepsis.

Late Complications

In most accounts of late complications the follow-up is incomplete (see Table 4-8).[3,25,29,30] Most of these patients are elderly and information is usually obtained by questionnaire. Restudy of asymptomatic elderly patients is not warrented clinically. Escourrou et al[25] reported follow up of patients without prior cholecystectomy (Gp I) and with prior cholecystectomy (Gp II). The mean age of group I was 79 and that of group II was 66 years. There were 407 successful sphincterotomies with 6-month follow-up of 74% in group I and 68% in group II.

In group I, those patients that developed acute cholecystitis did so in a mean of 4 months. Seven were treated with cholecystectomy and one was treated medically with no mortality. Cholangitis appeared 1–9 months after the procedure and was related to failed clearance of the common duct. Three were operated on after a second failure of an endoscopic sphincterotomy to remove

Table 4-8 Late Complications

	No. patients	No. Compl.	%	Treatment Surg.	Treatment Endosc.
Escourrou (1984)					
GB in situ "I"	130	16	16	11	5
Cholecystitis		8	6.2	7	0
Cholangitis		5	3.8	3	2
Restenosis		2	1.5	0	2
GB cancer		1	0.7	1	0
Postchole. "II"	96	5	5.2	4	1
Cholangitis		4	4.1	3	1
Restenosis		1	1	1	0
Kawai (1983)	496	13			
Stone recurrence		6		2	4
Cholecystitis		4		3	1
Cholangitis		3		0	3

the stones, while the other two were treated successfully by endoscopic sphincterotomy. Restenosis was treated endoscopically.

In group II, when cholangitis appeared three of the four patients underwent surgical treatment. In the single instance of restenosis described there was actually a cancer of the pancreas underlying the obstruction.

A similar scope of complications has been reported by others.[30-32] Most cases of cholangitis are associated with retained or recurrent stones. The incidence of stones and/or stenosis appears to be on the order of 5–10% during the 5–10 years after sphincterotomy, with a suggestion that the majority of late complications occur during the first 2 years.[31] One report in which patients were reexamined annually found no cases of late stenosis or stones.[33] Very infrequently, cholangitis occurs without stenosis or stones.[31] With the possible exception of these rare patients, bactobilia resulting from duodenobiliary reflux does not appear to cause infectious sequelae when the sphincterotomy is patent and stones are absent. In most reports of late complications, patients with gallbladders in situ did well, with only a small percentage developing cholecystitis requiring surgical intervention (see Chapter 7).

There is a consensus that the incidence of late stenosis is substantially higher when sphincterotomy is performed for papillary stenosis than for choledocholithiasis.[24,32,34] Also notable are observations that acute complications are more common when sphincterotomy is performed for papillary stenosis.[3,24,35] In one study the procedure-related mortality was doubled in such patients.[35]

Conclusion

This survey of complications of endoscopic sphincterotomy reflects the experience of tertiary referral centers and may not be totally applicable to less experienced endoscopists. There is a definite improvement in the complication rate with experience. On the other hand, all of the reports reviewed start with the first cases done. This biases the data toward the complications that occurred early in the investigator's experience. With improved endoscopic equipment and techniques, it is our impression that the complication rate, especially for retroduodenal perforation, cholangitis, and trapped baskets is diminishing with time.

To quantitate the trend more data are needed. Some of the more experienced centers should compare the complication rates of their first 500 cases and their most recent 500 cases. We would not be surprised if the overall rate dropped to 2–3% with fewer patients requiring surgery. Experience favors success! Nontheless the reported figures compare quite favorably with surgical series of complications and mortality rates for choledocholithotomy.

References

1. Geenen JE, Vennes JA, and Silvis SE: Resume of a seminar on endoscopic sphincterotomy (ERS). *Gastrointest Endosc* 1981;27:31–38.
2. Safrany L: Duodenoscopic sphincterotomy and gallstone removal. *Gastroenterology* 1977;72:338–343.
3. Cotton PB: Endoscopic management of bile duct stones; (apples and oranges). *Gut* 1984;25:587–597.
4. Cotton PB: Non-operative removal of bile duct stones by duodenoscopic sphincterotomy. *Br J Surg* 1980;67:1–5.
5. Safrany L, and Cotton PB: Endoscopic management of choledocholithiasis. *Surg Clin N A* 1982;62:825–836.
6. Silverstein FE, Deltenre M, Tytgat G, Martin RW, Lesterhuis W, Burette A, and Gilbert DA: An endoscopic Doppler probe: preliminary clinical evaluation. *Ultrasound Med Biol* 1985;11:347–353.
7. Grimm H, and Soehendra N: Unteerspritzung zur behandlung der papillotomieblutung. *Deutsch Med Wochen* 1983;108:1512–1514.
8. Leese T, Neoptolemos JP, and Carr-Locke DL: Successes, failures, early complications and their management following endoscopic sphincterotomy: Results in 394 consecutive patients from a single centre. *Br J Surg* 1985;72:215–219.
9. Staritz M, Ewe K, and Zumbüschenfelde M: Ballontamponade der akuten blutung nach endoskopischer papillotomie. *Schweiz Rundsch Med Prax* 1986;75:252–254.
10. Saeed M, Kadir S, Kaufman SL, Murray RR, Milligan F, and Cotton PB: Bleeding following endoscopic sphincterotomy; management by transcatheter embolization. *Gastrointest Endosc* (in press).
11. Rozler MH, and Campbell WL: Post-ERCP pancreatitis: association with urographic visualization during ERCP. *Radiology* 1985;157:595–598.
12. Sarr MG, Fishman EK, Milligan FD, Siegelman SS, and Cameron JL: Pancreatitis or duodenal perforation after peri-Vaterian therapeutic endoscopic procedures: Diagnosis, differentiation, and assessment. *Surgery* 1986;100:461–466.
13. Thatcher BS, Sivak MV Jr, Tedesco FJ, Vennes JA, Hutton SW, and Achkar EA: Endoscopic sphincterotomy for suspected dysfunction of the sphincter of Oddi. *Gastrointest Endosc* 1987;33:91–95.
14. Neoptolemos JP, Carr-Locke DL, Fraser I, and Fossard DP: The management of common bile duct calculi by endoscopic sphincterotomy in patients with gallbladder in situ. *Br J Surg* 1984;71:69–71.
15. Ferguson D, and Sivak MV Jr: Indications, contraindications, and complications of ERCP. In: Sivak MV Jr, ed.: *Gastroenterologic Endoscopy*. Philadelphia, W. B. Saunders, 1987, p. 581.
16. Helm EB: Direct choledochography and related diagnostic methods. Part 3: ERCP and biliary infections. *Clin Gastroenterol* 1983;12:115–123.
17. Allen JI, O'Connor-Allen M, Olson MM, Gerding DN, Shanholzer CJ, Meier PB, and Vennes JA: Pseudomonas infection of the biliary system resulting from use of a contaminated endoscope. *Gastroenterology* 1987;92:759–763.

18. Classen DC, Jacobson JA, Burke JP, Jacobson JT, and Evans RS: Serious Pseudomonas infections associated with endoscopic retrograde cholangiopancreatography. *Am J Med* 1988;84:590–596.
19. Haagenmuller F, and Classen M: Therapeutic endoscopic and percutaneous procedures. In: Popper H, Schaffner F, eds. New York, Grune and Stratton, p. 299.
20. Dunham F, Bourgeois N, Gelin M, Jeanmart J, Toussaint J, and Cremer M: Retroperitoneal perforation following endoscopic sphincterotomy: clinical course and management. *Endoscopy* 1982;14:92.
21. Byrne P, Leung JWC, and Cotton PB: Retroperitoneal perforation during duodenoscopic sphincterotomy. *Radiology* 1984;150:383–384.
22. Mustard R, MacKenzie R, Jamieson C, and Haber GB: Surgical complications of endoscopic sphincterotomy. *Can J Surg* 1984;27:215–217.
23. Neuhaus B, and Safrany L: Complications of endoscopic sphincterotomy and their treatment. *Endoscopy* 1981;13:197–199.
24. Classen M: Endoscopic papillotomy—new indications, short and long-term results. *Clin Gastroenterol* 1986;15:457–459.
25. Escourrou J, Cordova JA, Lazorthes F, Frexinos J, and Ribet A: Early and late complications after endoscopic sphincterotomy for biliar lithiasis with and without the gallbladder "in situ." *Gut* 1984;25:598–602.
26. Cotton PB: 2–9 year follow-up after sphincterotomy for stones in patients with gallbladders. *Gastroint Endosc* 1986;32:157 (abstract).
27. Siegel JH, Safrany L, Pullano W, and Cooperman A: The significance of duodenoscopic sphincterotomy in patients with gallbladders in situ: 11 year follow-up of 1272 patients. *Gastrointest Endosc* 1987;33:159 (abstract).
28. Davidson BR, Neoptolemos JP, and Carr-Locke DL: Endoscopic sphincterotomy for common bile duct calculi in patients with gallbladder in situ considered unfit for surgery. *Gut* 1988;29:114–120.
29. Tedesco FJ, Vennes JA, and Dreyer M: Endoscopic sphincterotomy: The USA experience. In: Okabe H, Honda T, Ohshiba S, eds: *Endoscopic Surgery*. Elsevier Science, 1984, pp. 41–46.
30. Kawai K, and Nakajima M: Present status and complication of EST in Japan. *Endoscopy* 1983;15:169–172.
31. Hawes R, Vallon AG, Holton JM, and Cotton PB: Long term follow-up after duodenoscopic sphincterotomy (DS) for choledocholithiasis in patients with prior cholecystectomy. *Gastrointest Endosc* 1987;33:157 (abstract).
32. Riemann JF, Lux G, Forster P, and Altendorf A: Long-term results after endoscopic papillotomy. *Endoscopy* 1983;15:165–168.
33. Rosseland AR, and Solhaug JH: Primary endoscopic papillotomy (EPT) in patients with stones in the common bile duct and the gallbladder in situ: A 5–8 year follow-up study. *World J Surg* 1988;12:111–116.
34. Seifert E: Long-term follow-up after endoscopic sphincterotomy (EST). *Endoscopy* 1988;20:232–235.
35. Seifert E, Gail K, and Weismuller J: Langzeitresultate nach endoskopischer sphinkterotomie: Follow-up studies aus 25 zentren in der Bundesrepublik. *Deutsche Med Wochen* 1982;107:610–614.
36. Strunk E, Kautz G, and van Husen N: Die Behandlung der komplilationen nach endoskopischer papillotomie. *Deutsche Med Wochensch* 1978;103:742–744.
37. Cotton PB, and Vallon AG: British experience with duodenoscopic sphincterotomy for removal of bile duct stones. *Br J Surg* 1981;68:373–375.
38. Reiertsen O, Skjoto J, Jacobsen CD, and Rossel AR: Complications of fiberoptic gastrointestinal endoscopy—five years experience in a central hospital. *Endoscopy* 1987;19:1–6.
39. Goodall RJR: Bleeding after endoscopic sphincterotomy. *Ann Roy Coll Surg Engl* 1985;67–87.

Chapter 5

Management of Bile Duct Stones Retained After Sphincterotomy

Stephen E. Silvis, M.D.

Prior to 1975, the size of common bile duct stones did not affect their treatment. Before that time, when common duct stones were treated, they were removed during surgical exploration of the abdomen and opening of the duct. The size of the common duct stones made only minimal difference. With the advent of endoscopic retrograde sphincterotomy (ERS)[1,2] there were rather marked limitations of the size of common duct stones that could be removed by this method. This chapter will describe variations in techniques that are available for the successful removal of the stones. It should be borne in mind that surgical removal of common duct stones is still a very viable option and should be considered in all patients, particularly patients who represent a satisfactory surgical risk.

Clinical Manifestations of Common Bile Duct Stones

The size of stones in the bile duct does not significantly influence their presentation. Biliary colic and/or jaundice are common manifestations of these stones. Infection within the biliary tree (cholangitis) occurs most often with common duct stones. However, it can occur with anything that obstructs or retards the flow of bile from the biliary tree such as benign or malignant strictures, compression of the bile duct by extrinsic masses or lymph nodes, or parasites within the bile duct. Although cholangitis is usually rather mild, there is a form of the disease described as suppurative cholangitis in which the patient is extremely ill. Charcot's triad, consisting of pain, jaundice, chills, and/or fever, is a classic, though inconstant, feature of the disease. About 70% of the severely ill patients have all of the triad. Fever is present in 95% and pain in 90%, but clinical evidence of jaundice may be absent in up to 20% of patients.[3-6] When suppurative cholangitis is suspected, prompt drainage of the biliary tree is essential. Milder forms of cholangitis will respond to nasogastric suction and antibiotic therapy. Common bile duct stones are a well-defined cause of pancreatitis. The pancreatitis may present without signs of biliary disease. Alcoholic pancreatitis may present in combination with alcoholic liver disease, making it difficult at times to separate biliary from alcoholic pancreatitis.[7-9]

Less frequently, common bile duct stones may present as one of the remote complications of diseases such as liver abscess. Any long-term obstruction of the common duct may produce biliary cirrhosis. This is an extremely unusual manifestation of common duct stones. In addition, elderly patients may present with weight loss with or without jaundice, anorexia, or vague abdominal complaints, suggesting an abdominal malignancy caused by common duct stones.

Laboratory Findings in Choledocholithiasis

Patients with asymptomatic common bile duct stone(s) may have entirely normal laboratory findings. Typical laboratory findings are that of increased direct-reacting bilirubin in the range of 2–15 mg%.[10] Values above 15 mg% generally are associated with liver disease or nearly complete obstruction. Serum alkaline phosphatase rises[11] as does the 5-nucleotidase. The serum glutamic oxaloacetic transaminase (SGOT) is usually only modestly elevated during stone obstruction. Occasionally, very elevated transaminases are found immediately after a high-grade obstruction.[12] They come down and approach normal within 1 or 2 days. The prothrombin time may be increased but is usually only slightly altered, and it is corrected by the administration of intravenous vitamin K. The abnormal serum bilirubin may be quite brief in gallstone obstruction. The serum amylase transiently rises with the passage of stone through the common duct. The blood counts are normal except in the presence of cholangitis, when the white count may be markedly elevated.

Differential Diagnosis of Common Bile Duct Stones

A classical history and physical examination makes the diagnosis of common duct stone(s) straightforward. However, a great many diseases may mimic the findings of ductal stones. The patient who has had the gallbladder removed will often describe the pain of common duct stones as similar to the attacks suffered with cholelithiasis. Renal and intestinal pain may be confused with biliary colic. Renal pain is usually in the flank and radiating down to the groin and to the inner aspect of the thigh. Intestinal colic is crampy and is more midline, centering around the umbilicus and frequently provoking emesis. The abdomen tends to distend with high-pitched bowel sounds. Hepatic abscess may be caused by choledocholithiasis. Amoebic or pyogenic hepatic abscess may stimulate cholangitis caused by choledocholithiasis. Patients with a solitary abscess have right upper quadrant pain which is often sudden in onset. Hepatic tenderness is quite apparent and the liver may be palpable. It is impossible to differentiate cholangitis from hepatic abscess unless the abscess is visualized on ultrasound or computerized axial tomography (CT).

Important in the differential diagnosis of the common duct stone is the fact that the pain of acute myocardial infarction and the pain of biliary colic may at times be very similar. Slight jaundice may follow a myocardial infarction, but it is less common than with a biliary calculus. It usually does not appear until several days after the infarction, rather than immediately, as in biliary calculus disease. Elevation of the (SGOT) may occur in both conditions. It rarely exceeds 100–150 units in myocardial infarction. Elevation of the serum glutamic pyruvic transaminase (SGPT) will be noted in choledocholithiasis but does not occur in myocardial infarction.

Congestive heart failure can produce right upper quadrant pain with distention of the liver, tenderness in that area, elevation of liver enzymes, and even jaundice. In patients with congestive heart failure the temperature is normal and the white count remains normal. The patient usually has obvious signs of congestive heart failure, particularly right-sided heart failure or tricuspid valve disease. The only difficult question is, does the patient have both biliary disease and congestive heart failure? It is occasionally difficult to separate the acute pancreatitis associated with common duct stone(s) from acute pancreatitis of other eitiology. This may require X ray of the common duct to exclude a common duct stone.[13-16]

Diagnosis of Common Duct Stones

The ultimate diagnosis of common duct stones is their removal either by surgery or endoscopic methods. Criteria for exploring the common duct at the time of surgery have been established in the surgical literature for many decades as follows: (1) history of cholangitis, (2) pancreatitis, (3) jaundice, (4) dilated common duct, and (5) palpable stones within the common duct.[17,18] Many surgeons routinely obtain operative cholangiograms; therefore, these are relative indications for common duct exploration.[19-21] With the advent of endoscopic retrograde cholangiopancreatography (ERCP)[22-25] and good scanning techniques, the diagnosis of common duct stones has usually been made preoperatively. The reliability of ultrasound in identifying a stone is not good unless a clear shadow is seen.[25] Computerized axial tomography is somewhat better.[26]

There is now a consensus that the patient with jaundice generally should have cholangiographic demonstration of the cause of the jaundice prior to surgical treatment. This may be done by percutaneous transhepatic cholangiogram (PTC) or by ERCP. The choice of which test to perform is based on the local expertise and whether endoscopic retrograde sphincterotomy (ERS) will be done if a common duct stone is found (see also Chapter 2). When dilated ducts are seen on ultrasound or CT scanning techniques, PTC is almost certain to be successful. Bile duct dilation does not influence the results of the ERCP. The success rate of ERCP with Billroth II gastrectomy drops to 65–70% from a 95% success rate in other situations.[27-31] In most centers at present, ERCP is chosen first for patients with suspected stones or with distal biliary obstruction. PTC may be preferred in patients with proximal obstruction (eg, suspected Klatskin tumors) if surgery is being contemplated and the proximal anatomy requires optimal definition.

In both ERCP and PTC care must be taken not to introduce air bubbles within the biliary tree. The air bubbles form round, radiolucent filling defects which may be difficult to distinguish from common bile duct stones. In most situations they can be distinguished because stones will have at least one flattened edge. Calculi will move down and bubbles will move up or coalesce if the

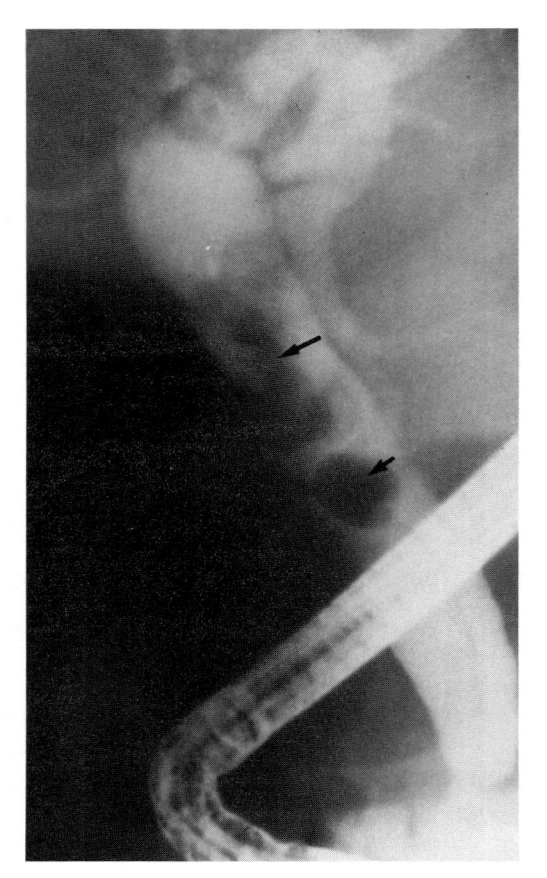

Figure 5-1 The cholangiogram of this patient demonstrates multiple calculi, the largest of which is about 1 cm (long arrow) above the balloon (short arrow). The filling defect (at the long arrow) is an aggregation of stone. This frequently cannot be determined with certainty before attempts at removal have been made. This film was taken after the sphincterotomy had been completed and as the stones were being extracted with a balloon. All of the stones were removed. The patient, who had a previous cholecystectomy, had no further symptoms in the following 4 years.

patient is placed in the upright position. As one begins to fill the common duct, it is frequently wise to switch to less dense contrast media; otherwise small filling defects are likely to be hidden in the dense contrast.

Multifaceted stones in the common duct make the unequivocal diagnosis (Figure 5-1). At times common duct stones may become impacted in the distal sphincter area. If this is a solitary common duct stone there may be a question of a distal tumor of the bile duct. On occasion this cannot be resolved until either sphincterotomy with removal of the stone is accomplished or surgery with exploration of the area is done.

Treatment of Common Duct Stones

Until very recently surgery represented the only successful therapy for common duct stone disease. It is frequently done at the same time cholecystectomy is performed. The gallbladder is removed and a longitudinal incision is made in the common duct, usually at its midportion. The duct is probed with baskets and extracting forceps until no further stones can be removed. Many surgeons advocate intraoperative choledochoscopy. Following exploration and stone extraction, a T tube is inserted into the common duct and X ray(s) are taken to determine if stones are still present. If the X rays are negative the patient is closed and a T-tube cholangiogram repeated before it is removed, usually in 10–14 days. Both Martin et al[32] and McSherry et al[33] showed that common bile duct exploration adds significantly to the morbidity and mortality of cholecystectomy.

Since the first endoscopic retrograde sphincterotomy (ERS),[1-2] the success rate of the procedure has increased to 85–90%. ERS has become the procedure of choice for removing common duct stones in patients with prior cholecystectomy.[23,34-48] Briefly, the technique of endoscopic retrograde sphincterotomy consists of passing a cannula, which has a short segment of wire exposed at the tip, into the common bile duct. This wire may be flexed by pulling on the handle at the proximal end to form a bowstring. The wire is retracted back into the duodenum so that its position can be determined and aimed toward the duodenal lumen. Radiofrequency current is applied to the wire, and a cut is produced extending through the sphincter and into the distal common bile duct. The size of the sphincterotomy should be tailored to the size of the stone. The technique of standard sphincterotomy and variations are discussed in detail in Chapter 3, and complications of sphincterotomy are discussed in Chapter 4.

In the present context, it should be emphasized that the size of the sphincterotomy should be tailored to the size of the stone. One should be able to see an impression of the common duct in the duodenal wall for the length that one wishes to make the sphincterotomy. It is important to determine the length of the incision before the sphincterotomy is begun because once cutting begins edema develops, and it is much harder to determine landmarks. When cutting has reached the predetermined extent, the papillotome is flexed and the size of the orifice is measured. The length of the incision does not determine the diameter of the sphincterotomy because the duct runs tangentially through the duodenal wall.

If the sphincterotomy appears large enough, the papillotome is removed and replaced with a balloon. The first step is to measure the papillary orifice with a balloon the size of the largest common duct stone. If a balloon which is the size of the stones will pull through the sphincterotomy, the stones can usually be removed (Figure 5-1). If the balloon does not come through and there is additional common bile duct in the duodenal wall, the balloon is removed and the sphincterotomy is extended. Extending the sphincterotomy probably increases the complication rate of both bleeding and perforation. Extensive edema may develop around the incision following the sphincterotomy. If one is unsuccessful in removing the stones at that time, a nasobiliary tube may be inserted to allow drainage. After waiting 2–5 days for the edema to subside, a repeat attempt to remove the stones is often successful.

Before sphincterotomy is attempted one should review the risk and prospects for success.[49] If the stones are extremely large, a stricture is present, or the bile duct passes almost straight through the duodenal wall, the prospect of removing the stones by endoscopic sphincterotomy may be markedly reduced. Under these circumstances the patient should again be considered for surgical stone removal.

Table 5-1 Management of Large Bile Duct Stones Retained After Sphincterotomy: Present and Potential Options

1. Reattempt in several days as edema subsides
2. Surgery
3. Placement of endoprosthesis
4. Monooctanoin infusion
5. Mechanical lithotripsy
6. Extracorporeal shockwave lithotripsy
7. Electrohydraulic lithotripsy
8. Laser
9. Percutaneous transhepatic ultrasonic lithotripsy
10. Methyl tert-butyl ether
11. EDTA

Problems of the Large Common Bile Duct Stone

The average common bile duct stone is 8–10 mm.[50] This is well within the range that can be removed readily by sphincterotomy. However, some stones reach a size considerably beyond that and may be as large as 2–3 cm, which is clearly beyond the size that most sphincterotomies can be safely done. Various approaches to extraction of large bile duct stones are listed in Table 5-1.

Our usual method of removing stones following sphincterotomy is by balloon extraction. Balloons that will inflate from 8 to 14 mm in diameter are currently available and, as indicated above, are useful in measuring the size of the sphincterotomy as well as extracting the stones. There are two major problems when extracting stones with a balloon. If the duct is very dilated, the stone can slip around the balloon instead of being pulled down through the sphincterotomy, even when the opening is large enough to allow passage of the stone. The other problem is that the balloons tend to be rather fragile and frequently break, either in the sphincterotomy or by striking the scope. If the stones cannot be removed in a few attempts with balloon extraction, it is common to place a nasobiliary tube in the duct, allow a 2- to 3-day period for the edema to subside, and then attempt extraction.

One of the problems is in a relative or absolute stenosis of the distal common duct. In Figure 5-2, the patient has huge stones in a markedly dilated bile duct. The stone then lodges in the widely dilated portion. Often this distal duct is distensible and will yield, allowing the stone to be pulled through.[51]

The major alternative to balloon catheters for the extraction of duct stones after sphincterotomy is baskets. One problem with baskets is the difficulty in trapping some stones within them. Frequently, the basket will not open wide enough to catch the stone. This problem occurs particularly with very large or impacted stones. The second problem with baskets is that if a large stone is trapped within the basket, but the sphincterotomy is not wide enough to allow passage of both stone and basket, they may become impacted. In this situation, if there is additional room to extend the sphincterotomy the basket can be cut off and the endoscope removed. The endoscope is reinserted and a papillotome passed alongside the basket to extend the sphincterotomy, allowing the release of the entrapped basket. In some of these patients surgical removal is necessary.

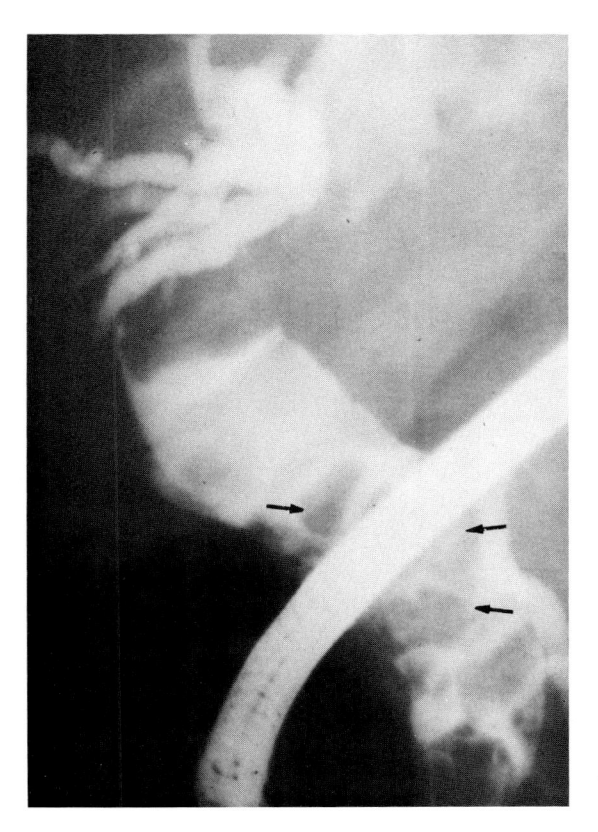

Figure 5-2 This cholangiogram shows massive dilation of the bile duct. The endoscope is approximately on the same plane as the bile duct; therefore, it can be used as a measuring device. The bile duct is over four times the size of the endoscope or greater than 4 cm in diameter. There are huge filling defects within the bile duct on this film. It is difficult to be certain as to which of these were single stones and which were aggregations of multiple stones. Obviously, the filling defect behind the endoscope (short arrow) is too large to remove from the bile duct in a single piece. This was actually a soft conglomeration of stones and was removed with a standard sphincterotomy and a balloon extraction. The sphincterotomy was somewhat longer than usual; however, there was a long segment of intraduodenal common bile duct. Although no complications occurred in this patient, a long sphincterotomy has increased complications. We prefer not to make a long sphincterotomy. These patients will be candidates for various methods of lithotripsy when they become effective.

Mechanical lithotripters[51-55] are a modification of the previously used Dormia baskets (Figure 5-3). The stone is entrapped in the wire basket, and the wires are pulled down under great pressure by the mechanical screw device to produce a fracturing of the stone. In recent models, the endoscope and Teflon sheath of the lithotripsy basket are removed after the stone has been entrapped. A metal spiral sheath is advanced over the basket wires to the papilla. The extruding portion of the basket wire outside the patient is connected to a cranking device. With cranking, the stone is pulled against the metal sheath at the papilla and crushed by the strong wires of the basket. The fragments of the stone produced by mechanical lithotripsy are removed either with the basket or with a balloon. If the entire stone can be grasped in the mechanical lithotripter it can be crushed. Often only the edge of the stone can be grasped, and closing the basket may produce some shaving of the stone, reducing its size enough to remove the stone with a balloon. Some studies report success rates of up to 75–100% for mechanical lithotripsy.[54-56] However, Classen found that with very large stones, over 25 mm, the success rate falls considerably.[56]

Stent placement and drainage[57] can be the treatment of choice in the patient with very large stones that cannot be removed by any of the endoscopic methods and who is at extremely high surgical risk (Figure 5-3). In this situation a pigtail stent is placed so that one limb of the stent is above the stone and the other is

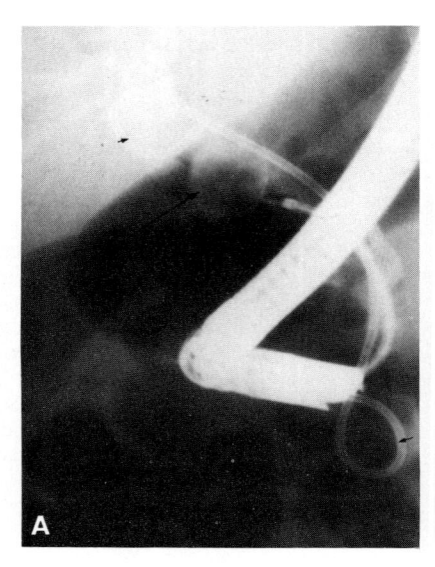

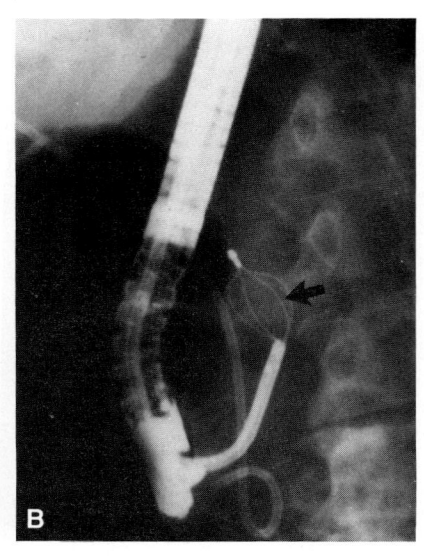

Figure 5-3 This cholangiogram shows a large stone (long arrow). At the time of the sphincterotomy it was not possible to extract it; therefore, a pigtail stent (short arrow) was placed to allow drainage around the stone. **(A)** A mechanical lithotriptor is being passed into the duct. **(B)** The stone has been captured within the mechanical lithotriptor (large arrow) and is being extracted. Afterward the pigtail stent was also removed. Allowing time for edema of the sphincterotomy to disappear will frequently facilitate the removal of very large stones. A small number of patients have been treated with the pigtail stent to bypass the stone(s). There is a limited amount of data on these patients[58]; they generally seem to do quite well.

in the duodenum. Although the stents clog within months, long-term drainage occurs because the stents prevent stone impaction. It is my feeling that this should be done only in the patient whose risk for surgery is high because the foreign bodies may potentially produce recurrent biliary infection. Most authors have treated only a small number of patients in this manner and have the general impression that they are doing quite well. Of 17 patients treated with long-term stent placement by Cotton *et al*[58] and followed for a mean of 39 months, biliary sepsis occurred in 2, while 5 died of nonbiliary diseases and 8 were alive and well. Pigtail stents were used early, but subsequent results were equally good with straight stents, which did not migrate. Ursodeoxycholic acid failed to dissolve any of eight patients' bile duct stones. The authors were encouraged by their results with stents but emphasized their preliminary nature. As lithotripsy techniques are perfected, the need for long-term stenting should become less frequent.

Other Fragmentation Techniques

Electrohydraulic lithotripsy has been used for about a decade, primarily to fracture stones within the urinary tract.[59-61] Its basic principle is that of discharging very short electrical sparks of milliseconds duration into a fluid medium which produces an acoustic shock. This acoustic shock wave does not cause injury to structures that have elasticity, but will fracture crystalline structures such as calculi. A modified electrohydraulic lithotripter has been produced which is passed through a catheter (Figure 5-4). This allows close contact with the stone but requires the balloon to keep the catheter away from the duct wall to avoid

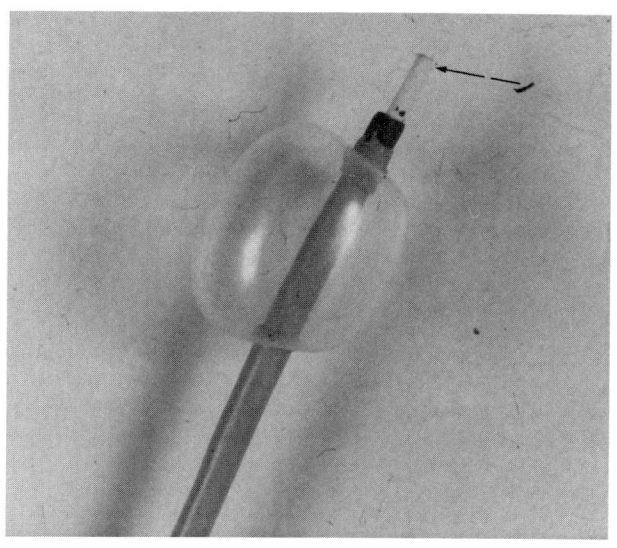

Figure 5-4 This shows the tip of the electrohydraulic lithotriptor with the balloon inflated and the lithotriptor probe extended (arrow). This is a bipolar probe that transmits a very brief electric spark across the tip of the instrument. When it is placed in fluid an acoustical shock wave is generated which fractures nonelastic materials (such as stones) in its path. The catheter is necessary to inject contrast to visualize the stones and to inject saline to allow propagation of the shock waves. The presently available probe is 9 French and requires a 4.2-cm channel scope for utilization. Maximum efficiency is reached when the lithotriptor probe is directly aligned and very close to the stone. However, it will fracture stones at a significant distance (6–10mm) and also will fracture stones that are not directly in front of the probe.

mucosal bleeding or perforation. With short electrical discharges, the fluid shock waves fragment the stone.[62–65]

Electrohydraulic lithotripsy has been performed via the percutaneous transhepatic route through a cholangioscope under direct vision.[56,66–68] The technology may soon be available to perform electrohydraulic lithotripsy via the retrograde route through a peroral cholangioscope. In the future, direct endoscopic control will probably be preferred over fluoroscopic monitoring.[56] Electrohydraulic lithotripsy has been applied to relatively few patients, is not widely available at present, and must still be considered investigational.

There is growing experience with extracorporeal focused shock wave lithotripsy for the treatment of common duct and especially gallbladder stones.[69–75] For common duct stones patients have undergoone sphincterotomy and placement of nasobiliary tubes after the stones proved unextractable. The fragments produced by lithotripsy usually must be removed endoscopically. Preliminary success rates for clearance of the duct of 70% to over 90% have been reported.[71,73,74] In the largest series yet reported, a multicenter group described complete stone clearance in 86% of 113 patients following one or, infrequently, two or more shockwave lithotripsy sessions. Minor adverse effects occurred in 29% of patients, with more serious complications in 8% including septic temperatures, biliary pain, fall in hemoglobin, gallbladder empyema, and a ruptured juxtapapillary diverticulum after endoscopic manipulation.[74] These are expensive devices that are not yet widely available and at this time must be considered experimental. If extracorporeal shock wave lithotripsy proves to merit the currently intense public interest in it and becomes widespread, it may eventually be used in many centers for unextractable common bile duct stones, particularly if mechanical lithotripsy has failed or is unavailable.

Percutaneous transhepatic ultrasonic lithotripsy has been utilized for both gallbladder and bile duct stones.[76,77] This requires producing a straight tract which will admit a 12 French instrument. General anesthesia is necessary and two of the reported cases were unsuccessful because of failure to introduce the instrument. This procedure may cause rupture or leakage of the gallbladder which necessitates surgical intervention. It will take considerable observation and time to show that these procedures are better than surgical treatment.

A small number of cases have been reported using lasers, which generally require direct vision of the stone through either a choledochoscope or through a scope passed up the papilla and into the bile duct.[78–81] A pulsed neodynium-YAG laser has been used via a peroral cholangioscope.[78] Another type of laser attracting particular interest is the tunable dye laser. This laser has the advantage of generating little heat and, because of the small size of its quartz fiber, should prove well suited to narrow cholangioscopes. The potential utility of tunable dye lasers was established in vitro, and experience with its successful use in patients has begun to accumulate.[82] Whether or not laser fracturing of gallstones will become widely useful has yet to be determined.

Dissolution Techniques

When sphincterotomy has been performed and a large stone demonstrated in the bile duct which cannot be removed by the usual methods, the physician must decide whether to do surgery, attempt to break the stone, or attempt to dissolve it. Monooctanoin has been used for a number of years. It is available clinically; however, it has only a 40–60% success rate and a rather high percentage of patients are intolerant to the diarrhea it sometimes produces.[83–89] Even in the patients who can tolerate the infusion of the monooctanoin through a transhepatic or nasobiliary catheter, usually 4–7 days is necessary to produce dissolution.

Recent preliminary studies have described the dissolution of gallstones by perfusion of methyl tert-butyl ether, or MTBE.[90–97] This ether dissolves gallstones in a few hours and does not injure the bile duct or gallbladder. Although not absorbed from the biliary tree, it is well absorbed from the small intestine. It injures the duodenum. The ether is an anesthetic producing sedation. At high levels the adverse effects are general anesthesia, irritation of the lung and bowel, and hemolysis.

Results with MTBE for radiolucent bile duct stones have been mixed. One group[96] was unable to dissolve stones in three patients given MTBE through a T tube, and all three had adverse effects. In contrast, another group[97] described dissolution of duct stones in all of six patients given MTBE, three via a percutaneous biliary drain and three via a nasobiliary tube. Side effects, eg, drowsiness and nausea, were relatively mild despite the presence of a sphincterotomy in most of these patients, which would presumably increase duodenal exposure to the ether. Despite this favorable experience, methods will probably be required to confine this material to the biliary tree if it is to be generally effective and safe in dissolving bile duct stones.

An important limitation of MTBE is that it dissolves only cholesterol stones.

Many common duct stones are formed primarily of calcium bilirubinate. There is some evidence to suggest a potential role for ethylene diamine tetraacetic acid (EDTA) in the dissolution of such stones.[98] In a group of 32 Asian patients with recurrent pyogenic cholangitis, which is usually associated with calcium bilirubinate stones in the bile duct, infusion of EDTA via nasobiliary tube, supplemented by manual or mechanical lithotripsy, resulted in duct clearance in half the patients.[99] Further studies with EDTA are needed.

Conclusion

Endoscopic sphincterotomy is the preferred method for removing gallstones from the common bile in patients who have had their gallbladder removed. It is also used in patients who are acutely ill with suppurative cholangitis or pancreatitis and in patients with severe extrabiliary diseases. The majority of patients with common bile duct stones do not have extremely large stones. Stones up to 1 cm in diameter can be removed with a standard sphincterotomy. Large stones in the common duct seen at our institution will have a sphincterotomy performed with an attempt to remove the stones first with a balloon and then by basket crushing. Mechanical lithotripsy baskets have recently been very markedly improved. It is difficult to be certain whether the filling defect in the common duct is a single stone or an aggregate of stones that have been fused together. This can usually be determined only after the sphincterotomy has been performed and the stone manipulated. If we are unable to remove the stones at the time of sphincterotomy, a nasobiliary tube is inserted and the patient observed for 2–3 days. After the edema around the sphincterotome has subsided, a second attempt at removal of the stones will be performed. If this is unsuccessful, the patient is either sent to surgery or has a stent placed to prevent impaction of the stone in the sphincterotomy. As extracorporeal shock wave lithotripsy becomes available we should be able to break these stones so that the fragments can be removed by balloon or basket techniques. Monooctonoate has not been used in recent years in our institution. It is quite cumbersome and requires extended hospitalization. It may be considered in the patient who has had trouble with a stent and is not a candidate for surgery.

References

1. Koch H, Classen M, Schaffner O, and Demling L: Endoscopic papillotomy: Experimental studies and initial clinical experience. *Scand J Gastroenterol* 1975;10:441–444.
2. Koch H, Rösch W, Schaffner O, and Demling L: Endoscopic papillotomy: *Gastroenterology* 1977;73:1393–1396.
3. Boey JH, and Way LW: Acute cholangitis. *Ann Surg* 1980;191:264.
4. Thompson JL Jr, Tompkins RK, and Longmire WP, Jr: Factors in management of acute cholangitis. *Ann Surg* 1982;195:137–145.
5. O'Connor MJ, Schwartz ML, McQuarrie DG, and Sumner HW: Acute bacterial cholangitis: An analysis of clinical manifestation. *Arch Surg* 1982;117:437–441.
6. Coelho JC, Buffara M, Pozzobon CE, Altenburg FL, and Artigas GV: Incidence of common bile duct stones in patients with acute and chronic cholecystitis. *Surg Gyn Obstet* 1984;158:76.

7. Stone HH, Fabian TC, and Dunlop WE: Gallstone pancreatitis: Biliary tract pathology in relation to time of operation. *Ann Surg* 1981;194:305–312.
8. Kelly TR: Gallstone pancreatitis. Local predisposing factors. *Ann Surg* 1984;200:479–485.
9. Kelly TR, and Swaney PE: Gallstone pancreatitis: The second time around. *Surgery* 1982;92:571–575.
10. Pellegrini CA, Thomas MJ, and Way LW: Bilirubin and alkaline phosphatase values before and after surgery for biliary obstruction. *Am J Surg* 1982;143:67–73.
11. Kiechle FL, Weisenfeld MS, Karcher RE, and Epstein E: Alkaline phosphatase in the assessment of choledocholithiasis before surgery. *Am J Emerg Med* 1985;31:556–560.
12. Fortson WC, Tedesco FJ, Starnes EC, and Shaw CT: Marked elevation of serum transaminase activity associated with extrahepatic biliary tract disease. *J Clin Gastroenterol* 1985;7:502–505.
13. Siegel JH, Tone P, and Menikeim D: Gallstone pancreatitis: Pathogenesis and clinical forms: The emerging role of endoscopic management. *Am J Gastroenterol* 1986;81:774–778.
14. Neoptolemos JP, London N, Bailey I, Shaw D, Carr-Locke DL, Fossard DP, and Moossa AR: The role of clinical and biochemical criteria and endoscopic retrograde cholangiopancreatography in the urgent diagnosis of common bile duct stones in acute pancreatitis. *Surgery* 1986;100:732–742.
15. Jones BA, Salsberg BB, Mehta MH, and Bohnen JM: Common pancreaticobiliary channels and their relationship to gallstone size in gallstone pancreatitis. *Ann Surg* 1987;205:123–125.
16. Lee MJ, Choi TK, Lai EC, Wong KP, Ngan H, and Wong J: Endoscopic retrograde cholangiopancreatography after acute pancreatitis. *Surg Gyn Obstet* 1986;163:354–358.
17. Moss AA, Filly RA, and Way LW: In vitro investigation of gallstones with computed tomography. *J Comput Assist Tomogr* 1980;4:827–831.
18. Hampson LG, Fried GM, Stets J, Ayeni OR, and Bourdon-Conochie F: Common bile duct exploration: Indications and results. *Can J Surg* 1981;24:455–457.
19. Wilson TG, Hall JC, and Watts JM: Is operative cholangiography always necessary? *Br J Surg* 1986;73:637–640.
20. Kitahama A, Kerstein MD, Overby JL, Kappelman MD, and Webb WR: Routine intraoperative cholangiogram. *Surg Gyn Obstet* 1986;162:317–322.
21. Reiss R, Deutsch AA, and Nudelman I: Clinical significance of choledochal diameter and hyperbilirubinemia in acute cholecystitis. *Int Surg* 1985;70:129–132.
22. Silvis SE, Rohrmann CA, and Vennes JA: Diagnostic accuracy of endoscopic retrograde cholangiopancreatography in hepatic, biliary and pancreatic malignancy. *Ann Int Med* 1976;84:438–440.
23. Geenen JE, Vennes JA, and Silvis SE: Resume on endoscopic sphincterotomy seminar. *Gastroint Endosc* 1981;27:31–38.
24. Lasser RB, Silvis SE, and Vennes JA: The normal cholangiogram. *Am J Dig Dis* 1978;23:586–590.
25. O'Connor HJ, Hamilton I, Ellis WR, Watters J, Lintott DJ, and Axon AT: Ultrasound detection of choledocholithiasis: Prospective comparison with ERCP in the postcholecystectomy patient. *Gastroint Radiol* 1986;11:161–162.
26. Jeffrey RB, Federle MP, Laing F, *et al*: Computed tomography of choledocholithiasis. *Am J Roentgenol* 1983;140:1179–1183.
27. Osnes M, Rosseland AR, and Aabakken L: Endoscopic cholangiography and endoscopic papillotomy in patients with a previous Billroth II resection. *Gut* 1986;27:1193–1198.
28. Bedogni G, Bertoni G, Contini S, Fabbian F, Pedrazzoli C, and Ricci E. Endoscopic sphincterotomy in patients with Billroth II partial gastrectomy: Comparison of three different techniques. *Gastroint Endosc* 1984;30:300–304.
29. Siegel JH, and Yatto RP: ERCP and endoscopic papillotomy in patients with a Billroth II gastrectomy: Report of a method. *Gastroint Endosc* 1983;29:116–119.

30. Rosseland AR, Osnes M, and Kruse A: Endoscopic sphincterotomy (EST) in patients with Billroth II gastrectomy. *Endoscopy* 1981;13:19–24.
31. Safrany L, Neuhaus B, Portocarrero G, and Krause S: Endoscopic sphincterotomy in patients with Billroth II gastrectomy. *Endoscopy* 1980;12:16–22.
32. Martin JK, and Van Heerden JA: Surgery of the liver, biliary tract and pancreas. *Mayo Clin Proc* 1980;55:333–337.
33. McSherry CK, and Glenn F: The incidence and causes of death following surgery of nonmalignant biliary tract disease. *Ann Surg* 1980;191:271–275.
34. Ihre T, Lönn M, and Kager L: Long-term effects of papillotomy. *Endoscopy* 1984;16:109–111.
35. Cotton PB, and Vallon AG: British experience with duodenoscopic sphincterotomy for removal of bile duct stones. *Br J Surg* 1981;68:373–375.
36. Rösch W, Riemann JF, Lux G, and Linder HG. Long-term follow-up care after endoscopic sphincterotomy. *Endoscopy* 1981;13:152–153.
37. Classen M, and Safrany L: Endoscopic papillotomy and removal of gallstones. *Br Med J* 1975;4:371–374.
38. Zimmon DS, Falkenstein DB, and Kessler RE: Endoscopic papillotomy for choledocholithiasis. *N Engl J Med* 1975;293:1181–1182.
39. Safrany L: Duodenscopic sphincterotomy and gallstone removal. *Gastroenterology* 1977;72:338–343.
40. Siegel JH: Endoscopic papillotomy in the treatment of biliary tract disease: 258 procedures and results. *Dig Dis Sci* 1981;26:1057–1064.
41. Passi RB, and Raval B: Endoscopic papillotomy. *Surgery* 1982;92:581–588.
42. Geenen JE: New diagnostic and treatment modalities involving endoscopic retrograde cholangiopancreatography and esophagogastroduodenoscopy. *Scand J Gastroenterol (Suppl)* 1982;77:93–98.
43. Siegel JH: Endoscopy and papillotomy in disease of the biliary tract and pancreas. *J Clin Gastroenterol* 1980;2:337–340.
44. Cotton PB: Nonoperative removal of bile duct stones by duodenoscopic sphincterotomy. *Br J Surg* 1980;67:1–5.
45. Kozarek RA, and Sanowski RA: Nonsurgical management of extrahepatic obstructive jaundice. *Ann Intern Med* 1982;96:743–745.
46. Safrany L, and Cotton PB: Endoscopic management of choledocholithiasis. *Surg Clin N A* 1982;62:825–836.
47. Silvis SE: Current status of endoscopic sphincterotomy. *Am J Gastroenterol* 1984;79:731–733.
48. Vennes JA: Management of calculi in the common duct. *Semin Liver Dis* 1983;3:162–171.
49. Silvis SE, and Vennes JA: Endoscopic retrograde sphincterotomy. In *Therapeutic Gastrointestinal Endoscopy*. Silvis SE, ed. Igaku-Shoin, New York, 1985, p. 198.
50. Stave R, and Osnes M: Endoscopic gallstone extraction following hydrostatic balloon dilatation of stricture in the common bile duct. *Endoscopy* 1985;17:159–160.
51. Koch H, Rösch W, and Walz V: Endoscopic lithotripsy in the common bile duct. *Gastrointest Endosc* 1980;26:16–18.
52. Riemann JF, Seuberth K, and Demling L. Mechanical lithotripsy through the intact papilla of Vater. *Endoscopy* 1983;15:111–113.
53. Demling L, Seubarth K, and Riemann JF. A mechanical lithotriptor. *Endoscopy* 1982;14:100–101.
54. Riemann JF, Seuberth K, and Demling L: Mechanical lithotripsy of common bile duct stones. *Gastrointest Endosc* 1985;31:207–213.
55. Staritz M, Ewe K, and Meyer zum Büschenfelde KH. Mechanical gallstone lithotripsy in the common bile duct: In vitro and in vivo experience. *Endoscopy* 1983;15:316–318.
56. Classen M, Haagenmuller F, Knyrim K, and Frimberger E: Giant bile duct stones: Nonsurgical treatment. *Endoscopy* 1988;20:21–26.

57. Siegel JH, and Yatto RP: Biliary endoprostheses for the management of retained common bile duct stones. *Am J Gastroenterol* 1984;79:50–54.
58. Cotton PB, Forbes A, Leung JWC, and Dineen L: Endoscopic stenting for long-term treatment of large bile duct stones: 2- to 5-year follow-up. *Gastrointest Endosc* 1987;33:411–413.
59. Reuter HJ, and Kern E: Electronic lithotripsy of ureteral calculi. *J Urol* 1973;110:181–183.
60. Raney AM: Electrohydraulic lithotripsy: Experimental study and case reports with the stone disintegrator. *J Urol* 1975;113:345–347.
61. Mitchell ME, and Kerr WS, Jr: Experience with the electrohydraulic disintegrator. *J Urol* 1977;117:159–160.
62. Tanaka M, Yoshimoto H, Ikeda S, Matsumoto S, and Guo RX: Two approaches for electrohydraulic lithotripsy in the common bile duct. *Surgery* 1985;98:313–318.
63. Sievert CE, and Silvis SE: Evaluation of electrohydraulic lithotripsy on human gallstones. *Am J Gastroenterol* 1985;80:854 (abstract).
64. Silvis SE, Siegel JE, Katon RM, Hughes R, Sievert CE, and Sivak MV: Use of electrohydraulic lithotripsy to fracture common bile duct stones. *Gastroint Endosc* 1986;32:155 (abstract).
65. Sievert CE, and Silvis SE: Evaluation of electrohydraulic lithotripsy as a means of gallstone fragmentation in a canine model. *Gastroint Endosc* 1987;33:233–235.
66. Liguory CL, Bonnel D, Canard JM, *et al:* Intracorporeal electrohydraulic shock wave lithotripsy of common bile duct stones; preliminary results in 7 cases. *Endoscopy* 1987;19:237–240.
67. Mo L, Hwang M, Yueh S, *et al:* Percutaneous transhepatic choledochoscopic electrohydraulic lithotripsy (PTCS-EHL) of common bile duct stones. *Gastrointest Endosc* 1988;34:122–125.
68. Ponchon T, Valette PJ, and Chavaillon A: Percutaneous transhepatic electrohydraulic lithotripsy under endoscopic control. *Gastrointest Endosc* 1987;33:307–309.
69. Sackman M, Delius M, Sauerbruch T, Holl J, Weber W, Hagelauer U, Hepp W, Brendel G, and Paumgartner G: Extra-corporeal shock wave lithotripsy of gallstones: Results of 101 treatments. *Gastroenterology* 1987;92:1608 (abstract).
70. Sauerbruch T, Delius M, Paumgartner G, Holl J, Wess O, Weber W, Hepp W, and Brendel W: Fragmentation of gallstones by extracorporeal shock waves. *N Engl J Med* 1986;314:818–822.
71. Staritz M, Rambow A, Bork K, *et al*: Second generation extracorporeal shock wave lithotripsy for therapy of selected bile duct stones: 18 months of clinical experience. *Gastroenterology* 1988;94:A594.
72. Gelfand DW, McCullough DL, Myers RT, D'Sousa VJ, Leinbach LB, and Faust KB: Choledocholithiasis: Successful treatment with extracorporeal lithotripsy. *Am J Radiol* 1987;148:1114–1116.
73. Delhoye M, Vandermeeren A, and Cremer M: Extracorporeal shock wave lithotripsy (ESWL) for gallstones. *Gastroint Endosc* 1988;34:186 (abstract).
74. Sauerbruch T, Stern M, and the Study Group for Shock-Wave Lithotripsy of Bile Duct Stones: Fragmentation of bile duct stones by extracorporeal shock waves: a new approach to biliary calculi after failure of routine endoscopic measures. *Gastroenterology* 1989;96:146–152.
75. Silvis SE: The role of lithotripsy in biliary stone disease. *Gastroint Endosc* 1987;33:328–329.
76. Hwang MH, Mo LR, Chen GD, Yang JC, Lin C, and Yueh SK: Percutaneous transhepatic cholecystic ultrasonic lithotripsy. *Gastroint Endsoc* 1987;33:301–303.
77. Hwang MH, Mo LR, Yang JC, and Lin C: Percutaneous transhepatic cholangioscopic ultrasonic lithotripsy (PTCS-USL) in the treatment of retained or recurrent intrahepatic stones. *Gastroint Endosc* 1987;33:303–306.
78. Lux G, Ell C, Hochberger J, Müller D, and Demling L: The first successful endoscopic retrograde laser lithotripsy of common bile duct stones in man using a pulsed neodymium-YAG laser. *Endoscopy* 1986;18:144–145.

79. Nishioka NS, Teng P, Deutsch TF, Anderson RR: Mechanism of laser-induced fragmentation of urinary and bladder calculi. *Las Life Sci* 1987;1:231–245.
80. Nishioka NS, Levins PC, Murray SC, et al: Fragmentation of biliary calculi with tunable dye lasers. *Gastroenterology* 1987;93:250–255.
81. Fujita R, Yamamura M, Fujita Y: Combined endoscopic sphincterotomy and percutaneous transhepatic cholangioscopic lithotripsy. *Gastroint Endosc* 1988;34:91–94.
82. Kozarek RA, Low DE, Ball TJ: Tunable dye laser lithotripsy: In vitro studies and in vivo treatment of choledocholithiasis. *Gastrointest Endosc* 1988;34:418–421.
83. Palmer KR, and Hofmann AF: Intraductal monooctanoin for the direct dissolution of bile duct stones: Experience in 343 patients. *Gut* 1986;27:196–202.
84. Thistle JL, Carlson GL, Hofmann AF, Larrusso NF, MacCarthy RL, Flynn GL, Higuchi WI, and Babayan VK: Monooctanoin, a dissolution agent for retained cholesterol bile duct stones: Physical properties and clinical application. *Gastroenterology* 1980;78:1016–1022.
85. Jarrett LN, Balfour TW, Bell GD, Knapp DR, and Rose DH: Intraductal infusion of monooctanoin: Experience in 24 patients with retained common duct stones. *Lancet* 1981;1:68–70.
86. Venu RP, Gennen JE, Toouli J, Hogan WJ, Kozlov N, and Stewart ET: Gallstone dissolution using monooctanoin infusion through an endoscopically placed nasobiliary catheter. *Am J Gastroenterol* 1982;77:227–230.
87. Tritapepe R, Di Padova C, Pozzoli M, Robagnati P, and Montorsi W: The treatment of retained biliary stones with monooctanoin: Report of 16 patients. *Am J Gastroenterol* 1984;79:710–714.
88. Sharp KW, Gadacz TR. Selection of patients for dissolution of retained common duct stones with monooctanoin. *Ann Surg* 1982;196:137–139.
89. Train JS, Dan SJ, Cohen LB, and Mitty HA: Duodenal ulceration associated with monooctanoin infusion. *Am J Radiol* 1983;141:557–558.
90. Thistle JL, May GR, LeRoy AJ, et al: Dissolution of cholesterol gallbladder stone by methyl tert-butyl ether administered by percutaneous transhepatic catheter. *New Engl J Med* 1989;320:633–639.
91. Allen JM, Borody TJ, and Thistle JL: In vitro dissolution of cholesterol gallstones: A study of factors influencing rate and a comparison of solvents. *Gastroenterology* 1985;89:1097–1103.
92. Allen JM, Borody TJ, Bugliosi TF, May GR, LaRusso NF, and Thistle JL: Rapid dissolution of gallstones by methyl tert-butyl ether: Preliminary observations. *N Engl J Med* 1985;312:217–220.
93. Allen JM, Borody TJ, Bugliosi TF, May GR, LaRusso NF, and Thistle JL: Cholelitholysis using methyl tertiary-butyl ether. *Gastroenterology* 1985;88:122–125.
94. Zakko SF, and Hofmann AF: Micropressor assisted solvent transfer system for infusion of methyl tert-butyl ether (MTBE) or other gallstone (GS) solvents into the gallbladder. *Gastroenterology* 1987;92:1794 (abstract).
95. Zakko SF, Hofmann AF, Schteingart C, vanSonnenberg E, and Wheller HO. Percutaneous gallbladder stone dissolution using a microprocessor assisted solvent transfer (MAST) system. *Gastroenterology* 1987;92:1794 (abstract).
96. Di Padova C, Di Padova F, Montorsi W, and Tritapepe R: Methyl tert-butyl ether fails to dissolve retained radiolucent common bile duct stones. *Gastroenterology* 1986;91:1296–1300.
97. Bonardi L, Gandini G, Gabasio S, and Fascetti E: Methyl-Terbutyl ether (MTBE) and endoscopic sphincterotomy. A possible solution for dissolving gallstones. *Endoscopy* 1987;18:238–239.
98. Leuschner U, Wurbs D, Baumgartel H, and Helm EB: Alternating treatment of common bile duct stones with a modified glyceryl-l-monooctonoate preparation and a bile acid-EDTA solution by nasobiliary tube. *Scand J Gastroenterol* 1981;16:497–503.
99. Leung JWC, Chung SCS, Mok SD, and Li AKC: Endoscopic removal of large common bile duct stones in recurrent pyogenic cholangitis. *Gastrointest Endosc* 1988;34:238–241.

Chapter **6**

ERCP in Acute Cholangitis and Pancreatitis

John P. Neoptolemos, M.A., M.B., B.Chir. (Cantab), M.D. (Leics), F.R.C.S.(Eng), and David L. Carr-Locke, M.A., M.B., B.Chir. (Cantab), F.R.C.P.(UK)

Introduction

Endoscopic retrograde cholangiopancreatography (ERCP) has, in the relatively short time since its introduction,[1,2] had a major impact on the assessment of patients with pancreaticobiliary disorders.[3] The subsequent development of endoscopic sphincterotomy (ES)[4,5] with associated ancillary techniques has been a further therapeutic advance, particularly in the elective management of certain groups of patients with common bile duct (CBD) stones[6,7] and malignant obstruction of the biliary tree.[8,9] There has, however, been a reluctance to extend ERCP and ES to patients in the "emergency" situation. Although this has been based on the fear of unacceptably high complication rates initially reported with ERCP/ES, improvements in patient management and familiarity with these techniques have now made it possible to tackle such patients.[10] The recent view that ES is only indicated in the "*very* high risk anaesthetic patient who does not have acute pancreatitis and/or cholangitis"[11] can no longer be supported.

Acute Cholangitis
Definition and Clinical Features

In 1877 Charcot[12] described a "form of intermittent symptomatic fever, which is not associated with actual hepatic colic, but which sometimes accompanies either calculus obstruction of the bile duct, or intrahepatic biliary lithiasis." He went on to say that "it can occur with all the typical characteristics in cases of longstanding or persistent bile duct obstruction from whatever cause, such as fibrous stricture, cancer of the head of the pancreas, etc."

The features of acute cholangitis are obstructive jaundice, a swinging pyrexia of 38°C or greater, chills, and pain and tenderness over the liver. These features are the mainstay of diagnosis. The finding of pus in the bile ducts in the absence of one or other of these features is also diagnostic. Attempts to undermine this approach should be firmly resisted. To define acute cholangitis

Table 6-1 Types of Acute Cholangitis of Increasing Severity as Defined by Pitt and Longmire[16]

Type	Description
1	Acute cholangitis associated with acute inflammation of gallbladder without duct obstruction
2	Acute nonsuppurative cholangitis
3	Acute suppurative cholangitis
4	Acute obstructive suppurative cholangitis*
5	Acute suppurative cholangitis with intrahepatic abscess

* There is *complete* obstruction in type 4 compared to partial or intermittent obstruction in types 2 and 3.

as fever greater than 38.3°C or a history of rigors in the presence of stones in the CBD would seem to us too liberal a definition.[13] Similarly, it is difficult to conceive that over 20% of patients with acute cholangitis are not clinically jaundiced[14]; in our own experience this accounts for less than 2% of cases.

Acute cholangitis represents a disease with a wide range of severity, from the mildest form, which may resolve quickly with conservative measures, to one which is refractory to all treatment and is rapidly fatal.

Reynolds and Dargan in 1959[15] described a particularly lethal variety which they called *acute suppurative cholangitis* in which shock, mental confusion, and lethargy were additional features. Pitt and Longmire,[16] among others, chose to divide acute cholangitis into five types according to the degree of obstruction and the presence or absence of pus in the biliary tree (Table 6-1), and suggested that these types have a direct relevance to severity and outcome. While such a classification is useful in understanding the progress of the disease, its value from a practical point of view is less apparent. Usually, in individual cases such a classification can only be made retrospectively. Furthermore, we doubt whether the first form (in which there is no biliary obstruction) represents a true form of cholangitis. What this classification misses is the relationship between the virulence of the organisms and the effectiveness of host resistance. We have observed patients presenting in a moribund state with little or no jaundice in whom there is pus but no stones (presumably passed) in the biliary tree. On the other hand, patients with pus in the bile ducts may be relatively well on admission, whereas others, without any pus present, may present in an extreme state of shock. Boey and Way concluded that "suppurative cholangitis is an unsatisfactory synonym for severe cholangitis because the correlation between biliary suppurative and clinical manifestations in cholangitis is inexact."[14] Similarly, Connor and colleagues[17] reported no significant correlation "between liver histology and clinical presentation, laboratory data, or mechanism of biliary obstruction" and that "the clinical presentation of patients with mechanical biliary obstruction fails to correspond uniformly to either gross or microscopic pathologic findings in the biliary tree."

Etiology

By far the commonest cause is stone(s) in the bile duct occurring in around 80% of unselected cases.[17-22] Acute cholangitis is said to develop in 6–9% of

Table 6-2 Causes of Acute Cholangitis

Stones in the main bile ducts
Malignant obstruction
Iatrogenic stricture
Papillary stenosis
Choledochoduodenostomy
Choledochojejunostomy
Sclerosing cholangitis
Congenital abnormalities

patients admitted with gallstone disease.[22,23] In our own experience of over 2,500 patients undergoing surgery for gallstones over a recent 5-year period, 438 were found to have CBD stones (18%), of whom only 50 also had acute cholangitis. This represents 11% of patients with CBD stones or just 2% of patients requiring surgery for gallstones.

Malignant obstruction of the biliary tree from cancer of the pancreas or bile ducts themselves constitutes about 10% of cases. Twelve percent or more of cases of ampullary carcinoma present with acute cholangitis.[24] Five percent or less are caused by a miscellany of other conditions (Table 6-2). The sump syndrome, which occurs in about 3% of patients with choledochoduodenostomy rarely gives rise to acute cholangitis.[25]

Pathogenesis

In Western cholangitis obstruction of the biliary tree with bile stasis is probably the primary event followed by subsequent overgrowth of bacteria. Positive bile cultures are found in 80–100% of patients with CBD stones[26–28] compared with only 10–25% of those with malignant obstruction.[28,29] Why this should be so is not entirely clear. One possibility is that CBD stones cause intermittent and subclinical bile duct obstruction over a protracted period of time, thereby promoting bacterial overgrowth, compared with the relative short period of progressive obstruction in cancer.

Organisms probably reach the bile ducts via the portal circulation[30–33] in the majority of cases, although direct extension from the duodenum, lymphatic spread, and systemic arterial spread are alternative routes.[26] The organisms are typically those derived from the gut and can be grown from the bile in the majority of cases (Table 6-3). Blood cultures are less frequently positive, but this probably relates to intermittent showers of bacteria entering the systemic circulation. A rise in bile duct pressures in excess of 25 cm of H_2O is sufficient to force bile bacteria and endotoxins across the sinusoids into the systemic venous circulation.[33,34] The severity of the subsequent clinical syndrome will then depend on the degree of endotoxemia and bacteremia, the virulence of the organisms, and the degree of host resistance.

Management

Investigations

Once the clinical diagnosis has been made or is suspected, immediate investigations should include a full hematologic and biochemical profile and blood

Table 6-3 Bacteria Grown from Bile and Blood Cultures in Patients with Acute Cholangitis

---

Escherichia coli
Klebsiella spp
Streptococcus faecalis
Pseudomonas spp
Proteus spp
Streptococcus viridans
Staphylococcus albus
Staphylococcus aureus
Microaerophilic streptococci
Anaerobic streptococci
Clostridium perfringens
Bacteroides fragilis

---

cultures. Ultrasonography (US) is useful in helping to indicate the obstructive nature of the jaundice and may also detect hepatic abscesses, though these are usually small. The detection of stones in the CBD by US is not always reliable.[35] A mass at the lower end of the CBD may be due to tumor or an impacted stone with surrounding tissue edema. Dilation of the biliary tree may not be present, either because of early stone passage or because of the rapid development of symptoms before dilation can occur. CT scanning is highly accurate in diagnosing carcinomas of the head of the pancreas, but it is less accurate at identifying CBD stones and tumors of the ampulla of Vater. Even if not providing a clear-cut diagnosis, these techniques can provide a working diagnosis and allow the initiation of appropriate treatment measures. Nevertheless, in our own clinical practice we would ultimately wish to undertake an ERCP in the great majority of cases.

ERCP has the unique advantage of providing an immediate diagnosis of all the causes of acute cholangitis. ERCP can also detect hepatic microabscesses not detectable by other means.[36] The typical ERCP features of microabscesses are multiple small "dilations" of the smaller intrahepatic biliary radicles; communications with larger cavities also readily occur, representing sonographically detectable abscesses. Spontaneous passage of CBD stones may be revealed by the presence of empty ducts in the presence of a widely gaping papilla (sometimes draining pus) and allow bile to be obtained for culture.

Medical Treatment

All patients require the immediate institution of resuscitative measures (IV crystalloids, parenteral vitamin K, nil by mouth, broad-spectrum antibiotics) and regular monitoring. Although for milder cases a second or third generation cephalosporin with metranidazole is sufficient, severe cases will require at least triple therapy—a useful combination being benzylpenicillin, gentamicin, and metronidazole. Prolonged IV administration will be required in cases of associated liver abscesses.[37,38] Oxygen, IV colloids, inotropic agents, and the insertion of a nasogastric tube, urinary catheter, central venous line, and a Swan–Ganz catheter are additional measures to be used in more severe cases.

The majority of patients should see some improvement with these measures, allowing for a semielective approach to biliary decompression. Failure to improve after initial resuscitation is an indication for further action *without delay*. The outcome for those patients with continued conservative management is invariably fatal.[20,21,23,29] Decompression may be achieved by surgery, percutaneous transhepatic biliary drainage (PTBD), or endoscopic methods.

Surgical Decompression

Rogers in 1903 was the first to attempt decompression of the biliary tree using a glass tube.[40] T-tube decompression after CBD stone clearance is usually satisfactory but it may not be as effective as internal drainage. We would strongly recommend choledochoduodenostomy provided the CBD is sufficiently dilated (1.5 cm or more).[41,42] Cholecystostomy without a widely patent cystic duct is fraught with difficulties[43] and is frankly dangerous.

The mortality following early surgical decompression varies from 7 to 40%.[18-21,23,39,44-46] Bismuth and colleagues suggested that patients with advanced renal failure can be treated with renal dialysis before surgical intervention.[47] Of 281 patients with cholangitis, 21 (7.4%) had established renal failure. Eight of these patients died (38%). Although six of the patients were dialyzed preoperatively, three of them ultimately succumbed.

Percutaneous Transhepatic Biliary Drainage

PTBD has become popular since the introduction of the "skinny needle" by Molnar and Stockum in 1974.[48] Gould *et al* reported a limited success with PTBD in seven patients with acute cholangitis of whom two died (29%).[49] Kadir *et al* reported good results in 18 patients of whom three died (17%).[50] Pessa *et al* reported a series of 42 patients with two deaths (5%)[51]—only 86% of these patients with "acute cholangitis" were jaundiced, however.

The best study of PTBD came from Kinoshita and colleagues from Osaka, in which a retrospective attempt was made to define the type of cholangitis in relation to the type of treatment received.[33] Although the limitations to this approach have been discussed above, this was important as it showed that the distribution of the suppurative types of cholangitis was similar between those undergoing surgery and those having PTBD (Table 6-4). However, the difference in outcome between these two types of treatment *was not statistically different*.

PTBD should not normally be used as the definitive treatment. Obstruction due to malignancy can be managed in some cases by the percutaneous insertion of an internally draining biliary stent.[49-51] The percutaneous route may occasionally be used to eliminate CBD stones. Stones may be extracted along the tract following dilation using a Dormia basket, if necessary crushing the stones.[33,49-51] Alternatively, stones may be pushed through the ampulla of Vater before crushing, particularly larger stones which cause undue liver trauma.[52,55] The latter procedure may be assisted by catheter dilation of the sphincter of Oddi.[56] Chemical dissolution using monooctanoin[57] or methyl tert-butyl ether[58,59] may also be used either alone or in combination with percutaneous extraction.[55]

Table 6-4 Outcome of Treatment Using Conservative Treatment, Urgent Surgical Biliary Decompression, and Percutaneous Transhepatic Biliary Decompression in 125 Patients with Acute Cholangitis Reported by Kinoshita et al[33]

Type of Cholangitis	Conservative treatment Total	Conservative treatment Deaths	Emergency surgery Total	Emergency surgery Deaths	PTBD Total	PTBD Stress
Nonsuppurative	54*	4	15	2	15	1
Suppurative	1	0	12	1	9	0
Suppurative/obstructive	—	—	8	4	11	4
Total (% Deaths)	55	4 (7.3)	35	7 (20.0)	35	5 (14.3)

* It was noted that none of these patients had pus and/or obstruction on the basis of clinical criteria alone.

Endoscopic Sphincterotomy

In 1982 Vallon, Shorvon, and Cotton reported remarkable success in 14 patients with gallstone-associated acute cholangitis treated by ES.[60] Endoscopic drainage was achieved in all cases and all stones were removed or drainage achieved by a nasobiliary catheter (NBC) with dramatic improvement. Large stones could not be removed in two cases; one had uneventful surgery, but the other was totally unfit for surgery and died. Similarly, encouraging results were also reported by Delmotte et al.[61]

In a recent study, we reported our results of 94 patients with acute cholangitis, 82 (87%) of whom had gallstones as the cause.[18] Of those with noncalculous disease, six had malignant obstruction, two had papillary stenosis, one had an iatrogenic stricture, one had sclerosing cholangitis, and two had had a previous choledochoenterostomy. There were 12 deaths in the gallstone group (14.6%) compared with three in the acalculous group (25%)—one following PTHC.

Factors associated with mortality were a low serum albumin, high urea, high bilirubin, and the medical risk factor (MRF) score (Table 6-5). A high serum creatinine was also significantly associated with mortality when only those patients with gallstones were considered. Several attempts have been made previously to define risk factors in patients undergoing biliary surgery but none have been specifically related to acute cholangitis.[62–64] Our laboratory risk factors correlated best with the Glasgow group, who found that serum albumin and creatinine had independent significance in predicting mortality.[64] None of these other studies, however, looked at the role of medical risk factors despite the major influence these have on postoperative outcome, particularly for those aged 65 years or more.[65] In previous studies of acute cholangitis in whom the mean age of the patients was 47–62 years, the mortality was 2.7–14%.[13,19,41,44] In contrast, in studies in whom the patients were much older, the mortality was 22–47%.[20–22,45] In our own study, the mean age was 70 years. The system we used to define medical risk was to allocate a score of one point for any adverse chronic medical condition requiring active therapy, the main categories being heart disease, hypertension, chronic lung disease, and any condition requiring long-term steroids. No attempt was made to weight these factors.

The management and subsequent mortality of the 82 patients with gallstones is shown in Figure 6-1. Only seven patients settled completely with antibiotics

Table 6-5 Comparison of Risk Factors in Relation to Mortality in 94 Patients with Acute Cholangitis*

Risk factor	Survived ($N = 79$)	Died ($N = 15$)	Correlation
Age (years)	70 (25–88)	78 (60–84)	NS
Medical risk factors	2 (0–5)	3 (1–4)	$p < 0.05$
Systolic BP <100 mm Hg	11/79 (4%)	4/15 (27%)	NS
Blood culture	28/55 (51%) (0.9–4.0)	5/12 (42%) (0.68–1.35)	NS
Prothrombin ratio	1.11 (0.94–4.0)	1.2 (0.68–1.35)	
WBC ($\times 10^9$/L)	12.2 (1.2–38.5)	15.0 (5.0–31.0)	NS
Serum bilirubin, μmol/L	110 (20–520)	171 (40–660)	$p = 0.06$
Serum alkaline phosphatase units/L	474 (105–2400)	631 (251–2178)	NS
Serum γ-GT units/L	379 (22–1170)	445 (122–1926)	NS
Serum ALT units/L	151 (29–895)	114 (30–520)	NS
Serum albumin (g/L)	34 (24–44)	29 (25–35)	$p < 0.005$
Serum urea (mmol/L)	6.1 (2.1–34.9)	10.3 (2.2–56.5)	$p < 0.05$
Serum creatinine (μmol/L)	90 (30–500)	137 (60–600)	NS
Serum glucose (mmol/L)	6.8 (4.2–19.8)	6.6 (3.5–10.7)	NS

* Values are median (range); NS = not significant.
Modified from Leese et al[18] with permission from the *British Journal of Surgery*.

alone (8.5%). This is lower than that reported by previous series (18–41%).[19,33] This probably reflects our strict diagnostic criteria and the poorer response rate to conservative measures among the more elderly patients. Four patients were moribund on admission and died before they could be stabilized for biliary decompression. Of the remainder, 28 underwent urgent or early* surgery with six deaths (21.4%) and 43 had endoscopic biliary decompression with only two deaths (4.7%). The number of patients developing post-ES complications (27.9%) was also significantly less compared with those who underwent surgery (57.1%)

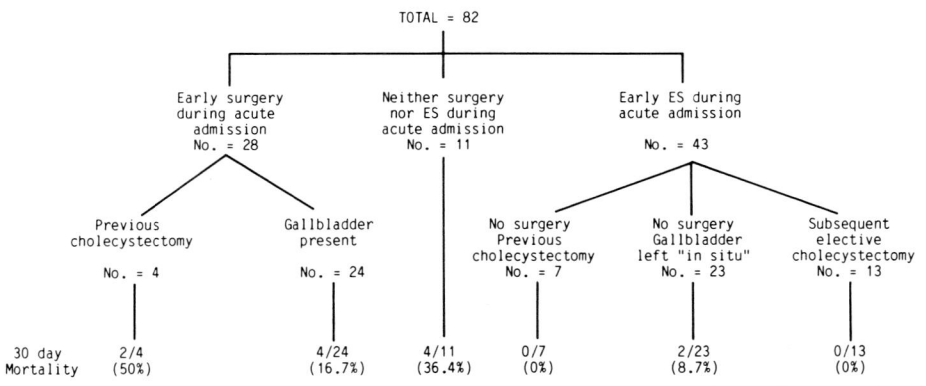

Figure 6-1 Outcome in relation to treatment in 82 patients with acute cholangitis associated with common bile duct stones (ES = endoscopic sphincterotomy). (From Leese et al[18] with permission of the of *Br J Surg*.)

---

* In this chapter, investigations or treatment undertaken within 72 hours of admission are referred to as "urgent"; "early" = from 72 hours to 30 days; "delayed" = following the first hospital admission.

Table 6-6 Comparison of Complications Following Early ES or Surgical Decompression of the Biliary Tree in Gallstone Cholangitis

Endoscopic sphincterotomy (N = 43)		Surgery (N = 28)	
Complication	Number	Complication	Number
Hemorrhage	5	Multisystem failure	8
Recurrent cholangitis	4 (1*)	Respiratory failure	1
Acute pancreatitis	1	Blood loss (transfused)	7
Gallstone ileus	1 (1*)	Wound infection	7 (2*)
Death	2	Biliary leak	4
Number of patients with complications =	12 (27.9%)	Burst abdomen/incisional hernia	2 (1*)
		Retained CBD calculi	3 (1*)
		Death	6
		Number of patients with complications =	16 (57.1%)

Source: Modified from Leese et al.[18] with permission from the *British Journal of Surgery*.
* requiring sugery.

(Table 6-6). These differences could not be accounted for by the distribution of risk factors; indeed, the ES patients were older and had a higher MRF score (Table 6-7). Although this was a retrospective study, the results were strikingly in favor of ES. Our standard approach had been for early surgery, but the initial results from ERCP and ES were such that these procedures became our treatment of choice in the latter part of the study.

Why should the results of ES be so superior to those of surgery? We recently undertook a multivariate analysis of nearly 450 patients undergoing surgery and/or ES for CBD stones in order to try to answer this question.[66] The results showed that the serum level of bilirubin was the most significant independent factor in predicting outcome. In patients undergoing surgery, the presence or absence of one (or more) MRF was also independently significant. In patients undergoing ES, however, the MRF score was of no relevance at all once the risk from other factors (bilirubin and albumin) had been accounted for.

Early complications following ES included hemorrhage from the sphincterotomy site, but only three of these required blood transfusion (2–4 units) and none required surgery. Three patients developed early exacerbation of preexisting cholangitis, all associated with initial incomplete clearance of large CBD stones. One of these patients (aged 72 years), whose general condition was so poor that surgery was ruled out, died from cholangitis and liver abscesses. A fourth patient with a persisting CBD stone developed a mild attack of cholangitis 5 months after initial resolution but was well enough to undergo successful surgery after a brief period of stabilization. One patient developed post-ES acute pancreatitis, but this was mild and settled on conservative management. Another developed gallstone ileus following endoscopic delivery of a large stone from the CBD but the patient's condition improved sufficiently to allow uneventful surgery.

Of the 36 patients with gallbladder in situ who underwent early ES, 13 were considered to be reasonably fit for surgery and all had successful surgery. The other 23 patients were considered to be at high surgical risk and were not initially

Table 6-7 Comparison of Risk Factors in Relation to Early Surgical or Endoscopic Biliary Decompression in Patients with Acute Cholangitis Due to Gallstones

Risk factor	Early surgery ($N = 28$)	Early endoscopic sphincterotomy ($N = 43$)	Comparison
Age (years)	66.5 (25–84)	75 (28–88)	$p < 0.02$
30-day mortality	6/28 (21%)	2/43 (5%)	$p < 0.02$
Hospital stay (days)	22.5 (6–60)	20 (5–90)	NS
Medical risk factors	1 (0–4)	2 (0–5)	$p < 0.05$
Systolic BP <100 mm Hg	3/28 (11%)	7/43 (16%)	NS
Blood culture positive	9/19 (47%)	17/30 (57%)	NS
Prothrombin ratio	1.08 (0.68–4.0)	1.13 (0.9–1.76)	NS
WBC ($\times 10^9$/L)	12.7 (5.1–31.0)	12.9 (1.2–38.5)	NS
Serum bilirubin (μmol/L)	94 (20–556)	118 (30–379)	NS
Serum alkaline phosphatase (U/L)	476 (107–1265)	474 (118–1766)	NS
Serum γ-GT (U/L)	357 (67–1045)	407 (116–1926)	NS
Serum ALT (U/L)	134 (30–690)	158 (36–895)	NS
Serum albumin (g/L)	33 (25–41)	33 (24–44)	NS
Serum urea (mmol/L)	6.2 (2.2–54.4)	7.3 (2.5–34.9)	NS
Serum creatinine (μmol/L)	106 (53–539)	108 (30–500)	NS
Serum glucose (mmol/liter)	6.6 (3.5–13.6)	6.7 (4.8–19.8)	NS

Source: Modified from Leese et al.[18] with permission from the *British Journal of Surgery*.

Values are median (range); NS = not significant.

considered for surgery (Table 6-8). This was, however, necessary in two cases, one because of subsequent cholangitis (mentioned above) and the other because of empyema of the gallbaldder. In addition to a death already referred to, the second death occurred in an 81-year-old who died from late bronchopneumonia and gastric erosions, with empty ducts and without evidence of persisting cholangitis at postmortem.

We recently recognized that empyema of the gallbladder is a particular problem of ES in patients with acute cholangitis, occurring in around 5% of cases.[67] Endoscopic sphincterotomy increases the risk of bacterobilia[68,69] and in particular may promote the growth of *Pseudomonas* spp.[69] Possibly this relates to the adequacy of endoscopic disinfection. Our standard practice has been to use antibiotics in patients with gallbladders who have had ES for cholangitis for 1 week at least or until there is complete resolution of symptoms. Recent results indicate that it may be advisable to continue with antibiotics for a longer period. Despite these drawbacks, if proper drainage of the biliary tree is achieved by adequate sphincterotomy with full clearance of the CBD stones, the risks of further problems are minimal.[67] Thus, it is important that clearance of all CBD stones be confirmed whenever possible.

In the present series we achieved complete clearance at the first endoscopic attempt in 30/43 patients (70%). Two or more attempts were required in 9/43 (21%) before adequate clearance was obtained. In three of these an NBC (7

Table 6-8 Comparison of Patients with CBD Stones and Gallbladders in Situ Undergoing Early Decompression for Acute Cholangitis

	Early surgery (N = 24)	Early ES → elective surgery (N = 13)	Early ES with gallbladder in situ (N = 23)
Age (years)	66 (25–84)	64 (28–82)	78 (65–87)*
30-day mortality	4/24 (16.7%)	0/13	2/23 (8.7%)
Hospital stay (days)	25 (6–60)	19 (15–70)	20 (6–90)
Medical risk factors	1 (0–4)	2 (0–3)	3 (0–5)**
Systolic BP <100 mm Hg	2/24 (8.3%)	2/13 (15.4%)	4/23 (17.4%)
Blood culture positive	7/16 (43.8%)	3/8 (37.5%)	8/16 (50%)
Prothrombin ratio	1.11 (0.93–4.0)	1.15 (0.94–1.42)	1.19 (1.04–1.76)
WBC ($\times 10^9$/L)	13.3 (5.1–31.0)	13.5 (6.9–22.8)	13.3 (1.2–38.5)
Serum bilirubin (μmol/L)	100 (20–556)	110 (30–225)	124 (32–379)
Serum alkaline phosphatase (IU/L)	424 (107–1192)	441 (118–1030)	487 (198–1710)
Serum γ-GT (IU/L)	357 (67–1045)	407 (156–1058)	432 (133–1926)
Serum ALT (IU/L)	117 (30–690)	253 (41–895)	130 (36–493)***
Serum albumin (g/L)	32 (25–41)	35 (24–44)	32 (25–42)
Serum urea (mmol/L)	6.2 (2.2–54.4)	5.9 (2.6–11.6)	7.3 (3.0–34.9)
Serum creatinine (μmol/L)	106 (53–539)	90 (30–155)	110 (61–500)
Serum glucose (mmol/L)	6.3 (3.5–13.6)	7.7 (5.6–19.8)	6.4 (4.8–14.6)

Note: Values are median (range).
* Gallbladder in situ group undergoing ES only significantly older than other two groups (both $p < 0.0002$).
** Gallbladder in situ group undergoing ES only had significantly more medical risk factors than other two groups ($p < 0.01$ and $p < 0.05$).
*** ES and elective surgery group had significantly higher serum ALT levels than other two groups ($p < 0.02$ and $p < 0.05$).

French) was inserted and monooctanoin infusion used to reduce the size of the stone. The progress of stone dissolution was followed by check cholangiography using the NBC. As complete dissolution with monooctanoin can take several weeks (and is often *not* completely successful),[70] we prefer to remove the stones endoscopically once their size has been reduced.

In the light of our recent experiences, we would recommend the wider use of NBCs and endoprostheses. An NBC may be inserted if not all stones can be removed, either as a temporary means of drainage prior to repeat attempts at endoscopic extraction, or with a view to dissolution therapy.

If stones cannot be eliminated, the insertion of a 10 French endoprosthesis is recommended.[71] Similarly, this should be inserted if there is incomplete removal of stones in the presence of pus while awaiting a repeat procedure. In general, however, we prefer to remove stones at the first attempt, as the incidence of complications rises significantly if this is not achieved.[67] While we are aggressive in attempting to remove CBD stones, we would not try to obtain a pancreatogram unless there was doubt about the diagnosis.

Although empyema of the gallbladder cannot be treated by antibiotics alone, surgery is not always necessary in high-risk cases. We recently treated two patients by percutaneous gallbladder aspiration and drainage.[72,73] One of these patients also had complete dissolution of a gallbladder packed with stones by cyclical instillation and aspiration using MTBE as previously recommended.[58,73–75] While awaiting the results of pus cultures, we recommend the direct instillation into the gallbladder of gentamicin in order to achieve high local bactericidal concentrations.

Overall, long-term follow-up of 21 patients with gallbladder in situ who were treated successfully by ES resulted in only two patients (9.5%) requiring surgery. This is similar to a larger series on which we reported[67] and to that reported by others.[76–78] Therefore the vast majority of elderly patients with gallbladder in situ treated by ES require no further treatment.

These results are in clear contrast to patients with PTBD, the majority of whom need to have additional procedures.[33,49–51] Endoprostheses, while acceptable in the elderly patient with malignant disease and a short prognosis, are not ideal in benign disease. The risk of blockage with recurrent cholangitis is high, although the results are better with the use of newer, larger prostheses.[71] Internal drainage can, of course, be achieved endoscopically but without the risks of intraperitoneal hemorrhage or bile leaks. In cases of advanced ampullary carcinoma, an excellent form of drainage is sphincterotomy through the tumor.[24]

If the necessary skills for performing ERCP/ES in patients with acute cholangitis are not available, then we prefer PTHC/PTBD, but this also depends on availability and expertise in the institution. We would encourage the use of these techniques in most patients presenting with acute cholangitis but in particular those very ill patients described by Reynolds and Dargan[15] and Bismuth et al.[47] Some patients will respond to conservative measures alone. Provided these patients are relatively young and are not high-risk surgical cases, they may proceed to surgery without recourse to ERCP. Alternatively, patients not responding to initial conservative measures within 24–48 hr, or those surgical high-risk cases who have responded, should proceed to ES.

Recurrent Pyogenic Cholangitis

First described by Digby in 1930[79] and characterized by Cook in 1954,[80] recurrent pyogenic cholangitis (RPC) is now recognized to be an extremely common condition in Hong Kong,[32] and parts of China, Japan, and South-East Asia.[81] It is also being increasingly recognized in Chinese immigrants in Canada[82] and the United States.[83]

The signs and symptoms during an acute attack are similar to those of Western cholangitis. Many of the patients will settle on conservative management but will continue to have chronic symptoms with superimposed recurrent acute attacks.[84] Cholangiography reveals multiple strictures in the intrahepatic and extrahepatic bile ducts with dilation.[85] Stones in the main bile ducts are only apparent in about 80% of cases and these are invariably of the soft brown pigment variety (calcium bilirubinate),[32] in contrast to the cholesterol-type stones frequently seen in the West.[75] Less than 20% of patients with RPC have stones in the gallbladder.[32]

The etiology of RPC is not certain but evidence suggests that it is a primary infective condition of the bile ducts with secondary gallstone formation. Both *E. coli* and *Clonorchis sinensis* have been implicated, either individually or in combination.[32,86]

Once the acute attack has resolved, good long-term results can be achieved

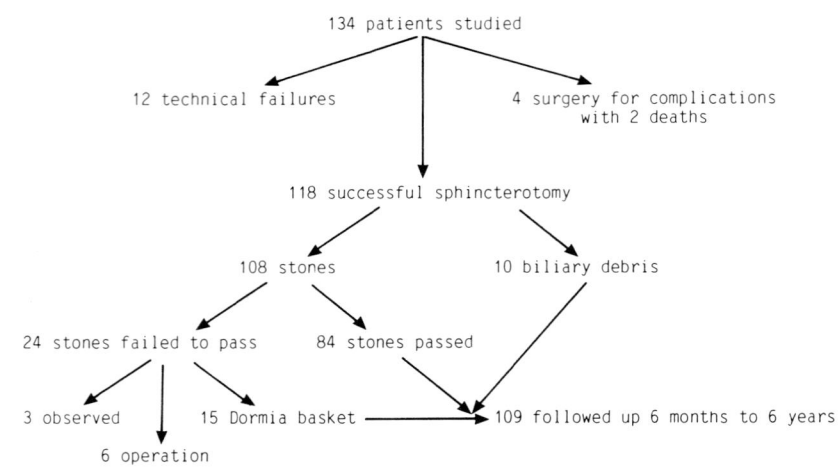

```
                        134 patients studied
                       /         |         \
       12 technical failures     |      4 surgery for complications
                                 |              with 2 deaths
                                 ↓
                    118 successful sphincterotomy
                       /                    \
                  108 stones              10 biliary debris
                  /        \
       24 stones failed   84 stones passed
       to pass    |            \
      /           |             \
  3 observed  15 Dormia basket ──→ 109 followed up 6 months to 6 years
              |
          6 operation
```

Figure 6-2 Results of ERCP and endoscopic sphincterotomy in 134 patients presenting with recurrent pyogenic cholangitis. (From Lam[81] with permission of the author and *Br J Surg*.)

in around 75–80% by choledocholithotomy, initially in combination with transduodenal sphincteroplasty and/or choledochojejunostomy.[87,88] Hepatic resection, hepatotomy, and transhepatic intubation are other surgical techniques which have been employed for intrahepatic strictures and calculi.[89] The mortality rates vary from 4.3 to 11.2% and are related to the severity of the acute attack rather than to the extent of surgery.[32,87–89] Recurrence rates are highest for transhepatic intubation (38%) and hepatotomy (75%) and lowest for hepatic resection (4%).[89]

ERCP has been an important advance in the assessment of these patients, permitting accurate identification of those requiring surgery as well as enabling surgical strategy to be planned.[84,85] Postprocedural cholangitis can be minimized by prophylactic antibiotics and the examination may be performed during the same admission following resolution of the acute attack.[85]

More recently, Lam[90] reported excellent results using ES in 134 patients with RPC *with stones confined to the CBD* (Figure 6-2). One hundred eighteen patients (88%) had successful ES, of whom 109 patients had complete ductal clearance. This represents 92% of those who had successful ES, or 81% of the total group. Complications occurred in 10 patients (7.5%) with emergency surgery in 4 (3%) and ensuing death in 2 (1.5%). Of interest is that 82 (61%) had had previous biliary surgery, 115 (86%) were aged greater than 60 years, and 55 (41%) had one or more medical risk factors. Though the long-term follow-up was short (median 2 years, range 0.5–6 years), only 5 patients had further symptoms—none due to recurrent calculi.

There is probably a limited role for interventional percutaneous biliary techniques in patients with postoperative recurrent intrahepatic calculi.[91] Short-term success has been reported in 8 of 14 patients in two recent series from the United States, but the long-term strategies are not clear.[92,93] It has been suggested that "routine drainage tube replacement and stone extraction should be performed every 3–4 months."[92] Given that these patients are young, surgery along the lines recommended by the Hong Kong group might be a better alternative.

Acute Pancreatitis

Definition

Acute pancreatitis is an acute inflammatory condition of the pancreas characterized by the *sudden* onset of severe upper abdominal pain and tenderness.[94,95] The serum amylase or lipase is always elevated in the acute phase. Values of at least three times the upper limit of the reference range of one or other of these enzymes are required for diagnosis. We use an amylase level greater than 1,000 IU/liter (Phadebas method; upper limit of normal = 300 IU/liter). A falsely low amylase may occur in hyperlipemias but clues to this condition are pseudohyponatremia and lipemic serum.[96] There are many other conditions which can give rise to a high amylase, but these can usually be determined by associated clinical features. The pancreas is abnormal on computerized tomography (CT) in more than 95% of cases diagnosed as having acute pancreatitis using these criteria.[97] We do not regard mild exacerbation of pain and elevation of serum amylase less than 1,000 IU/liter in patients with chronic pancreatitis as having acute pancreatitis.

Etiology and Pathogenesis

The list of conditions associated with acute pancreatitis is very long, but gallstones and excess alcohol account for over 80% of cases.[98–100] Acute pancreatitis is probably triggered by the activation of trypsinogen to trypsin (which is autocatalytic) which then activates many other pancreatic enzymes. This results in autodigestion of the gland, which may produce local necrosis and ultimately systemic toxicity.

In the present context, it is important to mention those factors by which gallstones can bring about enzyme activation. Opie in 1901 described a patient who died with a small stone impacted at the papilla of Vater; the stone was small enough for direct communication between the common bile and pancreatic ducts via a "common channel."[101] He then performed experiments in which he showed that hemorrhagic pancreatitis could be produced by injecting bile into the pancreatic duct. The role of bile reflux into the pancreatic duct in humans is still the subject of debate.

Reflux of contrast into the pancreatic duct during operative cholangiography occurs in about 60% of patients with a history of pancreatitis compared with about 15% of controls.[102–104] A long common channel (5 mm or more) has also been found in 72% of pancreatitis cases compared with only 20% of control subjects.[104]

Gallstones are found in the stools of 85–95% of patients during an attack of acute pancreatitis, while fecal stones are found in only 10% of those with gallstones but no pancreatitis.[105,106] Although there is no difference in the largest sized stones between those with and without pancreatitis, the former also have a larger number of smaller stones, often in association with a large cystic duct.[104,107]

The incidence of CBD stones at the time of urgent operation has been reported to be as high as 63–78% of cases.[108–110] In contrast, the proportion of patients with CBD stones operated on at a later time (either "early" or "delayed") varies from 3 to 33%.[104,108,110–113]

All these findings provide indirect evidence for Opie's hypothesis. An al-

Table 6-9 Ranson's Criteria Used to Predict Severity of Outcome in Acute Pancreatitis

Admission or diagnosis	During initial 48 hours
Age >55 years	Hematocrit fall >10%
WBC 16,000/mm³	BUN rise >5 mg/100 mL
Blood glucose >200 mg/100 mL	Serum calcium <8 mg/100 mL
Serum lactic dehydrogenase >350 IU/L	PaO_2 <60 mm Hg
SGOT >250 Sigma Frankel Units %	Base deficit >4 meq/L
	Fluid sequestration >6 L

Note: Mild attack = 0–2 factors; severe attack = 3–11 factors. This system has been reduced to 10 factors with alterations of six of the cutoff points in patients with known gallstones.[91]

ternative explanation is that patients who are prone to acute pancreatitis have a lax sphincter of Oddi, thereby facilitating the reflux of activated duodenal juice into the pancreatic duct.[114] This observation, however, could be entirely secondary to initial stone passage.

Clinical Course and Prediction of Severity

The large majority of patients fully recover within a week or so of the attack using conservative measures alone. However, there is a mortality of around 10% in unselected series,[98,113,115–118] but is double this if those cases diagnosed at postmortem are also included.[119] Local complications include pseudocysts, abscesses, and hemorrhagic necrosis; systemic complications include coagulopathies and failure of the respiratory, cardiac, and renal systems.

Means by which to predict severity of outcome are useful not only in permitting the clinician to anticipate complications, but also to allow objective comparison between different treatment modalities. Ranson from New York used 11 factors to predict severity (Table 6-9)[100] and Imrie and coworkers from Glasgow proposed a slightly simplified system.[116,120] The validity of these systems is now widely accepted.[121] We use a modified Glasgow system (Table 6-10), which differs from the "standard" system by including age greater than 55 years as originally proposed,[116] but not transaminase greater than 200 IU/liter. Our own studies (unpublished), as well as a recent report from Glasgow[122] and an

Table 6-10 Modified Glasgow Criteria Used to Predict Severity of Outcome in Acute Pancreatitis within 48 hours

Age	>55 years
WBC	>15 × 10⁹/L (15,000/mm³)
Blood glucose	>10 mmol/L (180 mg/dL) (no diabetic history)
Serum urea	>16 mmol/L (96 mg/dL) (no response to IV fluids)
PaO_2	<8 KPa (60 mm Hg) (no O₂ by mask for 15 min)
Serum calcium	<2.0 mmol/L (8 mg/dL) (uncorrected value)
Lactase dehydrogenase	>600 IU/L
Serum albumin	<32 g/L (3.2 g/dL)

Note: mild attack = 0–2 factors. Severe attack = 3–8 factors.

Table 6-11 Principles of Management in Patients with Acute Pancreatitis

Acute Phase

Assess severity
Modify acute attack
   supportive care
   ? specific therapeutic agents
   ? peritoneal lavage
   ? pancreatic resection
   remove common bile duct stones

Postacute Phase (Severe Attacks)

Continued supportive care
Treat local complications
   drain abscesses ± } open packing
   sequestrectomy ± } lavage
   drain symptomatic pseudocysts
   treat fistulae

Convalescent Phase

Identify cause and if possible treat to prevent current attacks

---

independent study from Leicester,[123] confirm the statistical significance of age in relation to outcome but not of transaminase. An alternative method is to assess the volume and color of peritoneal return lavage fluid.[124] This has the advantage of providing an immediate result but is not as sensitive for predicting the severity from gallstones as it is from alcohol.[99] Indium-labeled leukocyte scanning[125] and CT scanning[126] are other alternatives that have not been fully evaluated.

Management

The principles of management are summarized in Table 6-11. Immediate investigations should include those necessary to assess severity and anticipate major systemic complications. Arterial blood gas measurements need to be carefully monitored in the first 72 hours as respiratory failure can suddenly supervene. Erect chest X rays are important to reveal any large pleural effusions or free gas from a perforated abdominal viscus.

Treatment—Supportive Measures

Patients with a mild attack require to be kept nil by mouth and receive IV crystalloid solutions. Severe cases will require intensive care along the lines previously discussed in the section on acute cholangitis. We routinely administer a single-agent cephalosporin to patients with gallstone pancreatitis and all patients with severe attacks during the period of illness. Prospective studies of antibiotics have not shown a benefit in acute pancreatitis, but these were mostly mild cases. On the other hand, around 40% of patients with necrotizing pancreatitis have infections of the pancreas (excluding abscesses, etc.).[127]

Numerous specific therapeutic procedures have been proposed, including aprotinin, gabexate, mesylate (Foy), leupeptin, anticholinergics, glucagon, calcitonin, cimetidine, somatostatin, and thoracic duct drainage, but none has been shown to be of value. Among those agents under current consideration, including prostaglandin E_2, inhibitors of phospholipase A_2, dextran, and scavengers of free O_2 radicals, the use of high-dose fresh-frozen plasma seems most promising.[128,129] Although some authors remain convinced about the value of urgent peritoneal lavage, a recent prospective randomized trial has cast serious doubt on this.[130]

Urgent Diagnosis and Treatment of Gallstone Pancreatitis

Most patients with gallstones have a mild attack. In these instances gallstones in the gallbladder may be detected by US in about 80% of cases during the postacute phase.[131] Cholecystectomy during the same admission offers the optimum means of treatment as the postoperative morbidity is similar to that of elective cholecystectomy.[108,112,113,120,132] Peroperative cholangiography is mandatory to determine the presence of CBD stones. If the gallbladder is not removed, recurrent attacks will soon occur in 30–40% of cases, sometimes with fatal consequences.

However, severe cases are a different proposition. Between 30 and 60% of patients who die from gallstone pancreatitis have stones present in the CBD, although these are not always "lodged" in the ampulla of Vater.[118,119] The role of urgent surgical intervention in these cases is still controversial.

Acosta et al in 1978[133] reported only one death out of 46 patients (2.9%) treated urgently compared with 14 deaths out of 86 (16%) "control" patients treated at a later time. The validity of these data is questionable because of the use of an *historical* control group, and there were no objective criteria by which to assess the severity of the attack in each group.

Ranson, on the other hand, urged nonoperative intervention during the acute phase in patients with gallstone pancreatitis.[113] Out of 23 patients with predicted severe attacks, nine were operated on with four deaths, compared with none out of 14 who were not operated on. The conclusions of this study, however, were undermined by the fact that the mean prognostic severity score was 5.4 in those who had urgent surgery compared with 3.5 in those treated conservatively. Furthermore, those who died following surgery also had higher scores than those who survived after surgery. Other studies have also shown high mortality rates for urgent surgery, but these too were poorly controlled.[108,120,132]

Stone et al[110] undertook a prospective randomized study in 65 patients with one death out of 36 (2.8%) urgent operations and two deaths out of 29 (5.9%) patients who had early or delayed surgery. These differences were not statistically significant. The major defect of the trial was that no objective grading was used.

One of the biggest stumbling blocks in establishing any trial on gallstone pancreatitis is the urgent selection of those patients who actually have gallstones. In the acute phase, US can detect only about 60% of cases that are ultimately shown to involve gallstones.[131] CT has a low sensitivity for gallstones.[97] Radionuclide biliary scanning is of no value in distinguishing those with and without gallstones during the acute phase of pancreatitis.[131,134] Bio-

Table 6-12 Results of Endoscopic Sphincterotomy for Common Bile Duct Stones in Acute Pancreatitis in Eight Separate Studies

Authors	Number	Complications	Deaths
Classen et al. 1978[137]	17	0	0
Van Der Spuy 1981[138]	10	1	0
Safrany 1982[139]	28	3	2
Schott et al. 1982[140]	32	2	0
Kautz et al. 1982[141]	21	1	1
Reimann and Lux 1984[142]	15	0	0
Rosseland and Solhaug 1984[143]	29*	2	1
Neoptolemos et al. 1986[144]**	10	0	0
Total	162	9 (5.5%)	4 (2.4%)

* 15 patients had ES <48 hours; 14 at 1–8 weeks.
** Nontrial patients (vide infra).

chemical predictive tests are of assistance, particularly if the cutoff points are set relatively high and are then combined with US.[131] PTHC has been used in acute pancreatitis,[135] but we would not recommend it because of its high complication rate.

Over the past 10 years there have been sporadic reports of ES being undertaken in patients with acute pancreatitis and CBD stones (Table 6-12). There has been no particular problem from hemorrhage as once feared.[136] All the authors commented on how rapidly the patients improved following ES. Although these results are encouraging, there are important deficiencies in most of these studies including:

1. the method of selecting patients in the first instance;
2. the timing of ES in relation to the acute attack; many were done in the postacute phase when surgery is also safe;
3. the complications reported tend to be only those that the authors attributed to ES.

We ourselves have undertaken a 5-year prospective randomized trial to assess both the safety of ERCP and the efficacy of ES in the urgent situation.[145] From a total of 223 consecutive patients with acute pancreatitis of all causes, 131 patients with gallstone pancreatitis were randomized to either receive conventional treatment or to undergo urgent ERCP with ES and stone extraction only if stones were found in the CBD at the time of ERCP. Patients were selected if gallstones were suspected by biochemical prediction and/or US. The patients were stratified according to predicted severity. Ten of these patients were excluded because an alternative etiology was detected (malignancy, alcoholism, etc.). The results in the remaining 121 patients are shown in Table 6-13.

In order to minimize trauma to the ampulla of Vater, the sphincterotome was used to obtain cholangiography from the outset. If possible, the pancreatic duct was not filled with contrast, and injection of contrast was immediately stopped if this was the case. With careful readjustment of the tip of the sphincterotome, cholangiography was attempted again, but undue manipulation on the ampulla of Vater was avoided. The bile ducts were visualized in 80% of those

Table 6-13 Results of a Prospective Randomized Trial of Conventional Treatment versus ERCP ± ES in Suspected Acute Gallstone Pancreatitis

Group	Number	Complications Pseudocysts	Systemic	Deaths	Number of patients with complications
Mild–Conventional					
GS, confirmed	29	4	0	0	4 (14%)
GS, not confirmed	5	0	0	0	0
Mild–ERCP/ES					
GS, confirmed	28	3	1	0	4 (14%)
GS, not confirmed	6	0	0	0	0
Severe–Conventional					
GS, confirmed	24	6	9	3	13 (54%)
GS, not confirmed	4	2	3	2	4
Severe–ERCP/ES					
GS, confirmed	22	3	1	0	4 (18%)
GS, not confirmed	3	0	2	1	2

GS = gallstones.

predicted severe and 94% of those predicted mild. The respective figures for pancreatic duct filling (often incomplete) were 50 and 90%.

The four important findings were that (1) ERCP could be safely undertaken in acute pancreatitis, provided it was done by an experienced endoscopist. In particularly there were no undue complications whether or not CBD stones were present. (2) There was a significant reduction in the major complications of patients who underwent urgent ERCP/ES ($p = 0.03$). (3) The reduction in morbidity was only apparent in those with predicted severe attacks ($p = 0.007$). (4) Finally, there was a significant reduction in the hospital stay of those with severe attacks who had urgent ERCP ± ES (median 9.5 days versus 17.0 days; $p = 0.03$).

In the results we have included 18 patients in whom gallstones were never confirmed. These patients represent either cases of "true" idiopathic pancreatitis or, alternatively (as we suspect), cases who have passed all their stones by the time of investigation (or death).

No statistical difference in mortality was shown in this study. However, none was anticipated given the size of the trial, although there was a definite trend in favor of ERCP/ES. With an overall mortality of only 5% we may have needed to run the trial for perhaps another 10 years to achieve a statistical difference in mortality.

Of the three patients in the conventional group with confirmed gallstones who died, one had a postmortem and was found to have a gallstone impacted at the ampulla of Vater. We were unable to randomize another 13 patients with gallstones into the trial, and two of these died.

In the urgent ERCP/ES group, 63% of those who had a predicted severe attack had CBD stones compared with only 26% of those with a mild attack ($p = 0.0286$). In the conventionally treated group only 13% of cases were shown to have CBD stones. This latter figure may be artificially low because a postmortem was not carried out for two of the deaths and some others never had cholangiography for various reasons. Of further interest is that the CBD diameter of patients with severe attacks was significantly greater than those with mild attacks.

These results confirm the view that the majority of patients with acute pancreatitis pass their CBD stones. An additional hypothesis has also been proposed that patients with severe attacks have CBD stones for a longer period thereby prolonging the attack.[146] This may be because patients with severe attacks (1) have more stones to pass through the ampulla; (2) have large stones (as well as small ones); (3) have ampullae that are unduly resistant to the passage of stones. This provides the rational for urgent ERCP/ES and accounts for the reduction in both local and systemic complications when this approach is utilized.

Why, then, should the results of urgent ES differ from the results of some series of urgent surgery[108,112,113,120,132,147]? There are two possible explanations: (1) Surgery may provide inadequate decompression of the biliary tree using cholecystostomy.[113] (2) Perhaps of equal importance, outcome from ES is independent of associated medical risk factors, whereas that of surgery is not.[66]

The evidence to date leaves little doubt that ERCP and ES have important roles to play in the management of patients with *severe* attacks of gallstone acute pancreatitis. The sooner they can be performed the better. They should also be considered in the patient who presents with a mild attack but then fails to improve. They are, however, potentially dangerous techniques and should only be performed by a skilled endoscopist. We previously suggested that a patient with gallstone pancreatitis who has an admission serum bilirubin of greater than 40 μmol/liter is highly likely to have persisting CBD stones.[148] In the trial we reported above, the sensitivity of this biochemical marker for persisting CBD stones was 83%. This confirms our view that a serum bilirubin of more than 40 μmol/liter should prompt urgent ERCP/ES.

Pancreatic Surgery and the Role of ERCP

The place of urgent pancreatic resection for acute pancreatitis, which was first performed by Watts in 1963,[149] remains controversial. While some of the earlier supporters have lost their enthusiasm for this approach,[150–152] others remain convinced of its value.[153–155] Although many would agree that it may have a limited role, it will not receive general acceptance until there are clearly defined objective criteria for its use. A prospective randomized trial is pressingly required.

There is much more of a consensus regarding the role of sequestrectomy is *established* unremitting pancreatitis. This procedure is often combined with extensive debridement of necrotic peripancreatic tissue and drainage of abscesses. CT scanning is of great value in determining the sites and extent of these processes and is an unquestionable aid in clinical decision making.[155] What is perhaps still contentious is whether this should be followed by continuous peritoneal lavage[113] or open packing.[156] To some extent which to use will depend on the findings at surgery; our preference is for open packing in the worst sort of cases.

Gebhardt and colleagues from West Germany suggested a role for *preoperative ERCP* in planning surgical strategy.[157] These authors reported four types of pancreatograms in a series of eight severe cases of acute pancreatitis:

1. *Normal pancreatogram.* They suggested that in this situation there would

only be peripancreatitis and that only an "isolated necrosectomy" would be necessary. Clearly the decision to operate would be dependent on clinical factors and the CT findings.
2. *Isolated leakage of contrast medium.* The authors suggested that in this case resection of the distal pancreas to include the fistula was indicated. This is not always necessary, however, as illustrated by the case in Figure 6-3.
3. *Diffuse parenchymal staining.* What the authors refer to here is disruption of the pancreatic duct at numerous points. The authors suggest that there is total necrosis requiring a distal "resection." In our practice this is translated to a simple sequestrectomy rather than a formal pancreatectomy (Figure 6-4).
4. *Necrosis in the head of the pancreas.* The authors rightly recommend conservative treatment in this situation. Although both cases referred to by the authors were planned for surgery, their strategy was altered by the ERCP findings. We believe that this is a grave situation and agree that there is no place for surgery. Although both their patients survived, this has not been our experience (Figure 6-5).

This group from West Germany now has extensive experience with this technique.[158] There are, however, few centers combining large numbers of resection with preoperative ERCP, so that this approach still requires independent evaluation.

Role of ERCP in the Management of Complications

Pseudocysts may occur in up to 20% of cases of acute pancreatitis[97] but the majority of these are asymptomatic and a large proportion will resolve by 6 weeks.[159] The most accurate means of detecting these is by CT, although US is more practical in assessing their progress. Infection of a pseudocyst, or a pseudocyst which is rapidly enlarging, requires urgent treatment, and external surgical drainage may be most appropriate.

After 6 weeks large pseudocysts will require internal surgical drainage. Some authors have recommended routine ERCP, either for diagnosis or to plan surgery.[160-162] We believe that this sentiment is misplaced as ERCP is not superior to CT for diagnosis. Although the pancreatic duct is in communication with the pseudocyst in about 60–80% of cases, this has little bearing on surgical strategy.[156,163] There may, however, be indications for performing ERCP in patients also known to have a pseudocyst. In these cases care should be taken to avoid unnecessary filling of the pseudocyst with contrast. The endoscope should be properly sterilized and the patient should be receiving antibiotics. Even with these precautions there is a significant risk of infection.[162] In our opinion, with few rare exceptions (e.g., the mediastinal pseudocyst), there is no role for ERCP in the diagnosis of pseudocysts.

Technically, it is possible to aspirate pseudocysts endoscopically with a needle.[164] Endoscopically, they may also be drained directly into the stomach using a laser or a cutting diathermy knife[165]—a technique we have successfully used. It is important that the pseudocyst is bulging into the stomach and that it is preceded by aspiration to exclude a pseudoaneurysm. In one case we drained a pus-filled pseudocyst which was bulging into the second part of the duodenum with dramatic clinical improvement. Although such procedures are technically

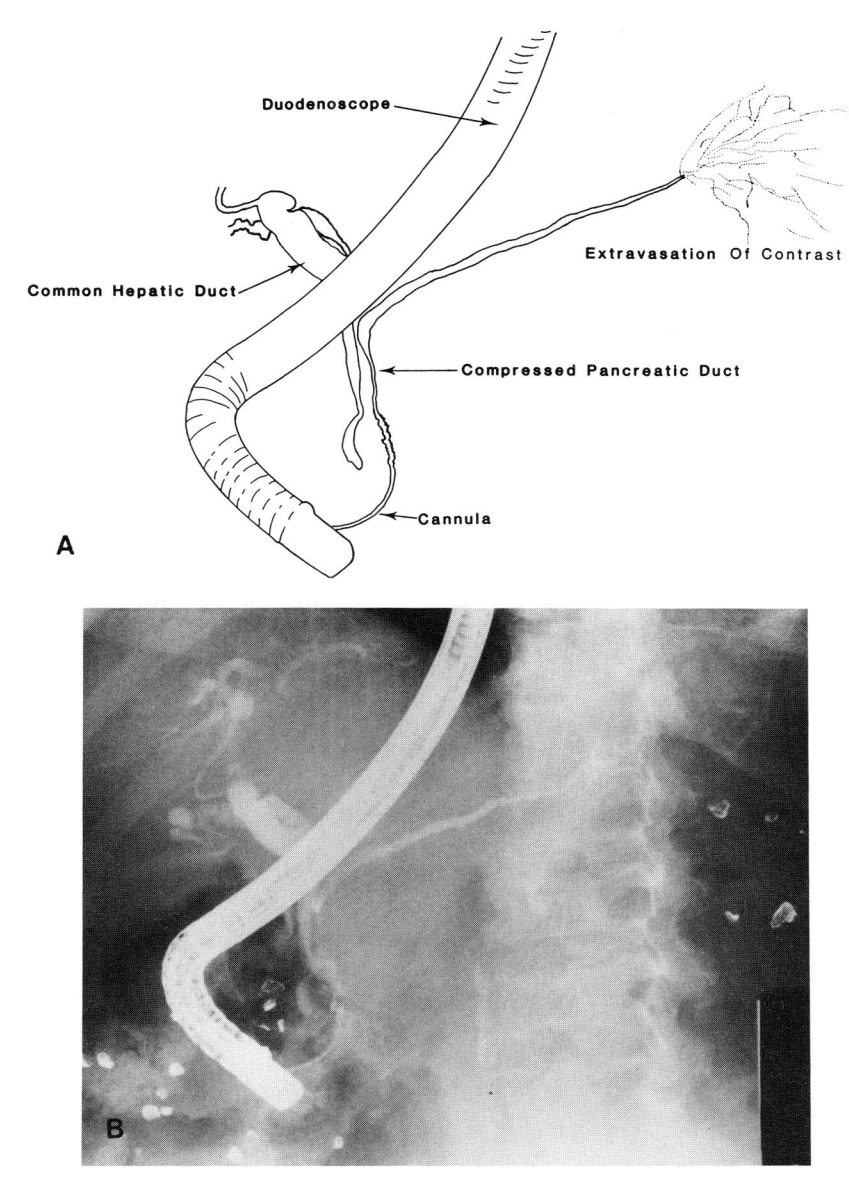

Figure 6-3 (A and **B).** The ERCP shows compression of the pancreatic duct by a noncommunicating pseudocyst and leakage of contrast from the tail of the pancreas into the peritoneal cavity. The patient, a 77-year-old alcoholic female, underwent laparotomy with simple aspiration of the pseudocyst (which was infected; cultures grew *E. coli*) and simple drainage of the fistula externally. Patchy necrosis was noted in the peripancreatic tissues but sequestrectomy was not performed. The patient made a full recovery and is asymptomatic at 12-month follow-up.

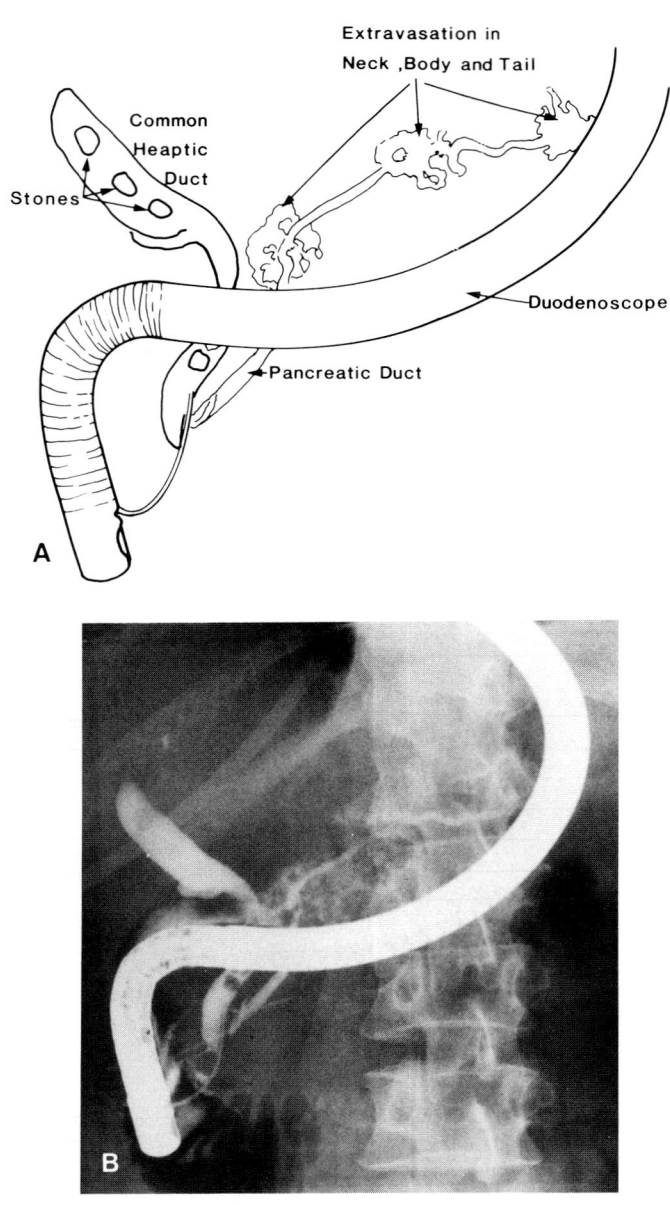

Figure 6-4 (A and B). This ERCP in a 52-year-old female with gallstone pancreatitis shows multiple areas of disruption along the course of the pancreatic duct. The patient required assisted ventilation on the ITU. She underwent laparotomy, cholecystectomy, and wide sequestrectomy. The patient improved rapidly and made a full recovery.

possible, they should not be used extensively because of the major risk of hemorrhage. Unless the patient represents a high surgical risk, the treatment of choice is operative.

ERCP may be helpful in identifying internal fistulae between the pancreatic duct and the peritoneal cavity, colon, and pleural cavity.[166-168] ERCP can be

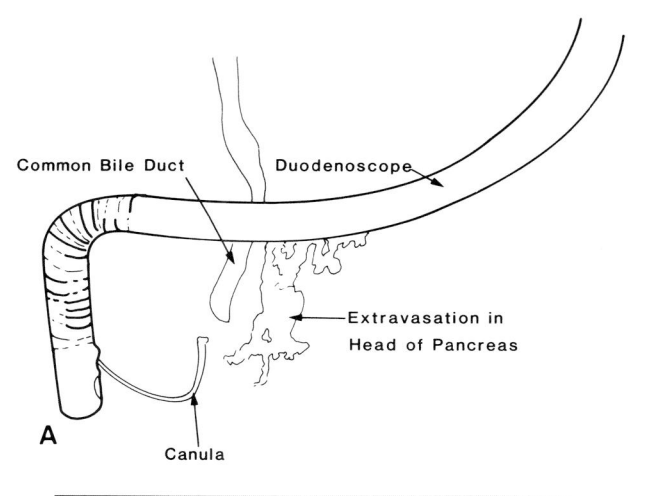

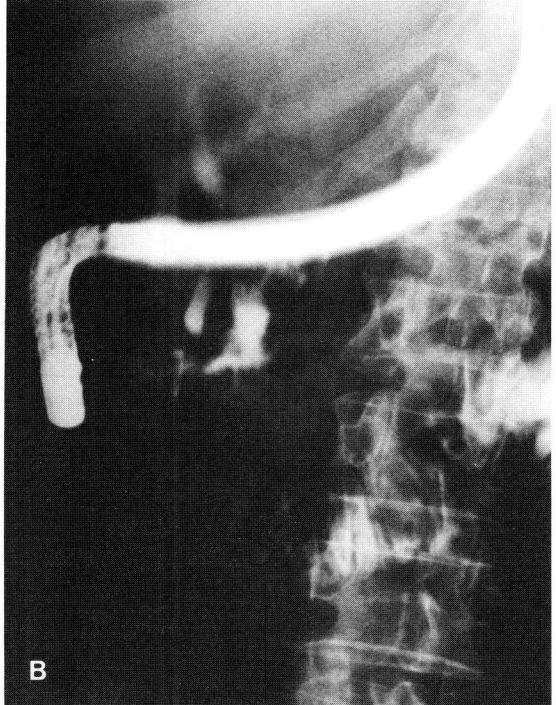

Figure 6-5 (A and B). This ERCP in a 78-year-old female shows complete disruption of the pancreatic duct in the head of the pancreas with necrosis of the parenchyma. Despite intensive care support she succumbed to the local and systemic effects of severe pancreatitis.

valuable in diagnosing and assessing the rare mediastinal pseudocyst.[169] Where there is direct communication between the pancreatic duct and the pseudocyst, conservative treatment may be successful, although the majority will require surgical drainage via the abdominal route.[170]

One of the obscure causes of upper gastrointestinal hemorrhage following acute pancreatitis is hemosuccus pancreaticus or pancreatorrhagia.[171-172] This usually occurs because of the rupture of an inflammatory pseudoaneurysm of the splenic artery (rarely the hepatic artery) into a pseudocyst or pancreatic duct.[173] Although bleeding from the ampulla of Vater may be seen by side-viewing duodenoscopy, this is often intermittent and the diagnosis may then only be made by ERCP when clots are observed along the pancreatic duct.[174]

Uncommonly, late jaundice may develop in patients with acute or chronic pancreatitis (usually alcoholic) resulting in a stricture of the lower CBD.[175] Rarely pancreatic duct strictures may follow an acute attack resulting in persistent or recurrent symptoms.[176] In both cases, ERCP is again indicated for diagnosis and allows surgery to be planned.

Prevention of Recurrent Attacks

Following the acute attack we would advocate cholecystectomy during the same admission or very soon afterward. If patients have had an ES we would also recommend cholecystectomy to avoid symptoms from the remaining gallbladder stones.[67] In high surgical risk cases, however, this need not necessarily be done; we have followed up over 50 patients with gallbladder in situ who have had ES for up to 10 years without a single instance of a recurrent attack.

Many patients following an attack of acute pancreatitis have no identifiable cause for their attack. Ultrasound should be repeated at least once[131] as there are often small gallstones which are difficult to detect.[177-179] In the absence of a diagnosis, patients should have an early ERCP[98]—the safety of this approach has been independently confirmed.[180] As well as detecting small stones which might be missed by US, other diagnoses which are readily treatable and can be diagnosed include ampullary tumors, carcinoma of the pancreas, lymphomas involving the pancreas, choledochal cysts, parasitic infestation, and pancreatic duct strictures.[24,98,180-183] Although there is a relatively high incidence of pancreas divisum among patients with idiopathic pancreatitis,[183] the management of this condition in the absence of obstruction or chronic pancreatitis[184] should be conservative. We have managed all our cases conservatively to date, and none has had a recurrent attack. Endoscopic sphincterotomy and insertion of a prosthesis of the accessory papilla has been used to treat patients with pancreatic duct obstruction associated with pancreas divisum, but the results are poor.[164] We repeat that *indiscriminate ES or surgical sphincteroplasty for pancreatitis in the absence of any objective evidence of obstruction is to be condemned.* Rarely there may be ampullary dysfunction due to papillary stenosis or ampullary dyskinesia; ERCP with manometry of the sphincter of Oddi is required to confirm the diagnosis.[185] Hydrostatic balloon dilation has been suggested as a form of treatment[186] but this has not been adequately evaluated and carries a high complication rate.

Gallstones may still be missed, however, even with numerous US and ERCP investigations.[98,186] This may be because the stones are very small; alternatively, the patients have passed *all* their stones, and with time the stones reform and can be detected. Bile crystal analysis may be another means by which patients with microlithiasis can be detected. Gallbladder bile may be readily obtained by endoscopic aspiration in the fasted patient using IV cholecystokinin. We recently had some success with this and we would recommend that this be included in the diagnostic workup of patients with "idiopathic" acute pancreatitis.[187]

Acute Cholangitis in Association with Acute Pancreatitis

There have been only sporadic reports of patients with coexisting acute cholangitis and acute pancreatitis from Western countries. Andrew and Johnson reported an incidence of acute pancreatitis of 24% in 17 patients with acute suppurative cholangitis, but the relevance of this was not discussed.[23] We found the incidence of acute pancreatitis to be 23% in 113 consecutive patients with acute cholangitis.[188] Conversely, we found the incidence of acute cholangitis to be 14.4% in 187 consecutive cases of gallstone pancreatitis.[188]

Ong et al reported 29 cases of acute pancreatitis in 237 patients (12.2%) with recurrent pyogenic cholangitis.[189] McFadzean and Yeung reported 36 cases of RPC out of 172 patients (20.9%) with acute pancreatitis of varying etiologies[190] compared with 8.5% in our own series.[188] Ong et al, in reviewing the Hong Kong experience of 163 patients with acute pancreatitis from biliary tract disease in 1979, reported gallstones alone in 36 (22.1%), gallstones and cholangitis in 50 (30.7%), and cholangitis without gallstones in 77 (47.2%).[147]

In our overall experience of 32 patients with both conditions, we found that the majority were elderly (median 76 years) and female (75%).[188] A higher proportion had predicted severe attacks (63%) than would normally be expected in patients with acute pancreatitis alone (30–40%).[122,123,144] The biochemical and clinical profile of patients with both conditions is similar to that of patients with acute cholangitis alone (Tables 6-14 and 6-15). Out of our 32 patients, 23 had ERCP ± ES with one death (4.3%) compared with three deaths in nine patients who were managed conservatively (33%).

Patients with both conditions had an overall complication rate of 38% and mortality rate of 12.5% compared with 23% and 4.4%, respectively, in those with acute pancreatitis alone (unpublished). Patients with coexisting conditions can

Table 6-14 Important Biochemical Features of Patients with Acute Cholangitis and Acute Pancreatitis Compared with Cholangitis Alone*

Feature	Acute cholangitis and acute pancreatitis ($N = 32$)	Acute cholangitis only ($N = 87$)
Serum amylase (IU/L)	2,940 (1,120–10,848)	160 (19–840)
White cell count ($\times 10^9$/L)**	15.9 (1.2–51.9)	12.7 (4.0–31.0)
Urea (mmol/L)	6.7 (2.6–28.7)	6.9 (1.9–56.5)
Blood glucose (mmol/L)	7.8 (2.1–36.1)	6.6 (1.4–19.8)
PaO$_2$ (KPa)	9.7 (4.0–14.1)	—
Calcium (mmol/L)	2.11 (1.31–2.46)	—
Lactate dehydrogenase (mmol/L)	445 (252–842)	—
Alkaline phosphatase (IU/L)	407 (97–2,365)	463 (29–2,178)
γ-glutamyl transpeptidase (IU/L)	465 (86–1,110)	357 (39–1,926)
Alanine transaminase (IU/L)	171 (36–614)	134 (12–895)
Bilirubin (μmol/L)	105 (8–240)	114 (20–379)
Total protein (g/L)	60.5 (50–76)	62.0 (47–83)
Albumin (g/L)	31.5 (22–44)	32.0 (22–47)

* Values are median (range).
** All differences are not statistically significant with the obvious exception of amylase and also the white cell count ($p < 0.05$).

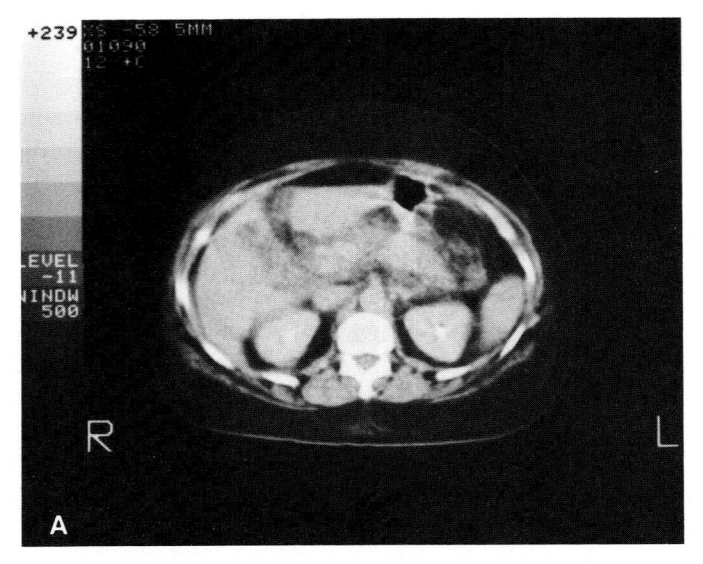

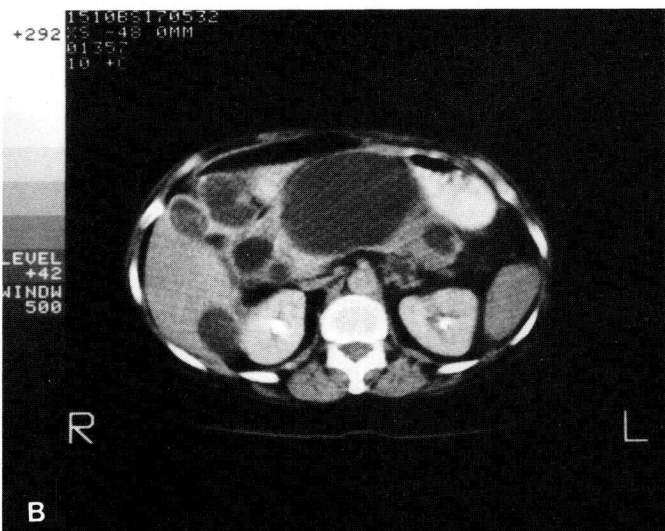

Figure 6-6 This series of CT films were taken from a 54-year-old patient who presented with severe acute pancreatitis. The admission CT scan (**A**) shows marked swelling of the pancreas with loss of pancreatic tissue planes. She soon progressed to acute cholangitis as well and developed abscesses in the pancreas, liver, and falciform ligament (**B**). A preoperative ERCP was performed which confirmed the presence of stones and pus in the common bile duct and an endoscopic sphincterotomy was performed. Laparotomy was then performed for external drainage of the abscesses, cholecystectomy, and sequestrectomy. The duodenum and extrahepatic bile ducts were engulfed by necrotic tissue, which would have made surgery on the bile ducts extremely hazardous. The patient made a full recovery (**C**).

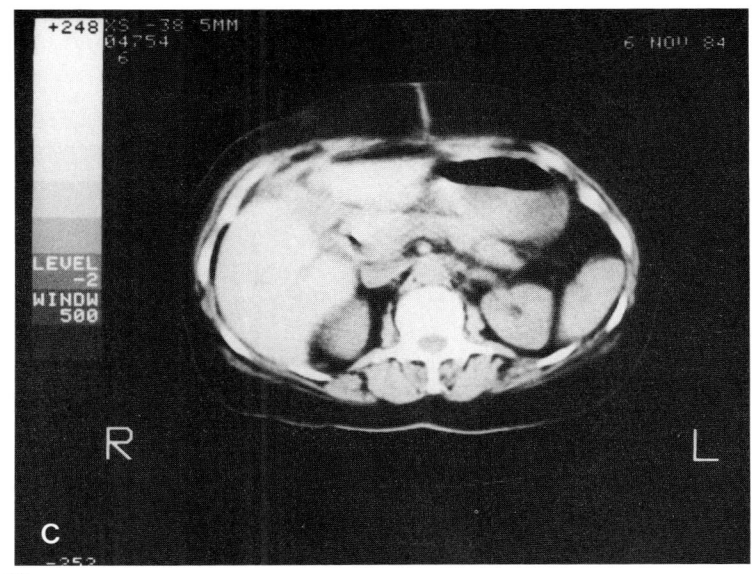

Figure 6-6C

develop the complications of each condition alone and need to be managed along appropriate lines. A combined medical, endoscopic, and surgical approach is mandatory (Figure 6-6). Usually patients present with conditions simultaneously but on occasions patients with either can develop the other after an intervening period of several days or even 1 or 2 weeks.

Ong et al reported an 8.3% mortality for those with gallstone pancreatitis compared with 10% for those with pancreatitis, gallstones, and cholangitis, and 13% for those with pancreatitis and cholangitis without gallstones.[147] These authors strongly recommended urgent biliary decompression by surgical means; the current approach must now be the use of ERCP ± ES.

As an aside, ERCP may also reveal parasitic infestation (common in Hong

Table 6-15 Clinical Features in Patients with Acute Cholangitis and Acute Pancreatitis Compared with Patients with Acute Cholangitis Only

	Acute cholangitis and acute pancreatitis ($N = 32$)	Acute cholangitis only ($N = 87$)
Median age (range) years	76 (52–87)	74 (25–88)
Females/males	24:8 (75%)	55:28 (63%)
Positive blood culture	9/14 (64%)	34/60 (57%)
Previous cholecystectomy	5 (15.6%)	7 (8.0%)
ERCP	24 (75%)	60 (69%)
Passed CBD stones*	8 (25%)	5 (5.7%)
ES performed	15 (47%)	40 (46%)
All deaths	4 (12.5%)	13 (14.9%)

* The difference is statistically significant ($p = 0.0028$).

Kong and some of the migrant Chinese community) as a cause for either acute cholangitis or acute pancreatitis.[190] Treatment may also be undertaken endoscopically either by ES or basket extraction following balloon dilation of the sphincter of Oddi.[191]

CONCLUSIONS

The role of ERCP and ES has moved from the elective field to the area of emergency diagnosis and treatment. The impressively good results are readily apparent to those who have witnessed them. More importantly, there has been a steady accumulation of objective data which show their worth in many, but by no means all, situations. The scientific approach (as opposed to simplistic data collection) must continue in this field in order to allow refinement of the indications as well as the techniques themselves.

In dealing with severely ill patients, including those requiring assisted ventilation, we have encountered surprisingly few difficulties in undertaking ERCP and ES. A support team of anesthetists and specialist nurses is, however, required to ensure the safe transfer of patients from the intensive therapy unit (ITU) or general wards to the X-ray screening room. It is essential for this support team to be present during the endoscopic procedures in order to maintain ventilation and continue monitoring. The presence of a screening room adjacent to the ITU may be helpful, but it is not essential and should not be viewed as a limiting factor to the wider use of these techniques in the emergency situation.

In this chapter we have sought to define the role of these techniques within the context of the overall management problems of acute cholangitis and pancreatitis. In this way we hope that readers will share our view that ERCP and ES are techniques which are not a substitute for either medical treatment or surgery. Rather, they should become incorporated into the routine management of all patients with acute pancreaticobiliary disorders. The days when endoscopists and surgeons acted independently of one another are gone.

References

1. McCune WS, Short PE, and Moscovitz H: Endoscopic cannulation of the ampulla of Vater: a preliminary report. *Ann Surg* 1968;167:752–756.
2. Oi I, Takemoto T, and Kondo T: Fibreduodenoscope. Direct observations of the papilla of Vater. *Endoscopy* 1969;1:101–103.
3. Cotton PB: Progress Report. ERCP. *Gut* 1977;18:316–341.
4. Kawai K, Akasaka Y, Murakami I, Tada M, Kohli Y, and Nakajima M: Endoscopic sphincterotomy of the ampulla of Vater. *Gastrointest Endosc* 1974;20:148–151.
5. Classen M, and Demling L: Endoskipische sphincterotomie der papilla Vateri und steinextraktion aus dem ductus choledochus. *Dtsch Med Wschr* 1974;99:469–476.
6. Safrany L: Endoscopic treatment of biliary tract diseases. *Lancet* 1978;2:983–985.
7. Cotton PB: Endoscopic management of bile duct stones; (apples and oranges). *Gut* 1984;25:587–597.
8. Huibregtse K, and Tytgat GNJ: Endoscopic placement of biliary prostheses. In: Salmon PR, ed. *Gastrointestinal Endoscopy: Advances in Diagnosis and Therapy*, Vol. 1 London; Chapman and Hall, 198:219–231.
9. Cotton PB: Endoscopic methods for relief of malignant obstructive jaundice. *World J Surgery* 1984;8:854–861.

10. Carr-Locke DL, and Cotton PB: Biliary tract and pancreas. *Br Med Bull* 1986;42:257–264.
11. Pitt HA: Is endoscopic sphincterotomy a safe and effective method for the management of stones in the distal common bile duct? In: Gitnick G, ed. London, Churchill-Livingstone, 1984, pp. 89–116.
12. Charcot JM: Lecons sur les maladies du foie, des voies biliares et des reins. Paris, Faculte de Medicine de Paris 1877:194–195.
13. Pitt HA, Postier RG, and Cameron JL: Consequences of preoperative cholangitis and its treatment on the outcome of operation for choledocholithiasis. *Surgery* 1983;94:447–452.
14. Boey JH, and Way LW: Acute cholangitis. *Ann Surg* 1980;191:264–270.
15. Reynolds BM, and Dargan EL: Acute obstructive cholangitis: A distinct clinical syndrome. *Ann Surg* 1959;150:299–303.
16. Pitt HA, and Longmire WP: Suppurative cholangitis. In: Hardy JD. ed. *Critical Surgical Illness.* 2nd ed. London, W.B. Saunders, 1980:380–408.
17. Connor MJ, Sumner HW, and Schwartz ML: The clinical and pathologic correlations in mechanical biliary obstruction and acute cholangitis. *Ann Surg* 1982;195:419–425.
18. Leese T, Neoptolemos JP, Baker AR, and Carr-Locke DL: The management of acute cholangitis and the impact of endoscopic sphincterotomy. *Br J Surg* 1986;73:988–992.
19. Saharia PC, and Cameron JL: Clinical management of acute cholangitis. *Surg Gynecol Obstet* 1976;142:369–372.
20. Welch JP, and Donaldson GA: The urgency of diagnosis and surgical treatment of acute suppurative cholangitis. *Am J Surg* 1976;131:527–532.
21. Hinchey EJ, and Couper CE: Acute obstructive suppurative cholangitis. *Am J Surg* 1969;117:62–67.
22. Saik RP, Greenburg AG, Farris JM, and Peskin GW: Spectrum of cholangitis. *Am J Surg* 1975;130:143–150.
23. Andrew DJ, and Johnson SE: Acute suppurative cholangitis, a medical and surgical emergency. *Am J Gastroenterol* 1970;54:141–54.
24. Neoptolemos JP, Talbot IC, Carr-Locke DL, Shaw DE, Cockleburgh R, Hall AW, and Fossard DP: Treatment and outcome in 52 consecutive cases of ampullary carcinoma. *Br J Surg* 1987;74:957–961.
25. Baker AR, Neoptolemos JP, Carr-Locke DL, and Fossard DP: Sump syndrome following choledocho-duodenostomy and its endoscopic treatment. *Br J Surg* 1985;72:533–535.
26. Edlung YA, Mollstedt BO, and Ouchterlony O: Bacteriological investigation of the biliary system and liver in biliary tract disease correlated to clinical data and microstructure of the gallbladder and liver. *Acta Chir Scand* 1959;116:461–476.
27. Keighley MRB, Flinn R, and Alexander Williams J: Multivariate analysis of clinical and operative findings associated with biliary sepsis. *Br J Surg* 1976;63:528–531.
28. Scott AJ, and Khan GA: Origin of bacteria in bile duct bile. *Lancet* 1967;2:790–792.
29. Flemma BJ, Flint LM, Osterhout S, and Shingleton WW: Bacteriological studies of biliary tract infection. *Ann Surg* 1967;166:562–572.
30. Schotton WE, Desprez JD, and Holden WA: A bacteriological study of portal vein blood in man. *Arch Surg* 1955;71:404–409.
31. Dineen P: The importance of the route of injection of experimental biliary tract obstruction. *Surg Gynecol Obstet* 1964;119:1001–1008.
32. Ong GB: A study of recurrent pyogenic cholangitis. *Arch Surg* 1962;84:199–225.
33. Kinoshita H, Hitohashi K, Igawa S, Nagata E, and Sakai K. Cholangitis. *World J Surg* 1984;8:963–969.
34. Huang T, Bass JAB, Williams RD, and Tex G: The significance of biliary pressure in cholangitis. *Arch Surg* 1969;98:629–632.

35. Einstein DM, Lapin SA, Ralls PW, and Halls JM: The insensitivity of sonography in the detection of choledocholithiasis. *Am J Roentgenol* 1984;143:725–728.
36. Neoptolemos JP, Macpherson DS, Holm J, and Fossard DP: Pyogenic liver abscess: a study of forty-four cases in two centres. *Acta Chir Scand* 1982;148:415–421.
37. Moore-Gillon JC, Eykyn S, and Phillips I: Microbiology of pyogenic liver abscess. *Br Med J* 1981;283:819–821.
38. Neoptolemos JP, and Macpherson DS: Pyogenic liver abscess. *Br J Hosp Med* 1981;26:47–51.
39. Furey AT: Ascending cholangitis. *NY J Med* 1966;66:1299–1303.
40. Rogers L: Biliary abscess of the liver with operation. *Br Med J* 1903;2:706–707.
41. Lygidakis NJ: Acute suppurative cholangitis: comparison of internal and external biliary drainage. *Am J Surg* 1982;143:304–306.
42. Baker AR, Neoptolemos JP, Leese T, and Fossard DP: Choledochoduodenostomy and transduodenal sphincteroplasty and sphincterotomy for calculi of the common bile duct. *Surg Gynecol Obstet* 1987;164:245–251.
43. Saik RP, Greenburg AG, and Peskin GW: Cholecystotomy hazard in acute cholangitis. *J Am Med Assoc* 1976;235:2421–2413.
44. Thompson JE, Tompkins RK, and Longmire WP: Factors in management of acute cholangitis. *Ann Surg* 1982;195:137–145.
45. Haupert AP, Carey LC, Evans WE, and Ellison EH: Acute suppurative cholangitis. *Arch Surg* 1967;94:460–468.
46. Lygidakis NJ, and Brummelkamp WH: The significance of intrabiliary pressure in acute cholangitis. *Surg Gynecol Obstet* 1985;161:465–469.
47. Bismuth H, Kuntziger H, and Corlette MB: Cholangitis with acute renal failure. Priorities in threapeutics. *Ann Surg* 1975;181:881–887.
48. Molnar W, and Stockum AE: Relief of obstructive jaundice through percutaneous transhepatic catheter: A new therapeutic method. *Am J Roentgenol* 1974;122:356–367.
49. Gould RJ, Vogelzang, Neimen HL, Pearl JG, and Politcha SM: Percutaneous biliary drainage as an initial therapy of the biliary tract. *Surg Gynecol Obstet* 1985;160:523–527.
50. Kadir S, Baassiri A, Barth KH, Kaufman SL, Cameron JL, and White RT: Percutaneous biliary drainage in the management of biliary sepsis. *Am J Roentgenol* 1982;138:25–29.
51. Pessa ME, Hawkins IF, and Vogel SB: The treatment of acute cholangitis. Percutaneous transhepatic biliary drainage before definitive therapy. *Ann Surg* 1987;205:389–392.
52. Dotter CT, Bilbao MK, and Katon RM: Percutaneous transhepatic gallstone removal by needle tract. *Radiology* 1979;133:242–243.
53. Perez MR, Oleaga JA, Freiman DB, McLean GL, and Ring EJ: Removal of a distal common bile duct stone through percutaneous transhepatic catheterisation. *Arch Surg* 1979;114:107–109.
54. Fernstrom I, Delin NA, and Sundblad R: Percutaneous transhepatic extraction of common bile duct stones. *Surg Gynecol Obstet* 1981;153:405–407.
55. Clovise ME, and Falchuk KR: Percutaneous transhepatic removal of common duct stones: A report of ten patients. *Gastroenterology* 1983;85:815–819.
56. Centola CAP, Jander HP, Stauffer A, and Russinovich MAE: Balloon dilatation of the papilla of Vater to allow biliary stone passage. *Am J Roentgenol* 1981;136:613–614.
57. Mack E, Crummy AB, and Babayan VK: Percutaneous transhepatic dissolution of common bile duct stones. *Surgery* 1981;90:584–587.
58. Allen MJ, Borody TJ, Bugliosi TF, May GR, Larusso NF, and Thistle JL: Rapid dissolution of gallstones by methyl tert-butyl ether. *N Engl J Med* 1985;312:217–220.
59. Murray WR, Laferla G, and Fullarton GM: Choledocholithiasis: In vivo stone dissolution using methyl tertiary butyl ether (MTBE). *Gut* 1988;29:143–145.

60. Vallon AG, Shorvon PJ, and Cotton PB: Duodenoscopic treatment of acute cholangitis (Abstract). *Gut* 1982;23:A915.
61. Delmotte JS, Pommelet P, Houcke P, Desurmont P, Lisambert B, Lortot A, and Paris JC: Initial duodenoscopic sphincterotomy in patients with acute cholangitis or pancreatitis complicating biliary stones. (Abstract). *Gastroenterology* 1982;82:1042.
62. Pitt HA, Cameron JL, Postier RG, and Gadacz TR: Factors affecting mortality in biliary tract surgery. *Am J Surg* 1981;141:66–71.
63. Dixon JM, Armstrong CP, Duffy SW, and Davies CG: Factors affecting morbidity and mortality after surgery for obstructive jaundice: A review of 373 patients. *Gut* 1983;24:845–852.
64. Blamey SL, Fearon KCH, Gilmour WH, Osborne DH, and Carter DC: Prediction of risk in biliary surgery. *Br J Surg* 1983;70:535–538.
65. Seymour DG, and Vaz FG: Aspects of surgery in the elderly: Pre-operative medical assessment. *Br J Hosp Med* 1987;37:102–112.
66. Neoptolemos JP, Shaw DE, Davidson BR, and Carr-Locke DL: Multivariate analysis of risk factors in patients undergoing treatment for common bile duct stones: Implications for treatment. *Ann Surg* 1989;209:157–161.
67. Davidson BR, Neoptolemos JP, and Carr-Locke DL: Endoscopic sphincterotomy for common bile duct calculi in patients with gallbladder in situ considered unfit for surgery. *Gut* 1988;29:114–120.
68. Gregg JA, De Girolami P, and Carr-Locke DL: Effects of sphinteroplasty and endoscopic sphincterotomy on the bacteriologic characteristics of the common bile duct. *Am J Surg* 1985;149:668–671.
69. Neoptolemos JP, Carr-Locke DL, and Fossard DP: Prospective randomised study of preoperative endoscopic sphincterotomy versus surgery alone for common bile duct stones. *Br Med J* 1987;294:470–474.
70. Palmer KR, and Hofmann AF: Introductal mono-octanoin for the direct dissolution of bile duct stones: Experience in 343 patients. *Gut* 1986;27:196–202.
71. Dias LM, Cairns SR, Salmon PR, and Cotton PB: Endoscopic prosthesis for common bile duct stones (abstract). *Gut* 1987;28:A1371.
72. Radder RW: Ultrasonically guided percutaneous catheter drainage for gallbladder empyema. *Diag Imag* 1980;49:330–333.
73. Van Sonnenberg E, Wittich GR, Casola G, *et al:* Diagnostic and therapeutic percutaneous gallbladder procedures. *Radiology* 1986;160:23–26.
74. Van Sonnenberg E, Hofmann AF, Neoptolemos JF, Wittich GR, Princenthal RR, and Wilson SN: Gallstone dissolution with methyl-tert-butyl ether via percutaneous cholecystostomy: Success and caveats. *Am J. Roentgenol* 1986;146:865–867.
75. Neoptolemos JP, Hofmann AF, and Moossa AR: Chemical treatment of stones in the biliary tree. *Br J Surg* 1986;73:515–524.
76. Cotton PB, and Vallon AG: Duodenoscopic sphincterotomy for removal of bile duct stones in patients with gallbladders. *Surgery* 1982;91:628–630.
77. Escourrou J, Cordova JA, Lazorthes F, Flexinos J, and Ribet A: Early and late complications after endoscopic sphincterotomy for biliary lithiasis with and without the gallbladder in situ. *Gut* 1984;25:598–602.
78. Martin DF, and Tweedle DEF: Endoscopic management of common duct stones without cholecystectomy. *Br J Surg* 1987;74:209–211.
79. Digby KH: Common duct stones of liver origin. *Br J Surg* 1930;17:578–591.
80. Cook J, Hou PC, and McFadzean AJS: Recurrent pyogenic cholangitis. *Br J Surg* 1954;42:188–203.
81. Nakayama F: Intraheptic stones: epidemiology and etiology. In: Okuda K, Nakayama F, Wong J. eds. *Intrahepatic Calculi*. New York, Alan R. Liss, 1984, pp. 17–28.
82. Ho CS, and Wesson DE: Recurrent pyogenic cholangitis in Chinese immigrants. *Am J Roentgenol Radium Ther Med* 1974;122:368–374.
83. Mage S, and Morel AS: Surgical experience with cholangiohepatitis (Hong Kong disease) in Canton Chinese. *Ann Surg* 1965;162:187–190.

84. Wong J, and Choi TK: Recurrent pyogenic cholangitis. In: Okuda K, Nakayama F, Wong J. eds. *Intrahepatic Calculi*. New York, Alan R. Liss, 1984, pp. 175–182.
85. Lam SK, Wong KP, Chan PKW, Ngan H, and Ong GB: Recurrent pyogenic cholangitis: A study by endoscopic retrograde cholangiography. *Gastroenterology* 1978;74:1196–1203.
86. Wong WT, Teoh-Chan CH, Huang CT, Cheng FCY, and Ong GB: The bacteriology of recurrent pyogenic cholangitis and associated diseases. *J Hyg Camb* 1981;87:407–411.
87. Choi TK, Wong J, Lam KH, Lim K, and Ong GB: Late result of sphincteroplasty in the treatment of primary cholangitis. *Arch Surg* 1981;116:1173–1175.
88. Choi TK, Wong J, and Ong GB: Choledochojejunostomy in the treatment of primary cholangitis. *Surg Gynecol Obstet* 1982;115:43–45.
89. Choi TK, Wong J, and Ong GB: The surgical management of primary intrahepatic stones. *Br J Surg* 1982;69:86–90.
90. Lam SK: A study of endoscopic sphincterotomy in recurrent pyogenic cholangitis. *Br J Surg* 1984;71:262–266.
91. Yamakawa T: Percutaneous transhepatic stone extraction technique for management of retained biliary tract stones. In: Okuda K, Nakayama F, Wong J. Eds. *Intrahepatic Calculi*. New York, Alan R. Liss, 1984, pp. 253–268.
92. Kerlan RK, Pogany AC, Goldberg HI, and Ring EJ: Radiologic intervention in oriental cholangiohepatitis. *Am J Roentgenol* 1985;145:809–813.
93. Van Sonnenberg E, Casola G, Glibberley DA, Halasz NA, Cabrera OA, Wittich GR, Mattrey RF, and Scheible FW: Oriental cholangiohepatitis: diagnostic imaging and interventional management. *Am J Roentgenol* 1986;146:327–331.
94. Sarner M, and Cotton PB: Classification of pancreatitis. *Gut* 1984;25:756–759.
95. Sarles H: Revised classification of pancreatitis: Marseille 1984. *Dig Dis Sci* 1985;30:573–574.
96. Dunne MJ, Shenikin A, and Imrie CW: Misleading hyponatraemia in acute pancreatitis with hyperlipidaemia. *Lancet* 1979;1:211–213.
97. London ND, Neoptolemos JP, Bailey I, and James R: Serial CT scanning in acute pancreatitis (abstract). *Gut* 1987;23:A369.
98. Goodman AJ, Neoptolemos JP, Carr-Locke DL, Finlay DBL, and Fossard DP: Detection of gallstones after acute pancreatitis. *Gut* 1985;26:125–132.
99. Corfield AP, Cooper MJ, Williamson RCN, Mayer AD, McMahon MJ, Dickson AP, Shearer MG, and Imrie CW: Prediction of severity in acute pancreatitis: A prospective comparison of three prognostic indices. *Lancet* 1985;2:403–407.
100. Ranson JHC: Etiologic and prognostic factors in human acute pancreatitis: A review. *Am J Gastroenterol* 1982;77:633–638.
101. Opie EL: The etiology of acute hemorrhagic pancreatitis. *Johns Hopkins Hosp Bull* 1901;121:182–188.
102. Cuschieri A, and Hughes JH: Pancreatic reflux during operative choledochography. *Br J Surg* 1973;60:933–936.
103. Kelly TR: Gallstone pancreatitis: Pathophysiology. *Surgery* 1976;80:488–492.
104. Armstrong CP, Taylor TV, Jeacock J, and Lucas S: The biliary tract in patients with acute gallstone pancreatitis. *Br J Surg* 1985;72:551–555.
105. Acosta JM, and Ledesma CL: Gallstone migration as a cause of acute pancreatitis. *N Engl J Med* 1974;290:484–487.
106. Kelly TR, and Swaney PE: Gallstone pancreatitis: The second time around. *Surgery* 1982;92:571–575.
107. McMahon MJ, and Shefta JR: Physical characteristics of gallstones and the calibre of the cystic duct in patients with acute pancreatitis. *Br J Surg* 1980;67:6–9.
108. Kelly TR: Gallstone pancreatitis. The timing of surgery. *Surgery* 1980;88:345–349.
109. Acosta JM, Pelligrini CA, and Skinner DB: Etiology and pathogenesis of acute biliary pancreatitis. *Surgery* 1980;88:118–25.

110. Stone HH, Fabian TC, and Dunlop WE: Gallstone pancreatitis: Biliary tract pathology in relation to time of operation. *Ann Surg* 1981;194:305–310.
111. Dixon JA, and Hillam JD: Surgery treatment of biliary tract disease associated with acute pancreatitis. *Am J Surg* 1970;120:371–375.
112. Paloyan D, Simonowitz D, and Skinner DB: The timing of biliary tract operations in patients with pancreatitis associated with gallstones. *Surg Gynecol Obstet* 1975;141:737–739.
113. Ranson JHC: The timing of biliary surgery in acute pancreatitis. *Ann Surg* 1979;189:654–662.
114. Cuschieri A, Cumming JGR, Wood RAB, and Baker PR: Evidence for sphincter dysfunction in patients with gallstone associated pancreatitis: Effect of ceruletide in patients undergoing cholecystectomy for gallbladder disease and gallstone associated pancreatitis. *Br J Surg* 1983;71:885–888.
115. MRC Multicentre Trial. Death from acute pancreatitis. *Lancet* 1977;2:632–635.
116. Imrie CW, Benjamin IS, Ferguson JC, et al: A single centre double blind trial of Trasylol therapy in primary acute pancreatitis. *Br J Surg* 1978;65:337–641.
117. Mayer AD, McMahon MJ, Benson EA, and Axon ATR: Operations upon the biliary tract in patients with acute pancreatitis: Aims, indications and timing. *Ann Royal Coll Surg Engl* 1984;66:179–183.
118. DeBolla AR, and Obeid ML: Mortality in acute pancreatitis. *Ann Royal Coll Surg Eng* 1984;66:184–186.
119. Corfield AP, Cooper MJ, and Williamson RCN: Acute pancreatitis: A lethal disease of increasing incidence. *Gut* 1985;26:724–729.
120. Osborne DH, Imrie CW, and Carter DC: Biliary surgery in the same admission for gallstone-associated acute pancreatitis. *Br J Surg* 1981;68:758–761.
121. Williamson RCN: Early assessment of severity in acute pancreatitis. *Gut* 1984;25:1331–1339.
122. Blamey SL, Imrie CW, O'Neill J, Gilmour WH, and Carter DC: Prognostic factors in acute pancreatitis. *Gut* 1984;25:1340–1346.
123. Leese T, and Shaw D: Comparison of three Glasgow multifactor prognostic scoring systems in acute pancreatitis. *Br J Surg* 1988;75:460–462.
124. McMahon MJ, Pickford A, and Playforth MJ: Early prediction of severity in acute pancreatitis using peritoneal lavage. *Acta Chir Scand* 1980;146:171–176.
125. Anderson JR, Spence RAJ, Laird JD, Ferguson WR, and Kennedy TL: Initial experience with iridium-111 autologous leucocyte imaging in patients with acute pancreatitis. *Br Med J* 1983;287:637–638.
126. Nordestgaard AG, Wilson SE, and Williams RA: Early computerised tomography as a predictor of outcome in acute pancreatitis. *Am J Surg* 1986;152:127–132.
127. Beger HG, Bittner R, Block S, and Buchler M: Bacterial contamination of pancreatic necrosis. A prospective clinical study. *Gastroenterology* 1986;91:433–438.
128. Cuschieri A, Wood RAB, Cumming JRG, Meehan SE, and Mackie CR: Treatment of acute pancreatitis with fresh frozen plasma. *Br J Surg* 1983;70:710–712.
129. Leese T, Holliday M, Heath D, London N, Hall AW, and Bell PRF. A multicentre prospective trial of low volume fresh frozen plasma therapy in acute pancreatitis. *Br J Surg* 1987;74:907–911.
130. Mayer AD, McMahon MJ, Corfield AP, Cooper MJ, Williamson RCN, Dickson AP, Shearer MG, and Imrie CW. Controlled clinical trial of peritoneal lavage for the treatment of severe acute pancreatitis. *N Engl J Med* 1985;312:399–404.
131. Neoptolemos JP, Hall AW, Finlay DF, Berry JM, Carr-Locke DL, and Fossard DP. The urgent diagnosis of gallstones in acute pancreatitis: A prospective study of three methods. *Br J Surg* 1984;71:230–233.
132. Tondelli P, Stutz K, Harder F, Schuppisser JP, and Allgower M. Acute gallstone pancreatitis: Best timing for biliary surgery. *Br J Surg* 1982;69:709–710.
133. Acosta JM, Rossi R, Galli OMR, Pellegrini LA, and Skinner DB. Early surgery for acute

gallstone pancreatitis: Evaluation of a systematic approach. *Surgery* 1978;83:367–370.
134. Neoptolemos JP, Fossard DP, Berry JM. A prospective study of radionuclide biliary scanning in acute pancreatitis. *Ann Roy Coll Surg Engl* 1983;65:180–182.
135. Coppa GF, LeFleur R, Ranson JHC. The role of Chiba needle cholangiography in the diagnosis of possible acute pancreatitis with cholelithiasis. *Ann Surg* 1981;193:393–398.
136. Roesch W, and Demling L. Endoscopic management of pancreatitis. *Surg Clin N A* 1982;62:845–852.
137. Classen M, Ossenberg W, Wurbs D, Dammermann R, and Hagenmuller F. Pancreatitis: An indication for endoscopic papillotomy? (abstract). *Endoscopy* 1978;10:223.
138. Van Spuy DS: Endoscopic sphincterotomy in the management of gallstone pancreatitis. *Endoscopy* 1981;13:25–26.
139. Safrany L: Controversies in acute pancreatitis. In: Hollender LF. Ed. *Controversies in Acute Pancreatitis.* New York, Springer-Verlag, 1982, pp. 214–218.
140. Schott B, Neuhaus B, Portacarrero G, Krause S, and Saffrany L: Endoskopische papillotomie bei akuter bilaren pankreatitis. *Klinikarzt* 1982;11:52–54.
141. Kautz G, Kohaus H, Keferstein R-D, and Bunte H: Zur pathogenese und endoskopischen therapie der akuten bilaren pankreatitis. *Klinikarzt* 1982;11:1202–1212.
142. Riemann von JF, and Lux G: Therapeutische strategie bei der akuten pankreatitis (I). *Fortschr Med* 1984;102:179–182.
143. Rosseland AR, and Solhaug JH: Early or delayed endoscopic papillotomy (EPT) in gallstone pancreatitis. *Ann Surg* 1984;199:165–167.
144. Neoptolemos JP, London N, Slater ND, Carr-Locke DL, Fossard DP, and Moossa AR: A prospective study of ERCP and endoscopic sphincterotomy in the diagnosis and treatment of gallstone acute pancreatitis. *Arch Surg* 1986;121:697–702.
145. Neoptolemos JP, Carr-Locke DL, London NJ, et al: Controlled trial of urgent endoscopic retrograde cholangiopancreatography and endoscopic sphincterotomy versus conservative treatment for acute pancreatitis due to gallstones. *Lancet* 1988;2:979–983.
146. Neoptolemos JP: The urgent diagnosis and treatment of biliary (gallstone associated) acute pancreatitis. Hunterian Lecture presented at the Royal College of Surgeons of England, London, 1988.
147. Ong GB, Lakn KH, Lam SK, Lim TK, and Wong J: Acute pancreatitis in Hong Kong. *Br J Surg* 1979;66:398–403.
148. Neoptolemos JP, London N, Bailey I, Shaw D, Carr-Locke DL, Fossard DP, Moossa AR. The role of clinical and biochemical criteria and endoscopic retrograde cholangiopancreatography in the urgent diagnosis of common bile duct stones in acute pancreatitis. *Surgery* 1987;100:732–742.
149. Watts GT: Total pancreatectomy for fulminant pancreatitis. *Lancet* 1963;2:384–385.
150. Hollender LF, Meyer C, Kauffman JP, Keller P, Sequin J, and Pagliano G: Traitment chirgical des pancreatites aigues-hemorragiques. Etude analytique et deductions prospectives de 58 observations. *J Chir (Paris)* 1983;120:595–601.
151. Smadja C, and Bismuth H: Pancreatic debridement in acute necrotising pancreatitis: an obsolete procedure? *Br J Surg* 1986;73:408–410.
152. Nordback IH, and Auvinen DA: Long-term results after pancreas resection for acute necrotizing pancreatitis. *Br J Surg* 1985;72:687–689.
153. Kivilaakso E, Lempinen M, Makelainen A, Nikki P, and Schroder T: Pancreatic resection versus peritoneal lavage for acute fulminent pancreatitis. *Ann Surg* 1984;199(4):426–431.
154. Aldridge MC, Ornstein M, Glazer G, and Dudley HAF: Pancreatic resection for severe acute pancreatitis. *Br J Surg* 1985;72:796–800.
155. Block S, Maier W, Bittner R, Buchler M, Malfertheiner P, and Begber HG: Identification of pancreas necrosis in severe acute pancreatitis: Imaging procedure versus clinical staging. *Gut* 1986;27:1035–1042.

156. Bradley EL, and Fulenwider JT: Open treatment of pancreatic abscess. *Surg Gynecol Obstet* 1984;159(6):509–513.
157. Gebhardt CL, Riemann JF, and Lux G: The importance of ERCP for the surgical tactic in haemorrhagic necrotizing pancreatitis (preliminary report). *Endoscopy* 1983;15:55–58.
158. Gebhardt C: Indications for surgical intervention in necrotizing pancreatitis with extrapancreatic necrosis. In: Beger HG, Buchler M, eds. *Acute Pancreatitis.* Berlin, Springer-Verlag, 1987, pp. 310–313.
159. Bradley EL III: Pancreatic pseudocysts. In: Bradley EL III. Ed. *Complications of Pancreatitis: Medical and Surgical Management.* London, W.B. Saunders, 1982, pp. 125–153.
160. Sugawa C, and Walt A: Endoscopic retrograde pancreatography in the surgery of pancreatic pseudocysts. *Surgery* 1979;86:639–647.
161. Laxson LC, Fromkes JJ, and Cooperman M: Endoscopic retrograde cholangiopancreatography in the management of pancreatic pseudocysts. *Am J Surg* 1985;150:683–686.
162. O'Connor M, Kolars J, Ansel H, Silvis S, and Vennes J: Pre-operative endoscopic retrograde cholangiopancreatography in the surgical management of pancreatic pseudocysts. *Am J Surg* 1986;151:18–23.
163. Mitchell KG, Cotton PB, and Russell RCG: Pre-operative ERCP in patients with pancreatic pseudocysts (abstract). *Gut* 1985;26:A651.
164. Rogers BHG, Circurel NJ, and Seed RW. Transgastric needle aspiration of a pancreatic pseudocyst through an endoscope. *Gastroint Endosc* 1975;21:133.
165. Kozarek RA, Brayko CM, Harlan J, Sanowski RA, Cintora I, and Kovac A: Endoscopic drainage of pancreatic pseudocysts. *Gastroint Endosc* 1985;31:322–328.
166. Alsumant AR, Jabbar M, and Goresky CA: Pancreatico-colonic fistula: A complication of pancreatitis. *Can Med Assoc J* 1978;119:715–719.
167. Russell JC, Welch JP, and Clark DG: Colonic complications of acute pancreatitis and pancreatic abscess. *Am J Surg* 1983;146:558–564.
168. McLatchie GR, Meek D, and Imrie CW: The use of ERCP in the diagnosis of internal fistulae complicating severe acute pancreatitis. *Br J Radiol* 1985;58:395–397.
169. Leechawengwong M, Berger HW, and Romeu J: Spontaneous resolution of mediastinal pancreatic pseudocyst. *Chest* 1979;75:632–633.
170. Banks PA, McLellan PA, Gerzof SG, Splaine EF, Lintz RM, and Brown ND: Mediastinal pancreatic pseudocyst. *Dig Dis Sci* 1984;29:664–668.
171. Lower WE, and Farrell JI: Aneurysm of the splenic artery: Report of a case and review of the literature. *Arch Surg* 1931;23:182–190.
172. Sandblom P: Gastrointestinal hemorrhage through the pancreatic duct. *Ann Surg* 1970;171:61–66.
173. Cahow CE, Gusberg RJ, and Gottlieb LJ: Gastrointestinal hemorrhage from pseudoaneurysms in pancreatic pseudocysts. *Am J Surg* 1983;145:534–551.
174. Clay RP, Farnell MB, Lancaster JR, Weiland LH, and Gostout CJ: Hemosuccus pancreaticus. An unusual cause of upper gastrointestinal bleeding. *Ann Surg* 1985;202:75–79.
175. Warshaw AL, Schapiro RH, Ferrucci JT, and Galdabini JJ: Persistent obstructive jaundice, cholangitis, and biliary cirrhosis due to common bile duct stenosis in chronic pancreatitis. *Gastroenterology* 1976;70:562–567.
176. Laugier R, Camatte R, and Sarles H: Chronic obstructive pancreatitis after healing of a necrotic pseudocyst. *Am J Surg* 1983;146:551–557.
177. Freund H, Pfeffermann R, Durst AL, and Rabinovici N: Gallstone pancreatitis. Exploration of the biliary system in acute and recurrent pancreatitis. *Arch Surg* 1976;111:1106–1107.
178. Houssin D, Castaing D, Lemoine J, and Bismuth H: Microlithiasis of the gallbladder. *Surg Gynecol Obstet* 1983;157:20–24.

179. Farinon AM, Sianesi M, and Zanella A: Physiopathologic role of microlithiasis in gallstone pancreatitis. *Surg Gynecol Obstet* 1987;164:252–256.
180. Lee MJR, Lai ECS, and Wong J: Endoscopic retrograde cholangiopancreatography after acute pancreatitis. *Surg Gynecol Obstet* 1986;163:354–358.
181. Beshlian K, and Ryan JAB: Pancreatitis in teenagers. *Am J Surg* 1986;152:133–139.
182. Cooperman M, Ferrara JJ, Fromkes JJ, and Carey LC: Surgical management of pancreas divisum. *Am J Surg* 1982;143:107–111.
183. Cotton PB: Congenital anomaly of pancreas divisum as a cause of obstructive pain and pancreatitis. *Gut* 1980;21:105–114.
184. Russell RCG, Wong NW, and Cotton PB: Accessory sphincterotomy (endoscopic and surgical) in patients with pancreas divisum. *Br J Surg* 1984;71:954–957.
185. Toouli J, Roberts-Thomson IC, Dent J, and Lee J: Sphincter of Oddi motility disorders in patients with idiopathic recurrent pancreatitis. *Br J Surg* 1985;72:859–863.
186. Guelrud M, and Siegel JH: Hypertensive pancreatic duct sphincter as a cause of pancreatitis. Successful treatment with hydrostatic balloon dilatation. *Dig Dis Sci* 1984;29:225–231.
187. Neoptolemos JP, Davidson BR, Vallance D, Winder AF: The role of duodenal bile crystal analysis in the investigation of "idiopathic" pancreatitis. *Br J Surg* 1988;75:450–453.
188. Neoptolemos JP, Carr-Locke DL, Leese T, and James D: Acute cholangitis in association with acute pancreatitis: Incidence, clinical features, outcome and the role of ERCP and endoscopic sphincterotomy. *Br J Surg* 1987;74:1103–1106.
189. Ong GB, Adiseshiah M, and Leong CH: Acute pancreatitis associated with recurrent pyogenic cholangitis. *Br J Surg* 1971;58:891–894.
190. McFadzean AJS, and Yeung RTT. Acute pancreatitis due to clonorchis sinensis. *Trans R Soc Trop Med Hyg* 1966;60:466–470.
191. Leung JWX, Chung SCS, and King WWK: Round worm pancreatitis: endoscopic worm removal without papillotomy. *Br J Surg* 1986;73:925.

Chapter **7**

Endoscopic Sphincterotomy in Patients with Intact Gallbladders

Ira M. Jacobson, M.D.

Even in the absence of controlled trials comparing surgery to endoscopic sphincterotomy for the treatment of common bile duct stones, the widespread favorable experience with sphincterotomy has led to its present position as the treatment of choice in most centers for patients with choledocholithiasis who have had a cholecystectomy. Increasingly, however, endoscopic sphincterotomy is also being performed in patients with symptomatic duct stones who still have their gallbladders. Many such patients, particularly those considered poor operative candidates, have been followed after sphincterotomy in the hope that their gallbladders, which often still contain stones, will not cause illness.

There are now sufficient numbers of published reports to permit a quantitative analysis of the benefits and risks of this approach, which appears unlikely to abate in popularity. Indeed, if nonoperative treatments of cholelithiasis currently in evolution, such as shock wave lithotripsy, become well established, it is conceivable that increasing numbers of young, fit patients otherwise suitable for surgery may prefer endoscopic treatment of their symptomatic common duct stones followed by nonsurgical treatment of their gallbladder stones. Given the proven track record and safety of cholecystectomy,[1] such alternative approaches should be required to meet stringent tests of efficacy and safety.

Physiologic Considerations

Physiologic alterations in the biliary tract after sphincterotomy may potentially affect the risk of developing clinically overt gallbladder disease. The duration of any influence exerted on the gallbladder by the presence of a sphincterotomy will depend at least in part on how long the sphincterotomy remains patent. The observations of experienced endoscopists suggest that, in most patients, the sphincterotomy remains patent for years.[2-6]

Geenen *et al*[2] performed serial measurements of the size of their sphincterotomies and found a mean decrease from 11.6 mm immediately after the procedure to 6.5 mm 2 years later. Although manometric recordings showed a return of phasic contraction of the sphincter of Oddi, the pressure gradient normally present between the bile duct and duodenum remained absent, as did basal sphincter of Oddi pressure.

In one of the longest follow-ups of patients who underwent sphincterotomy postcholecystectomy, Hawes et al[3] studied 148 patients, most of whom had undergone sphincterotomy over 5 years previously. Fifteen had recurrent biliary symptoms, most of them within 1–2 years after the procedure. Ten of these had followup ERCP, as did 35 asymptomatic patients. Of these 45, 5 had sphincter stenosis with or without stones and 1 had stones without stenosis. Only 1 asymptomatic patient had an abnormal ERCP. It would appear from these and similar data from other centers[4–6] that only a small number of patients, ie, 10% or less, develop recurrent stones and/or stenosis for years after sphincterotomy. Given the infrequency of stenosis, any influence of a patent sphincterotomy on the risk of gallstone formation or cholecystitis can be expected to be longstanding.

Bacterial colonization of the bile, usually with enteric organisms, was common after sphincterotomy in two studies,[7,8] one of which[7] showed the bile to be sterile before sphincterotomy in all of a series of 45 patients with presumed papillary stenosis. Although these studies evaluated bile obtained by endoscopic aspiration from the bile duct, it is inevitable that bacterial colonization of gallbladder bile also occurs after sphincterotomy, as was demonstrated in a canine model in which gallbladder and hepatic bile flora were similar after surgical sphincteroplasty.[9]

Despite the prevalence of bactobilia, acute cholangitis did not occur in the two human studies cited above,[7,8] presumably because of free drainage of bile. Whether the risk of cholecystitis after sphincterotomy is increased by the consequent bactobilia is difficult to determine, particularly in light of the fact that most patients with duct stones, the commonest indication for sphincterotomy, already have contaminated bile.[10] So long as the cystic duct is patent, it seems doubtful that the bactobilia after sphincterotomy would predispose to cholecystitis any more than it does to cholangitis. Conceivably, however, the bactobilia could lead to a diminished capacity to tolerate transient periods of subsequent cystic duct obstruction, or chronic partial obstruction, before cholecystitis develops.

The composition of bile after sphincterotomy has been studied.[11,12] In patients with intact gallbladders there is a marked reduction in the bile acid pool size, in contrast to the absence of such a change in patients who have had a cholecystectomy. However, the cholesterol saturation of bile does not appear to increase in patients who have had sphincterotomies with intact gallbladders.[11]

Observations on the rate of gallstone formation after sphincterotomy have not been reported extensively. Following sphincterotomy, Tanaka et al[13] observed formation of new gallbladder stones in only 2 of 91 patients initially lacking gallbladder stones during a mean 3-year followup period. In both patients the stones were pigmented calcium stones. Their Oriental population had a preponderance of primary common duct stones (which are usually pigment stones), and is therefore not strictly analogous to Western populations in which cholesterol stones are prevalent. There is evidence to suggest that sphincterotomy may actually prevent gallstone formation and enhance the clearance of preexisting stones from the gallbladder. Hutton et al[14,15] showed that sphincterotomy prevented gallstone formation in prairie dogs fed a lithogenic diet. Sphincterotomy was associated with a more rapid turnover of gallbladder bile as measured with radiolabeled cholic acid, and gallbladder volume was reduced after sphincterotomy. In subsequent studies, these investigators demonstrated enhanced spontaneous passage of glass beads from the gallbladder of dogs subjected to sphincterotomy. This was associated with an increased ejection fraction after sphincterotomy, as measured by cholescintigraphy.[16] The authors concluded that sphincterotomy enhances gallbladder emptying, in large part due to the reduction in common bile duct pressure that follows sphincterotomy.[16] This would result in enhanced emptying of crystals or tiny stones before larger gallstones have a chance to form.

Studies on the fate of gallbladder stones after sphincterotomy are scarce. Cotton and Vallon[17] found that gallbladder stones had disappeared by the time of surgery in 2 of 11 patients undergoing cholecystectomy during the same admission after sphincterotomy, and that 1 stone remained in the gallbladder of a patient 4 months after sphincterotomy when multiple stones had been present initially. Moss et al[18] observed the passage of gallstones in 2 of 19 patients following sphincterotomy, and Rooseland and Solhaug[5] observed the same phenomenon in 9 patients. Studies comparing the fate of gallbladder stones of patients postsphincterotomy with a group of controls would be of interest.

In summary, there is no compelling reason to assume that sphincterotomy will increase the risk of cholecystitis. Increased lithogenicity of bile has not been reported after the procedure. Bacterial contamination of bile will not necessarily predispose to cholecystitis any more than it will to cholangitis. However, it can be argued that a few patients with severe gallbladder disease or an occluded cystic duct may have an increased risk of cholecystitis as a result of the bactobilia that follows ERCP and sphincterotomy. On the other hand, the apparently enhanced ability of the gallbladder to empty particulate matter may actually decrease the risk of future gallbladder-related illness.

Sphincterotomy with Intact Gallbladder: Experience to Date

As early as 1980, nearly half of patients in whom endoscopic sphincterotomy was being performed at some centers had intact gallbladders (Table 7-1).[17] In more recent years a number of follow-up studies have been interpreted as vindication of this approach in selected patients. Important issues still to be resolved are the degree to which this can reasonably be extended to all uncholecystectomized patients with symptomatic bile duct stones, and the determination of risk factors predictive of future gallbladder disease that might facilitate the selection of patients for whom sphincterotomy alone is appropriate.

The existence of a small subset of patients at risk for acute gallbladder disease shortly after sphincterotomy has been suggested by several authors. When this occurs, it is probably due at least in part to the presence of an already diseased gallbladder that cannot freely drain bacteria that reflux up the biliary tree after sphincterotomy or are injected in contaminated contrast material during the ERCP. A contributing role for the latter mechanism was suggested by the patients of Allen et al[19] with post-ERCP biliary infections associated with *Pseudomonas* introduced from the endoscope. One of these patients developed gangrenous cholecystitis, with bile cultures positive for *P. aeruginosa*, 1 day after sphincterotomy.

Of 70 patients with intact gallbladders undergoing sphincterotomy at the

Table 7-1 Long-Term Follow-up of Patients with Intact Gallbladders After Endoscopic Sphincterotomy (ES)

Authors	No. patients followed	Follow-up period	Gallbladder Complications	Comments
Escourrou[22]	130	6–66 mo (mean 22 months)	8 (6.2%)–cholecystitis 1 (0.8%)–gallbladder cancer	All cholecystitis occurred 1–9 mo after ES; 7/8 had cholecystectomy
Moss[36]	23	4–32 mo (mean 15 mo)	2 (8.7%)–cholecystitis 1 (4.4%)–pain	Both patients with cholecystitis had cholecystectomy
Cotton[25]	118	2–9 years (median 40 mo)	6 (5.1%)–elective cholecystectomy same admission as ES 6 (5.1%)–biliary pain	35% dead from nonbiliary causes; all 6 with late biliary pain had cholecystectomy
Martin[23]	70	To 44 mo	5 (7.1%)–elective cholecystectomy same admission as ES 4 (5.7%)–cholecystectomy for "persistent or recurrent symptoms" within 6 mo of ES	61 followed for 12–44 mo (mean 24 mo) without biliary symptoms; 18 died of nonbiliary causes
Tanaka[13]	122	6 mo–10 yr	5 (4.1%)–cholecystitis	Most patients had primary duct stones (presumably pigment, not cholesterol) and lacked GB stones; late cholecystitis correlated strongly with presence of GB stones or nonvisualization of GB
Siegel[21]	1272	0–11 years	109 (8.6%)–cholecystitis	All cholecystitis within 10 days of ES; many presented initially with cholangitis; incidence of late morbidity unclear

Jacobsen[26]	44	2–105 mo (median 35 mo)	0	Three developed late cholangitis
Miller[27]	34	Mean 28 mo	7 (20.6%)—cholecystitis or chronic symptoms	
Rosseland[5]	66	0–8 yr	11 (16.7%)—cholecystitis 3 (4.5%)—biliary pain	8/11 with cholecystitis had cholecystectomy, 3/3 with biliary pain; one additional patient had acute cholecystitis on day 1 after ES, with cholecystectomy 4½ mo later

Davidson[20]	105 total
	85 discharged
		1–8 yr (mean 29.6 mo)	5 (4.8%)—empyema of gallbladder
			8 (9.4%)—"gallbladder symptoms"
			  6—cholecystectomy
			  2—cholangitis
			  2—biliary colic
			  1—cholecystitis
			  1—prior cholecystostomy for empyema
				4/5 with empyema initially had cholangitis

Worthley[30]	20	0–42 mo (median 8 mo)	2 (10.0%)—early cholecystectomy for persistent or recurrent symptoms 3 (15.0%)—acute cholecystitis 1 (5.0%)—ruptured gallbladder 1 (5.0%)—cholecystocholedochal fistula with cholecystitis	All late complications occurred in patients with nonvisualized gallbladders at initial ERCP

Middlesex Hospital through 1980, 2 required emergent surgery for cholecystitis that developed within a week after the endoscopic procedure.[17] Rosseland and Solhaug[5] reported 1 of 75 patients who developed acute cholecystitis 1 day after sphincterotomy. Davidson et al[20] reported that 5 of 106 patients who underwent sphincterotomy developed empyema of the gallbladder within 30 days. Four of the 5 had presented with cholangitis initially. Most striking, perhaps, was a preliminary report of Siegel et al[21] indicating the occurrence of acute cholecystitis in 10 of 1,272 (8.6%) patients within 10 days after sphincterotomy. Many of their patients had cholangitis at presentation. One difficulty in analyzing such data is that some patients may already have had cholecystitis on admission which was masked by concomitant cholangitis or pancreatitis.

In some series, early cholecystitis was not reported in any patient after sphincterotomy.[18,22,23] Cotton[24] feels that postsphincterotomy cholecystitis and gallbladder empyema are very rare when antibiotics are given prophylactically. In the absence of formal trials to address this issue, it seems prudent to administer antibiotics before and for at least 24–48 hours after sphincterotomy to patients with intact gallbladders even if cholangitis was absent at presentation.

Of greater concern than the risk of immediate or early cholecystitis has been the incidence of gallbladder-related illness in the months and years after sphincterotomy. Although there is some variation in the frequency of biliary colic versus cholecystitis among different studies, ample available data indicate that gallbladder disease sufficient to warrant cholecystectomy occurs in a minority of patients, e.g., 5–20%, during the 5–10 years after sphincterotomy.

In the initial report from Cotton's group,[17] of 48 patients discharged without having cholecystectomy, 44 were followed and only 5 required subsequent operation, all for biliary symptoms, 3–12 months later. Longer term observations of a larger group of patients were even more favorable.[25] Of 112 patients undergoing successful sphincterotomy and discharged with the gallbladder in situ, no patient died of biliary disease during a 2- to 9-year (median 40 months) follow-up period, and only 6 underwent elective cholecystecomy for recurrent pain, while 29 patients died of nonbiliary causes. All the remaining patients were asymptomatic with regard to biliary disease. The experience of Martin and Tweedle was similar.[23] Of 65 patients discharged from the hospital, 4 required cholecystectomy for "persistent or recurrent symptoms" within 6 months. The remaining 61 were followed for 12–44 months (median 22 months). None of these had biliary symptoms during the follow-up period, although 18 died of nonbiliary causes.

Davidson et al[20] followed 85 patients for 1–8 years after sphincterotomy (mean 29.6 months). Six patients (7.1%) eventually had cholecystectomy, 2 during surgery for cholangitis related to retained bile duct stones, 2 for biliary colic, 1 for a prior gallbladder empyema, and 1 for cholecystitis. Two others had gallbladder symptoms but did not undergo cholecystectomy.

The long term incidence of cholecystitis, as opposed to biliary colic, has been somewhat higher in other studies. Eight of 130 patients (6.2%) followed by Escourrou et al[22] for a mean of 22 months developed cholecystitis, all in 1–9 months following endoscopic sphincterotomy. Seven of the eight underwent cholecystectomy. Gallbladder cancer developed in one other patient after 4 years. Five patients had cholangitis or symptoms related to retained or recurrent bile duct stones, and 2 had stenosis of the sphincterotomy. It is impossible to determine how often the recurrent common duct stones originated in the gallbladder in these patients. However, in this study and others,[26] the incidence of late complications involving the bile duct has not appeared higher in patients with intact gallbladders than in those who were postcholecystectomy.

A larger, but still relatively small, proportion of patients with late cholecystitis was reported in the longer term study of Rosseland and Solhaug.[5] Of 66 patients discharged from the hospital with intact gallbladders, 8 (12.1%) required cholecystectomy for cholecystitis during the next 7 years, and three others had cholecystitis which was treated conservatively. Cholecystitis occurred throughout the follow-up period. Three additional patients underwent cholecystectomy for recurrent pain attacks. One patient had carcinoma of the gallbladder after 1-½ years. Thirty patients died from nonbiliary causes during the follow-up period.

Miller et al[27] followed 34 patients for a mean of 28 months. Seven of them (21%) underwent subsequent cholecystectomy for either acute cholecystitis or chronic biliary symptoms. This is a higher incidence, at least within the time frame studied, of cholecystectomy after sphincterotomy than has been reported in most studies.

In many of these series a small number of patients had "elective" cholecystectomy after sphincterotomy during the same admission. These may have been patients with substantial preexisting gallbladder symptoms. Their exclusion from long-term analyses may introduce a slight downward bias in the estimates of how many patients will have gallbladder symptoms or cholecystitis after sphincterotomy. Moreover, a few patients in these series underwent cholecystectomy during the initial admission because surgery was required after sphincterotomy failed to clear the bile duct, as occurred, for example, in 4 of the 75 patients of Rosseland and Solhaug,[5] and 6 of the 105 patients of Davidson et al.[20] Like the possibility of complications or of long-term gallbladder disease, the possibility of failure must be considered when discussing treatment alternatives with patients whose gallbladders are intact. Indeed, the presence of a gallbladder is a relative argument against protracted endoscopic efforts to clear the bile duct when this proves technically difficult or appears to require maneuvers that entail added risk, such as precutting.

Risk Factors for Future Gallbladder-Related Illness

It has been suggested that obstruction of the cystic duct may predispose to a high risk of symptomatic gallbladder disease after sphincterotomy.[13,24,28,29] Tanaka et al,[13] for example, found that 2 of 6 patients with nonvisualization later developed cholecystitis, compared with 3 of 25 with visualizing gallbladder-containing gallstones and 0 of 91 with gallbladders containing no stones. In contrast, two groups were unable to demonstrate any association between filling of the gallbladder at ERCP and the risk of future gallbladder events.[20,23]

The use of nonvisualization of the gallbladder as a predictive factor is confounded by the absence of a uniform technique of filling the biliary tree at ERCP. Worthley and Toouli[30] addressed this by injecting sufficient contrast to opacify the extraheptic ducts densely and to till the tertiary intrahepatic radicles. Their findings provided strong evidence that nonvisualization predicted future cholecystitis. Of 20 patients who underwent sphincterotomy, 2 required cholecystectomy during the same admission for "continuing symptoms." Both of these patients had a patent cystic duct. Of the 18 patients discharged, 8 had nonvisualized gallbladders on ERCP. Six of these (75%) later required cholecystectomy: 3 had acute cholecystitis, 1 had a ruptured gallbladder, 1 had a cholecystocholedochal fistula with acute cholecystitis, and 1 had cholecystectomy during surgery for ampullary stenosis with cholangitis. Three patients died as a result of their gallbladder disease.

In marked contrast to the group with nonvisualized gallbladders, none of the 10 patients with visualized gallbladders had subsequent biliary problems. These authors therefore recommended cholecystectomy in patients with nonvisualized gallbladders at ERCP. The limitations of this study include the relatively small numbers of patients and the potential danger of overinjecting the biliary tree in patients presenting with cholangitis in the course of trying to fill the gallbladder. High filling pressures in this situation might precipitate bacteremia. Despite these considerations, it seems plausible on theoretical grounds, and likely from the available evidence, that patency of the cystic duct influences the chance of future cholecystitis. If adequate filling pressures are thought to have been applied during ERCP, visualization of the gallbladder might be used as one factor—if the decision is in question—in deciding whether a patient should have cholecystectomy after sphincterotomy.

A second potential predictive factor for future gallbladder-related illness is the presence, absence, or number of gallstones. As with gallbladder visualization, Davidson et al[20] found no correlation between the presence, absence, or number of stones and the risk of future problems. In contrast, in the Oriental patients of Tanaka et al,[13] the data cited above suggested a major relationship between residual gallstones and future cholecystitis. Again, because the patients usually had primary duct stones, a much higher proportion of them lacked gallbladder stones than is found in Western populations. Nevertheless, even in the latter group a significant minority of patients do not have detectable cholelithiasis,[20] and further data would be of interest.

Comparison with Risk of Gallbladder-Related Illness in the General Population

The risk of symptomatic gallbladder disease in patients who have had a sphincterotomy compares favorably with the risk in patients with gallbladder stones in the general population, although longer follow-up data are available for the latter group. In a compilation of cohort studies of patients with initially asymptomatic gallstones followed for up to 30 years, Gracie and Ransohoff[31] found that 16–36% developed overt biliary disease. The initial manifestation is almost always pain rather than a complication such as cholecystitis, cholangitis, or pancreatitis, although these can follow.[31,32] In some of the above-cited studies of patients who have had sphincterotomy, the distribution of manifestations was more even or weighted in several instances toward cholecystitis as opposed to biliary pain. On the other hand, cohorts of patients with painful gallstone disease have a risk of complications of about 30% during the 15–20 years of observation.[31]

Is There a Role for Sphincterotomy Prior to Cholecystectomy?

In light of the experience thus far, many old or systemically ill patients with symptomatic duct stones will continue to be treated with sphincterotomy alone. Others who are acutely ill with cholangitis or pancreatitis are also being treated endoscopically, with deferral of cholecystectomy till later (see Chapter 6). This leaves a large number of patients with symptomatic duct stones and intact gallbladders who are suitable candidates for surgery and in whom cholecystectomy is planned. It has been suggested that these patients first be treated by ERCP and sphincterotomy so that the surgeon need only perform cholecystectomy.[33] The rationale is to avoid the increment in operative morbidity and mortality attendant on common duct exploration, and save hospitalization time and cost. The obvious objection to the first argument is the morbidity and mortality associated with sphincterotomy itself.

Systematic evaluation of preoperative sphincterotomy has been limited. A prospective study of 64 patients aged 75 and over who underwent surgery for gallstone disease was conducted by Duron et al.[34] There were 33 patients with clinical, radiographic, or biochemical evidence of choledocholithiasis. Most of these patients underwent endoscopic sphincterotomy followed by cholecystectomy. There were no complications of sphincterotomy and the overall mortality was 6%. In the 31 patients who went directly to surgery, choledocholithiasis was discovered in 2, neither of whom died. The mortality rate in this group of 31 patients was 16%, not significantly different from the first group.

Nearly half the patients in each group had acute cholecystitis at surgery, which was undoubtedly a major factor in their initial presentation and is atypical for most patients who present with symptomatic duct stones. Compared with their historical controls, the mortality associated with the authors' approach of preoperative sphincterotomy in patients with suspected bile duct stones was substantially reduced. The authors therefore recommended preoperative ERCP "at the slightest suspicion of complicated biliary lithiasis in aged high-risk patients." However, due to the design of the study (patients with suspected bile duct stones were not prospectively randomized to preoperative sphincterotomy versus surgery alone), the superiority of preoperative sphincterotomy—when surgery is definitely planned—was not established conclusively.

There has been one prospective, randomized trial of sphincterotomy followed by cholecystectomy versus surgery alone.[35] In this study, in which 120 patients were randomized, the overall major complication rate for the sphincterotomy plus cholecystectomy group was 16.4% compared to 8.5% in the group treated only by surgery. The minor complication rates were 16.4% and 13.6%, respectively. Although these differences were not statistically significant, the study ended after the trend against preoperative sphincterotomy emerged. The only advantage of preoperative sphincterotomy was that hospitalization time was reduced. The authors pointed out that the exclusion of some of the highest risk patients, who were treated by sphincterotomy alone, may have affected the results. We still need to know whether there are predictive factors that can help to select patients for whom preoperative sphincterotomy is appropriate.

Although routine preoperative sphincterotomy in all patients appears to be unjustified, patients are encountered who undergo ERCP because the diagnosis is unclear. If the patient is a suitable candidate for cholecystectomy and ERCP reveals common duct stones not known to be present previously, should sphincterotomy be done or should the procedure be terminated? The course of action must be determined on the basis of a detailed discussion with the patient before the ERCP. Some patients will have a strong preference to defer cholecystectomy temporarily, while others who are motivated to have their gallbladders removed so that their biliary disease may be addressed definitively may actually prefer to have the surgeon do everything. For the remainder, it seems best to individualize these decisions and for the endoscopist to be able to exercise judgment during the procedure. If the bile duct can be cannulated easily with a standard sphincterotome, if there is nothing unusual about the papilla or intramural bile duct, and if the stones are small to medium in size, it seems reasonable to proceed with a sphincterotomy.

Nonsurgical Treatment of Gallbladder Stones after Sphincterotomy

With the availability of oral dissolution therapy, methyl tert-butyl ether, and extracorporeal shock wave lithotripsy, it is inevitable that nonsurgical therapy will be considered for many patients with intact gallbladders after sphincterotomy. Because of the reduced volume and accelerated emptying of the gallbladder after sphincterotomy, as well as the reduction in bile acid pool (discussed earlier), it is not obvious that bile acid dissolution therapy would be effective in these patients even if the stones were cholesterol-rich and of appropriate size for such treatment. However, Meier et al[37] showed that chenodeoxycholic acid and ursodeoxycholic acid did, in fact, significantly decrease the cholesterol saturation index of gallbladder bile in sphincterotomized patients. In 8 of their 9 patients, the gallbladder was either poorly visualized or nonvisualized on oral cholecystography, but the gallbladder failed to be visualized by cholescintigraphy in only 1 patient. This suggested that the poor cholecystographic visualization was due to decreased time for concentration of gallbladder bile rather than cystic duct obstruction. The rationale for dissolution therapy provided by this study must be tested in clinical trials. The rationale for studying shock wave lithotripsy in these patients is equally compelling, especially given the evidence that sphincterotomy may enhance the rate of clearance of small fragments from the gallbladder[16] and reduces the rate of stone formation in the gallbladder in experimental models.[15]

Conclusions

Accumulated experience supports the current practice of performing endoscopic sphincterotomy for symptomatic bile duct stones in elderly or high-risk patients, leaving the gallbladder in place if there is no acute gallbladder disease. In contrast, young patients with gallbladders should in general undergo surgery without preoperative sphincterotomy if the diagnosis is secure. Patients with intermediate risk factors for surgery can be offered alternative approaches but recommendations must be individualized. Surgery remains appropriate for many of these patients. The role of nonsurgical treatment for gallstones after sphincterotomy requires further evaluation.

References

1. McSherry CK, and Glenn F: The incidence and causes of death following surgery for nonmalignant biliary tract disease. *Ann Surg* 1980;191:271–275.

2. Geenen JE, Toouli J, Hogan WJ, et al: Endoscopic sphincterotomy: Followup evaluation of effects on the sphincter of Oddi. *Gastroenterology* 1987;87:754–758.
3. Hawes R, Vallon AG, Holton JM, and Cotton PB: Long term follow-up after duodenoscopic sphincterotomy (DS) for choledocholithiasis in patients with prior cholecystectomy. *Gastroint Endosc* 1987;33:157 (abstract).
4. Riemann JF, Lux G, Forster P, and Altendorf A: Long-term results after endoscopic papillotomy. *Endoscopy* 1983;15:165–168.
5. Rosseland AR, and Solhaug JH: Primary endoscopic papillotomy (EPT) in patients with stones in the common bile duct and the gallbladder in situ: A 5–8 year follow-up study. *World J Surg* 1988;12:111–116.
6. Kawai K, and Nakajima M: Present status and complications of EST in Japan. *Endoscopy* 1983;15:169–172.
7. Gregg JA, Girolami PD, and Carr-Locke DL: Effects of sphincteroplasty and endoscopic sphincterotomy on the bacteriologic characteristics of the common bile duct. *Am J Surg* 1985;149:668–671.
8. Classen M: Endoscopic papillotomy. In: Sivak, M.V., Jr., ed: *Gastroenterologic Endoscopy*, Philadelphia, W. B. Saunders, 1987, p. 645.
9. Cohn MS, Schwartz SI, Faloon WW, and Adams JT: Effect of sphincteroplasty on gallbladder function and bile composition. *Ann Surg* 1979;189:317–321.
10. Lygidakis N: Incidence of bile infection in patients with choledocholithiasis. *Am J Gastroenterol* 1982;77:12.
11. Saeurbruch T, Stellaard F, and Paungartner G: Effect of endoscopic sphincterotomy on bile acid pool size and bile lipid composition in man. *Digestion* 1983;27:87–92.
12. Stellaard F, Sauerbruch T, Brunholzl C, et al: Bile acid pattern and cholesterol saturation of bile after cholecystectomy and endoscopic sphincterotomy. *Digestion* 1983;26:153–158.
13. Tanaka M, Ikeda S, Yoshimoto H, and Matsumoto S: The long-term fate of the gallbladder after endoscopic sphincterotomy: complete follow-up study of 122 patients. *Am J Surg* 1987;154:505–509.
14. Hutton SW, Sievert CE, Jr, Vennes JA, and Duane WC: Inhibition of gallstone formation by sphincterotomy in the prairie dog: reversal by atropine. *Gastroenterology* 1982;82:1308–1313.
15. Hutton SW, Sievert CE, Jr, Vennes JA, and Duane WC: The effect of sphincterotomy on gallstone formation in the prairie dog. *Gastroenterology* 1981;81:663–667.
16. Hutton SW, Sievert CE, Jr, Vennes JA, Shafer RB, and Duane WC: Spontaneous passage of glass beads from the canine gallbladder: Facilitation by sphincterotomy. *Gastroenterology* 1988;94:1031–1035.
17. Cotton PB, and Vallon AG: Duodenoscopic sphincterotomy for removal of bile duct stones in patients with gallbladders. *Surgery* 1982;91:628–630.
18. Moss JG, Saunders JH, and Wild SR: Endoscopic papillotomy for removal of common bile duct stones without cholecystectomy. *J Royal Coll Surg Edinburgh* 1985;30:112–114.
19. Allen JI, O'Connor-Allen M, Olson M, et al: Pseudomonas infection of the biliary system resulting from use of a contaminated endoscope. *Gastroenterology* 1987;92:759–763.
20. Davison BR, Neoptolemos JP, and Carr-Locke DL: Endoscopic sphincterotomy for common bile duct calculi in patients with gallbladder in situ considered unfit for surgery. *Gut* 1988;29:114–120.
21. Siegel JH, Safrany L, Pullano W, and Cooperman A: The significance of duodenoscopic sphincterotomy in patients with gallbladder in situ: 11 year followup of 1272 patients. *Gastroint Endosc* 1987;33:159 (abstract).
22. Escourrou J, Cordova JA, Lazorthes F, et al: Early and late complications after endoscopic sphincterotomy for biliary lithiasis, with and without the gallbladder "in situ." *Gut* 1984;25:598–602.

23. Martin DF, and Tweedle DEF: Endoscopic management of common duct stones without cholecystectomy. *Br J Surg* 1987;74:209–211.
24. Cotton PB: Endoscopic management of bile duct stones (apples and oranges). *Gut* 1984;25:587–597.
25. Cotton PB: 2–9 year follow up after sphincterotomy for stones in patients with gallbladders. *Gastroint Endosc* 1986;32:157 (abstract).
26. Jacobsen O, and Matzen P: Long-term follow-up study of patients after endoscopic sphincterotomy for choledocholithiasis. *Scand J Gastroenterol* 1987;22:903–906.
27. Miller BM, Kozarek RA, and Ryan JA, Jr: Surgical versus endoscopic management of common bile duct stones. *Ann Surg* 1988;207:135–141.
28. Solhaug JH, Fokstuen O, Rosseland A, and Rydberg B: Endoscopic papillotomy in patients with gallbladder-in-situ. *Acta Chir Scand* 1984;150:475–478.
29. Buhler H, Deyhle P, Munch R, et al: Endoscopic papillotomy with preserved gallbladder. *Schweiz Med Wochenschr* 1983;113:1228–1231.
30. Worthley CS, and Toouli J: Gallbladder non-filling: An indication for cholecystectomy after endoscopic sphincterotomy. *Br J Surg* 1988;75:796–798.
31. Gracie WA, and Ransohoff DF: Natural history and expectant managment of gallstone diseases. In: Cohen S, Soloway RD, eds.: Gallstones. New York, Churchill-Livingstone, 1985, pp. 27–43.
32. Gracie WA, and Ransohoff DF: The natural history of silent gallstones: the innocent gallstone is not a myth. *N Engl J Med* 1982;397:798–800.
33. Siegel JH, Ramsey WH, and Pullano W: Cost effectiveness of 2 interventional endoscopic biliary procedures: Does anyone really care? *Gastroint Endosc* 1986;32:181 (abstract).
34. Duron JJ, Roux JM, Imbaud P, Dumont JL, Dutet D, and Validire J: Biliary lithiasis in the over seventy-five age group: A new therapeutic strategy. *Br J Surg* 1987;74:848–849.
35. Neoptolemos JP, Carr-Locke DL, and Fossard DP: Preoperative endoscopic sphincterotomy as an adjunct to cholecystectomy for common bile duct stones. *Br Med J* 1987;294:470–474.
36. Moss JG, Saunders JH, and Wild SR: Endoscopic papillotomy for removal of common bile duct stones without cholecystectomy. *J Royal Col Surg Edin* 1985;30:112–114.
37. Meier PB, Ansel HJ, Shafer RB, and Duane WC: Efficacy of chenodeoxycholic acid and ursodeoxycholic acid for lowering cholesterol saturation index of gallbladder in patients with a sphincterotomy. *Gastroenterology* 1988;95:1595–1600.

Chapter **8**

Function and Dysfunction of the Sphincter of Oddi

James A. Gregg, M.D.

Historical Perspectives

One hundred years ago, Oddi described the sphincter mechanism at the lower end of the common bile duct (CBD) which bears his name. Meltzer in 1917[1] and Berg in 1922[2] felt that biliary stasis might be the result of a functional disorder of the biliary sphincter. Berg demonstrated hypertrophy of the sphincter muscle in a patient who had biliary obstruction without any other documented abnormality in the biliary tree. In 1926 Del Valle and Donovan[3] presented the first classical description of true organic stenosis secondary to fibrosis of the biliary sphincter as a cause of recurrent biliary pain and recognized the need for identification of coexistent sphincter stenosis at the time of cholecystectomy. In 1936 McGowan et al[4] described postcholecystectomy biliary colic secondary to morphine and demonstrated by T-tube manometry that it was due to induced choledochal hypertension. Within the same decade, biliary sphincter dyskinesia in response to fat was described,[5] and Best and Hicken[6] showed cholangiographic evidence of sphincter of Oddi (SO) dysfunction. In 1941 Boyden[7] demonstrated pancreatic sphincter obstruction in a patient with SO hypertrophy and common duct stones.

In 1947, the first major review article on motor function and dysfunction of the biliary tract was written by Ivy,[8] presenting beyond a doubt the evidence for structural abnormalities of the sphincter of Oddi due to fibrosis and also the presence of functional disorders in which there appeared to be no cicatricial disease involving the sphincter. The existence of functional disorders of the gallbladder was also documented. The difficulties in determining whether or not a patient had true SO stenosis or sphincter dyskinesia became apparent, in some instances, both clinically and at surgery. Various histological studies of sphincters in cadavers and surgically resected specimens of sphincters gave different results, undoubtedly related in many instances to whether the patient had structural stenosis or a nonstructural dyskinesia. Because of the clinical difficulties in determining which of the two types of sphincter problems may cause biliary pain, the two terms are combined later in this chapter under the coinclusive term *biliary sphincter dysfunction*.

Surgical treatment by sphincterotomy for SO dysfunction was slow in evolution and by 1950 the two largest series in the United States[9,10] reported only eight patients, each with good relief of preoperative symptoms. Subsequently, much larger series appeared.[11–13] The majority of the 100 cases studied by Cattell et al[11] were postcholecystectomy and many had common duct stones. Diagnosis of stenosis was made at surgery by inability to pass a no. 3 Bakes dilator through the sphincter with ease, obvious induration of the sphincteric segment, and/or duct dilation. Sphincterotomy was done in 72 cases while 26 patients were treated by dilation of the sphincter with graded dilators. The majority of patients were symptom free in follow-up.

During these years, the diagnosis of sphincter dysfunction was established principally at surgery by sphincter calibration, peroperative manometry with passage pressures and flow rates, intraoperative cholangiography, or combinations of these methods. Preoperatively, intravenous cholangiography as described by Wise and O'Brien,[14] and to a lesser extent serial cholecystography as developed by Rose,[15] were helpful in detecting SO dysfunction. Finally, the sphincter challenge studies devised by Nardi and Acosta[16] provided a new preoperative approach to demonstrate pancreatic sphincter and probably common channel sphincter dysfunction.

The new era in the detection of sphincter dysfunction began with the advent of the duodenoscope, which permitted for the first time direct access to the biliary and pancreatic sphincters and their ductal systems. The subsequent development of endoscopic manometry, hepatobiliary scintigraphy, and ultrasound, with and without challenge tests, within the space of 10 years catapulted the nonsurgeon into a realm otherwise undreamed of, and for the first time gastroenterologists had the opportunity of firsthand experience with function and dysfunction of the biliary and pancreatic sphincters, problems with which knowledgeable surgeons had long been familiar.

Sphincter Motility in Man

The majority of the early manometric studies of the sphincter of Oddi[17–26] were done with a high-fidelity recording, low-compliance, pump perfusion system with either a single or multilumen side-hole cannula in the mildly sedated patient. Despite variations in technique and the use of meperidine and/or atropine by some, all studies demonstrated a gradient of pressure between bile duct, pancreatic duct, and duodenum. On station pull-through into the sphincter segment, a zone of tonic high pressure, called basal sphincter pressure (BSP), with superimposed phasic wave activity (PWA) was recorded. Some of the studies used more compliant systems, which have little effect on basal sphincter pressures and none on phasic wave frequency but do yield lower peak wave pressures.

The author performs manometric studies in the left lateral or semiprone position. We use a single side-hole cannula and measure duodenal pressures prior to and at the end of the study. Duct and sphincter pressures are referenced to duodenal pressure as 0. Others use a multilumen catheter to measure pressures in different segments of the sphincter simultaneously, believing that a high proportion of retrograde contractions is one determinant of SO dysfunction.[27]

To perform manometry the cannula is advanced through the sphincter into a duct. With gentle aspiration, the appearance of yellow bile locates the cannula in the CBD while the appearance of clear fluid signifies its location in the pancreatic duct. Carr-Locke and Gregg (personal observation) confirmed the validity of this method in conjunction with fluoroscopy in almost 200 cases. Others prefer to determine the precise location of the manometry catheter by flouroscopy with injection of contrast material in all patients. Pressures are measured within the duct, and the cannula is withdrawn slowly until maximal phasic wave activity is encountered in the sphincteric segment and the pressure characteristics of the sphincter recorded. Since one or both sphincters may be dysfunctional, it is important to measure pressures in both sphincters when possible. It is important that the cannula move freely within the sphincter segment and that sharp angulation be avoided to prevent spuriously high-pressure recordings. It is also important not to use meperidine, atropine, or medications other than diazepam since they can affect sphincter pressures and phasic wave frequency. Rarely minute amounts of glucagon (0.1 mg) may be used to facilitate cannulation but after this one must wait at least 15 minutes for its effects to subside.

Recordings from the biliary tract can be safely done for 5–10 minutes in the noncholecystectomized patient, provided that the bile is not infected due to an obstructing lesion in the biliary tract. Recording times in the pancreatic duct must be shorter. When possible, at least 2-min recordings from each sphincter should be obtained (after allowing the initial perfusate to drain from the duct) and the pressures averaged. It is imperative to know the anatomy of the pancreatic ductal system prior to manometry to prevent overfilling of a pancreatic duct, which can easily happen if the patient has pancreas divisum. When done in conjunction with ERCP, one must wait for emptying of contrast material prior to manometry. Any contrast material in the manometry cannula can produce artificially high duct or sphincter pressures. Pressures measured with contrast material in the duct will also give higher readings than if no contrast is present. The author prefers to do manometry as a separate study in the endoscopy unit, particularly if one is studying the effects of hormones and drugs on sphincter function since such studies require repeated manometric recordings. This increases the duration and risks of the procedure if done in conjunction with ERCP.

Duct pressures remain relatively stable during short recording periods but, if measured over long periods in the pancreatic duct, may show a gradual rise in pressure. Small fluctuations in duct pressure may occur during respiration in the common duct and may rise significantly with deep inhalation. Coughing or straining will produce marked rises in CBD pressures which may reach over 100 mm Hg. These rapid fluctuations in duct pressures are easily recognized. Respiration has little effect on pancreatic duct pressures.

In addition to perfused cannula systems for endoscopic manometry, endoscopic manometry has also been done using microtransducers.[28–29] A major problem with this method is that the endoscopist may not be able to determine in which duct or sphincter presure is being measured. However, transducer studies may give more reliable recordings than perfused cannula systems. Since the duct is not perfused, much longer recording periods can be used since there is never any possibility of "overfilling" a duct.

In addition to technical variations in the performance of manometry, another problem has been the selection of patients to serve as controls. Few studies have used normal volunteers as controls.[25,30–31] Such studies carry some ethical risk since pancreatitis may follow any endoscopic procedure involving the sphincters and ducts. Pressure studies in such subjects should be done either on the biliary sphincter alone or in those in whom pancreatic duct anatomy is known either through ERCP, which involves an element of risk, or based on an intraductal secretin test done previously. If normal secretory flow rates are present, pancreas divisum can be excluded and pancreatic sphincter manometry performed on a separate occasion. This precaution avoids measuring pressures in a short ventral duct and sphincter. In some of the reported studies, patients were used as controls. Some had pancreatic ducts up to 7 mm in diameter, and all had unexplained upper abdominal pain. Undoubtedly, some patients with pancreatitis were used as controls for these studies.

Normal Values

In studies of normal controls given no drugs other than diazepam, Carr-Locke and Gregg[25] found mean wave frequencies of 7.0 and 5.6 per min in the pancreatic and common duct sphincters, respectively. Maximum wave frequency was 10 per min. Similarly, Guelrud et al[30] found a frequency of 5.7 per min when both sphincters were considered together. In most studies involving no premedication other than diazepam, phasic wave activity has ranged from 3 to 7 per min. The author has seen only five cases in over 1,400 in whom no phasic wave activity was present on recordings of 2 min or longer. The endoscopic manometry of one such patient is contrasted with that of a normal control in Figure 8-1.

In studies on the relationship of SO phasic wave activity to phase of the migrating motor complex (MMC), the highest frequencies of PWA (10–12 per min) were recorded during phase III of the MMC as detected by concurrent duodenal manometry.[32] PWA over 8 per min was noted only during 3% of the recording time. The lowest rate of PWA occurred during phase I of the MMC, and during short periods of phase I there was no detectable PWA.

Despite the presence of relatively rapid activity under some physiologic circumstances, the majority of those with tachyarrhythmia seen by the author have also had elevated BSP and some have had prolonged periods of such rapid rhythms. Hogan et al[33] labeled such rapid rhythms "tachyoddia" and noted the disappearance of such rhythms, with relief of pain, after ESP. We have noted similar relief in some patients with persistent tachyarrthythmias. Rapid PWA presumably decreases diastolic time available to the spincter to permit either bile or pancreatic juice to enter the intestine and could increase duct pressure as a result. More prolonged recordings of sphincter pressures are necessary to determine the significance of tachyarrthythmias and for what duration a rapid rhythm may be part of the normal MMC. Until such time, studies that identify a rate of PWA over 7 per min as abnormal[27] are of questionable significance. Although principally antegrade propagation of PWA activity in the sphincters has been demonstrated by some,[34] others have found that most waves, when recorded with a triple lumen cannula, are simultaneous and not antegrade.[30]

Basal sphincter pressures in the pancreatic and common duct sphincters in normal controls were demonstrated to be 16.0 ± 8.1 and 15.2 ± 8.2 mm Hg, respectively, by Carr-Locke and Gregg.[25] These are remarkably similar to the composite pancreatic and biliary basal sphincter pressures of 14.8 ± 6.3 mm Hg found by Guelrud et al[30] in normal controls. The study of Carr-Locke and Gregg[25] is the only one in which pressures have been individually considered in both sphincters. The maximum value (mean ± 3 SD) in Guelrud's study was 35 mm Hg, a figure with which we concured in earlier and subsequent experience in which we employed a pump-perfused cannula with a low compliance system.

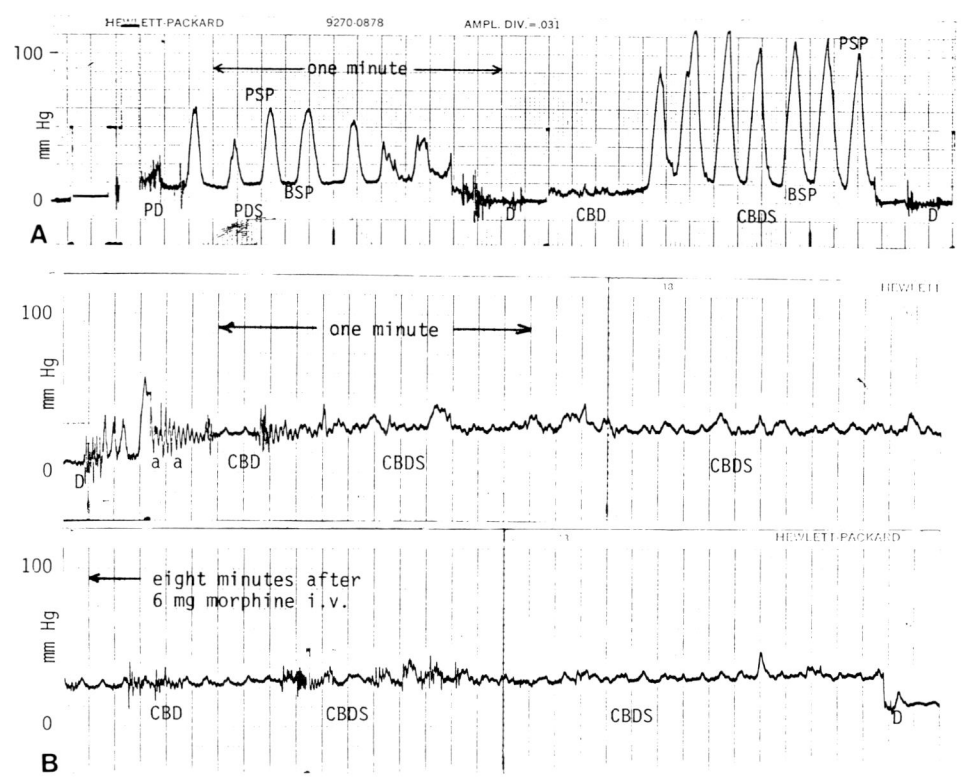

Figure 8-1 (A) Endoscopic biliary-pancreatic sphincter study of a normal control. D = duodenum, PD = pancreatic duct, PSP = peak sphincter pressure, BSP = basal (trough) sphincter pressure, CBD = common bile duct, CBDS = common bile duct sphincter. **(B)** Endoscopic biliary manometry study of patient with decompensated cirrhosis. There is an absence of phasic wave activity before and after morphine. a = artifact, CBD = common bile duct, CBDS = common bile duct sphincter.

There is much more variability in peak sphincter pressures. These are to a significant degree related to the type of pressure system used. The less compliant ones will demonstrate high peak pressures compared to ones with more compliant systems. More rapid infusion rates will also increase the height of PWA. The significance of elevated peak pressures in the presence of normal basal sphincter pressures is uncertain at this time.

In normal controls, Guelrud et al[30] demonstrated no significant difference in pressures in the CBD or PD, and pressures were 6.8 ± 1.7 mm Hg. We demonstrated lower CBD pressures of 3.0 ± 2.5 mm Hg and pancreatic duct pressures of 11.4 ± 3.0 mm Hg. Reported PD pressures of 10.9 mm Hg by Rosch[24] and 15.0 by Bar-Meir et al[26] using patient controls are similar to those in our normal population.

Our earlier studies documented a separate sphincter mechanism for the pancreatic and common bile ducts. Although both sphincters undoubtedly have some sphincter fibers in common, as demonstrated in the anatomic studies of Boyden,[35] the separate nature of the two sphincters was demonstrated by Carr-Locke and Gregg.[21] They found that ablation of the biliary sphincter did not significantly affect phasic wave activity and pressures recorded in the pancreatic sphincter segment. This demonstration of a separate pancreatic sphincter segment after either endoscopic sphincterotomy or sphincteroplasty of the choledochal sphincter has been demonstrated by the author in more than 200 subsequent patient studies. In addition, as discussed later, one sphincter may be dysfunctional while the other demonstrates a normal manometric profile.

Complications of Endoscopic Biliary-Pancreatic Sphincter Manometry

In most centers, SO manometry studies are done in conjunction with ERCP and the complication of pancreatitis is probably ascribed to ERCP. However, it has been suggested that concurrent manometry may increase the risk. Four of 21 patients developed pancreatitis when ERCP was combined with manometry in one study.[36] In our experience in which most manometry studies are not done in conjunction with ERCP, the complications of manometry can be identified separately. Pancreatitis due to manometry alone does occur. Usually it develops in patients with either pancreatic sphincter stenosis or in patients in whom repeat manometry is done to assess the effects of drugs on the sphincter or in whom cannulation of the ducts is difficult and there is more manipulation than usual. The incidence is less than that of ERCP alone but occurs in approximately 1 in 175 studies.

Effects of Gastrointestinal Hormones on the Human Sphincter of Oddi

Of the relatively few studies of hormonal effects on the human sphincter of Oddi, the majority are pharmacologic and usually only one hormone is studied. The complex and combined effects of multiple gastrointestinal hormones administered simultaneously in physiologic amounts has yet to be evaluated.

Cholecystokinin (CCK) normally inhibits sphincter of Oddi activity. Using pharmacologic bolus doses of CCK-OP, Toouli et al[37] demonstrated marked reduction in frequency of phasic wave activity and phasic wave amplitude and a slight drop in basal sphincter pressures. The usual antegrade sequence of the phasic wave was unaltered by the CCK-OP. In a physiologic study using graded infusions of CCK-OP, Carr-Locke and Bentley[38] found a marked decrease in rate of phasic wave activity, wave height, and basal sphincter pressures in both pancreatic and common bile duct sphincters, and that at pharmacologic doses there was total abolition of all PWA. Gregg and Chey (unpublished data) showed that cottonseed oil placed intraduodenally through an ERCP cannula during ERCP manometry released immunoreactive CCK in patients with normal and dysfunctional sphincters. This resulted in virtual abolition of all PWA in the common duct sphincter and a marked decrease in common duct pressure in control subjects. The abnormal responses encountered in some patients with sphincter disorders are discussed later.

Secretin infusions at physiologic ranges have been demonstrated by Carr-Locke et al[39] to significantly reduce both basal and peak pancreatic duct sphincter pressures. There was no significant change in pancreatic duct pressures except at pharmacologic infusion levels when the pressure increased significantly due to high rates of pancreatic secretion. There was no significant change in any manometric parameters in the biliary tract at either physiologic or pharmacologic infusion levels. Geenen et al[40] found that pharmacologic doses of secretin caused a transient increase in PWA and amplitude for several minutes followed by a decrease in PW amplitude and decrease in PWA.

Carr-Locke et al,[41] using graded infusions of glucagon, demonstrated significant reduction in height of bile duct phasic waves at physiologic infusion levels, but no other significant changes in sphincter function. Whether this has any physiologic significance is uncertain. Pharmacologic rates of infusion, however, resulted in a significant reduction in pancreatic and common duct pressures, and peak and basal pressures, as well as a decrease in PWA. These investigators (unpublished data) also found that glucagon reverses the effects of morphine on phasic wave activity and sphincter pressures.

Corazziari et al[42] studied the effects of a bolus dose of somatostatin on the SO. They demonstrated that it produced a marked increase in frequency of PWA, decreased phasic wave amplitude, and significantly decreased basal sphincter pressures during a short period of manometric observation.

Paradoxical Response of the SO and Pancreatic Sphincters to CCK-OP and Dietary Fat

Normally CCK, whether given intravenously or released endogenously in response to a meal, causes sphincter relaxation, which permits flow of bile and pancreatic juice into the duodenum. However, manometry has shown that some patients with biliary-pancreatic pain have an abnormal response.

Hogan et al[43] reported that 5 of 38 patients with suspected SO dysfunction and elevated basal SO pressures had a paradoxical response to CCK-OP with an increase in sphincter pressures. These patients all had either abnormal liver function tests and/or delayed drainage of contrast from the CBD after ERCP.

Toouli et al[27] described an increase in basal sphincter pressures or PWA after CCK-OP in 10 patients, all of whom had elevated basal SO pressures prior to CCK-OP. Mean basal sphincter pressures increased from 31 to 82 mm Hg. The majority of these patients experienced their typical biliary pain during the study.

Rolny et al[44] also reported a paradoxical response of the biliary sphincter to either cerulein or CCK-OP. Ten of 62 patients had an increase in basal sphincter pressures. Prestimulatory basal sphincter pressure was elevated in only 5 of the 10. The CCK-OP produced typical episodes of biliary pain in all 10 subjects. Endoscopic sphincterotomy in 7 and balloon dilation of the SO in 1 gave excellent initial relief; repeat sphincterotomy was required in 3 for restenosis. As in other studies, the paradoxical response of CCK was seen principally during the first 5 min after its administration and pharmacologic doses were used.

Response of the sphincter to physiologic increases in plasma CCK after a fatty meal is similar to that induced by pharmacologic doses but is longer lasting. Gregg studied the effects of a fatty meal on biliary and pancreatic sphincter pressures in 54 patients with severe recurrent biliary-pancreatic-like pain which was either entirely precipitated by a fatty meal or in whom more than 50% of these episodes were related to fatty meals. Sphincter response was abnormal

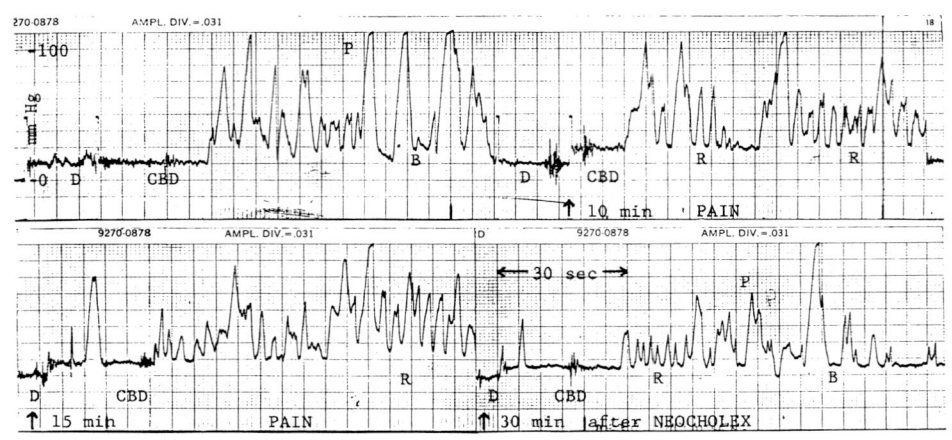

Figure 8-2 Effects of Neocholex on normal choledochal sphincter pressures of patient with sphincter dysfunctional for fat. There is a rapid transient increase in basal sphincter pressures associated with the rise in CBD pressures and obstructive pain after Neocholex. The low-amplitude phasic wave-like activity after Neocholex has been labeled "R waves," the source of which is unknown. If they were considered phasic wave activity, then the rate of PWA would be greater than the probable maximum 12 waves/min and this may be the reason that some endoscopic manometry studies reported PWA values of 16 and 18/min in the occasional patient. D = duodenum, BCD = common bile duct, P = peak sphincter pressure, B = basal sphincter pressure.

in all. More than 90% had elevated basal sphincter pressures. A fatty meal produced several different responses. These were (1) a decrease in elevated basal sphincter pressures to normal; (2) essentially no change in elevated basal sphincter pressures; (3) a paradoxical increase in already elevated basal sphincter pressures, and (4) in those with normal basal sphincter pressures, a paradoxical increase. The effects of a fatty meal on the basal sphincter pressures in these patients is illustrated in Figures 8-2 through 8-4.

The etiology of the paradoxical response of the sphincters to pharmacologic

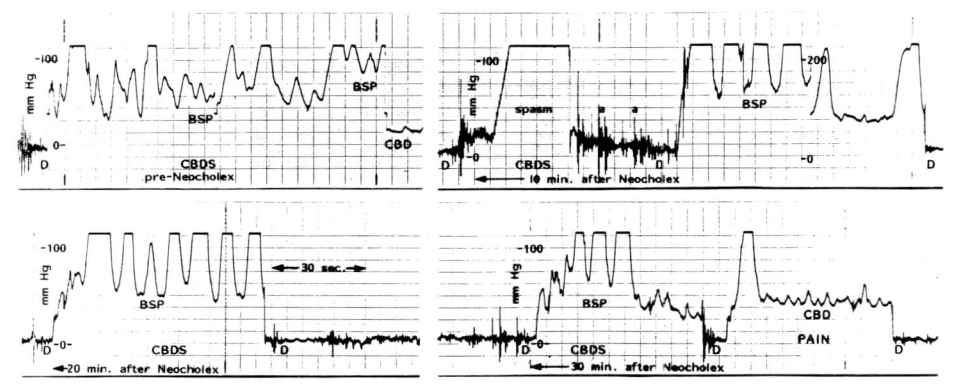

Figure 8-3 Effects of Neocholex on elevated sphincter pressures of patient with dysfunctional biliary sphincter. There is an increase in peak and basal sphincter pressures, no suppression of PWA, and a marked increase in CBD pressures with obstructive pain after Neocholex. D = duodenum, CBD = common bile duct, CBDS = common bile duct sphincter.

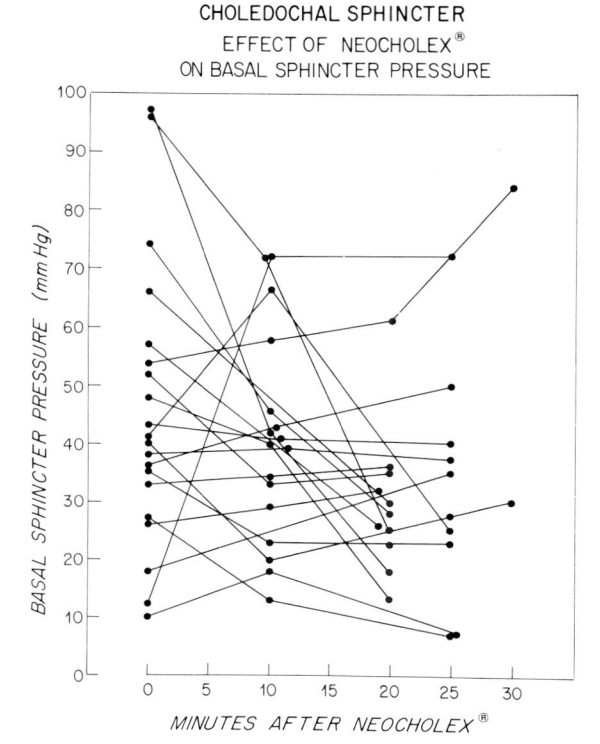

Figure 8-4 Effects of Neocholex on basal sphincter pressures in the choledochal sphincter in patients with fat-induced biliary-pancreatic-type pain. In most of these patients, basal sphincter pressure is either high at the outset or rises inappropriately.

and pharmacologic doses of CCK is probably related to abnormal innervation of the sphincter and parallels the studies of Behar and Biancani[45,46] in the cat. They demonstrated that the overall effect of CCK on the feline SO is an inhibitory one and is mediated via noncholinergic, nonadrenergic nerves. If, however, the neural pathway was blocked by tetrodotoxin, the resultant effect of CCK on the sphincter was a stimulatory one with sphincter contraction due to a direct effect of CCK on the SO musculature. Since cat SO resembles the human SO in its response to gastrointestinal hormones, it is likely that this same mechanism exists in man with failure of the nonadrenergic, noncholinergic neural pathway to oppose the direct effects of CCK on the SO musculature in patients with a paradoxical response to CCK.

Provocative Ultrasound and Quantitative Biliary Scintigraphy Using Fatty Meals or CCK-OP

Several studies assessed the potential role of provocative CCK-OP or fatty meal ultrasonography or HBS in the diagnosis of SO dysfunction. The principle underlying the sonographic approach is that CCK should cause dilation only of a structurally or functionally obstructed duct.

Aronchick et al[72] showed that duct dilation did not occur in a small number of normal controls and patients with biliary pain with normal ERCP and SO manometry. In contrast, in three patients with abnormal manometry and two with duct stones dilation did occur. Limitations of this study include the small number of patients and controls, and the definition of a 1-mm increase in CBD diameter as abnormal; we found that CCK-OP will increase CBD diameter up to 1 mm in normal controls.

Darweesh et al[73] compared quantitative hepatobiliary scintigraphy and fatty meal sonography in 22 asymptomatic subjects and 28 with symptoms suggestive of partial CBD obstruction after cholecystectomy. A positive test was an increase in duct diameter over 2 mm or a 45-min isotope clearance less than 63%. Each test was abnormal in 67%, increasing to 80% when both tests were combined. HBS had a specificity of 85% (all false positives had cirrhosis), while sonography had a specificity of 100%.

Gregg et al (manuscript in preparation) compared QHBS to endoscopic SO manometry in 49 noncholecystectomized patients presenting with biliary-pancreatic pain and 12 normal controls. Normal gallbladder ejection fractions by QHBS ranged from 35 to 91% after CCK-OP. Normal gallbladder ejection fractions after either CCK or a fatty meal (Neocholex) yielded similar ejection fractions ranging from 53 to 91%. Of 49 patients, 39 were demonstrated to have a poorly functioning gallbladder by QHBS and/or fatty meal ultrasound (FMUS). This was associated with abnormal SO manometry consisting of a poorly relaxing biliary and/or pancreatic sphincter and or elevated basal sphincter pressures in the majority of cases. The poorly functioning GB was an isolated abnormality in 8 but was more apt to occur in the presence of abnormal SO motility ($n = 26$). Figure 8-5 is the QHBS study of a normal control (right) and a patient with SO dysfunction (left). There is a very poor ejection fraction after CCK-OP in the patient with SO dysfunction compared to that of the normal control. The resected gallbladder demonstrated only mild cholecystitis. In only 2/49 patients was there an increase in CBD diameter greater than 2 mm and both had a dysfunctional sphincter by endoscopic manometry. Other associated abnormalities in these 49 patients were pancreas divisum, pancreatitis, and pancreatic sphincter stenosis. There was good correlation between GB emptying by FMUS and CCK-OP

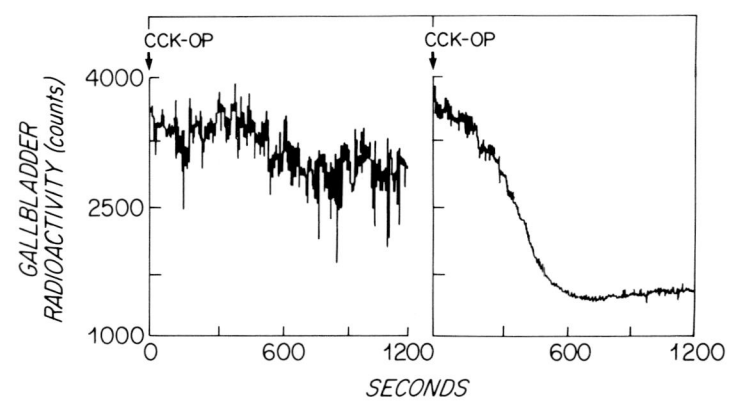

Figure 8-5 Quantitative HIDA scan showing normal gallbladder ejection fractions after CCK-OP (right), and very low ejection fractions (left) in patients with severe SO dysfunction.

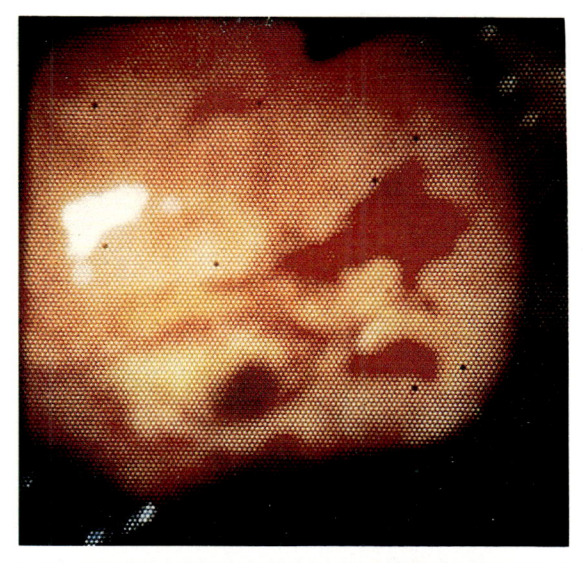

Plate 1 Endoscopic view of ampullary carcinoma (see Fig. 2-1A).

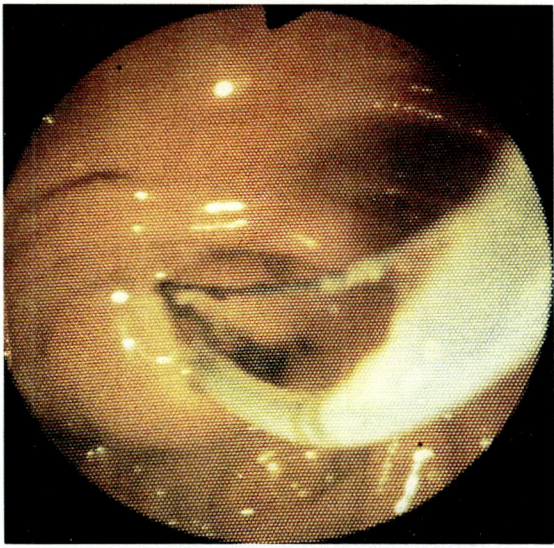

Plate 2 Endoscopic sphincterotomy (see Fig. 3-8A).

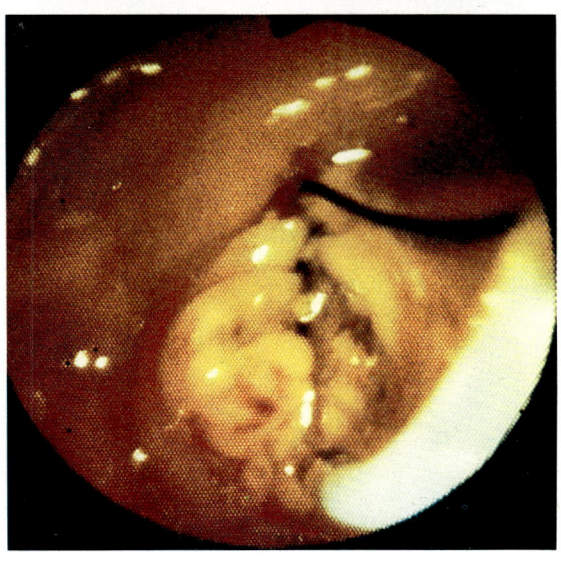

Plate 3 Endoscopic sphincterotomy (see Fig. 3-8B).

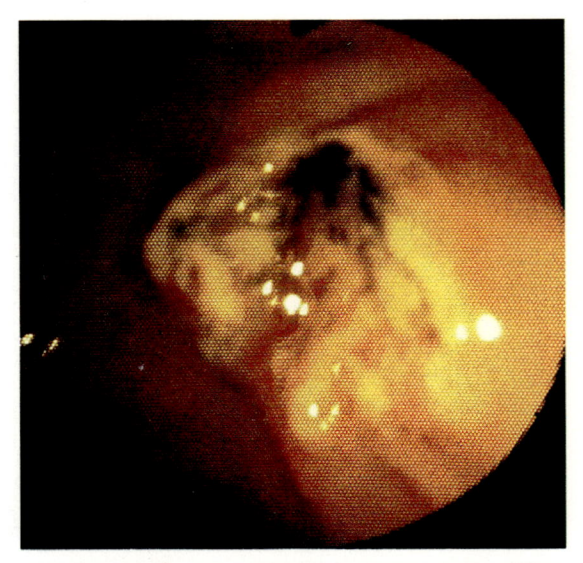

Plate 4 Endoscopic sphincterotomy (see Fig. 3-8C).

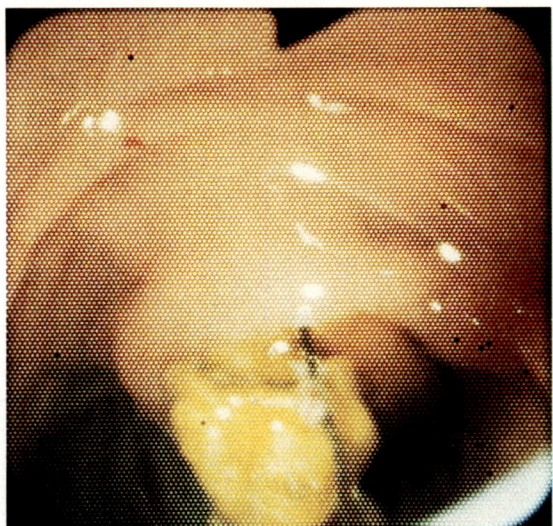

Plate 5 Endoscopic sphincterotomy (see Fig. 3-8D).

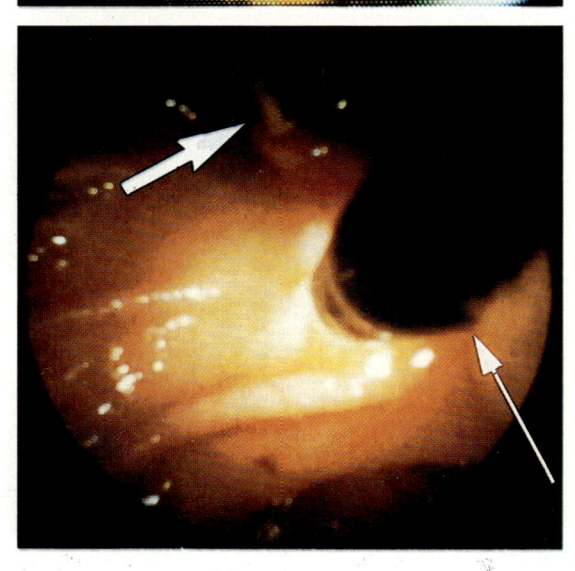

Plate 6 6 Fr miniscope (small arrow) at time of insertion into papilla (large arrow) (see Fig. 14-7).

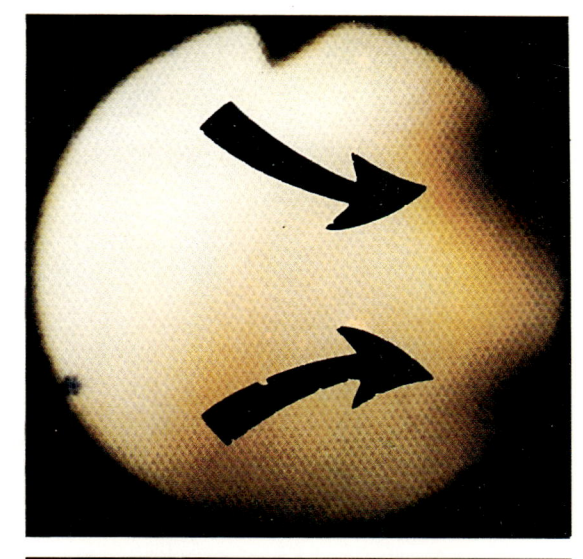

Plate 7 Bifurcation of common hepatic duct (arrows) seen with miniscope (see Fig. 14-9A).

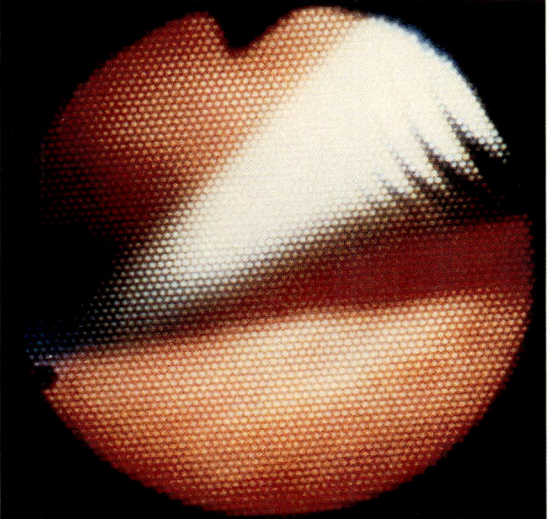

Plate 8 CBD seen through 8.7 Fr miniscope; note guidewire (see Fig. 14-9B).

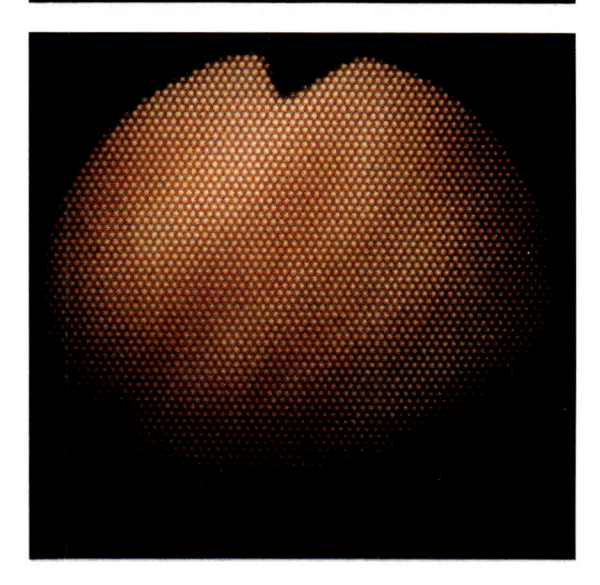

Plate 9 Pancreatic duct wall in patient with chronic pancreatitis; note ductal irregularity (see Fig. 14-9C).

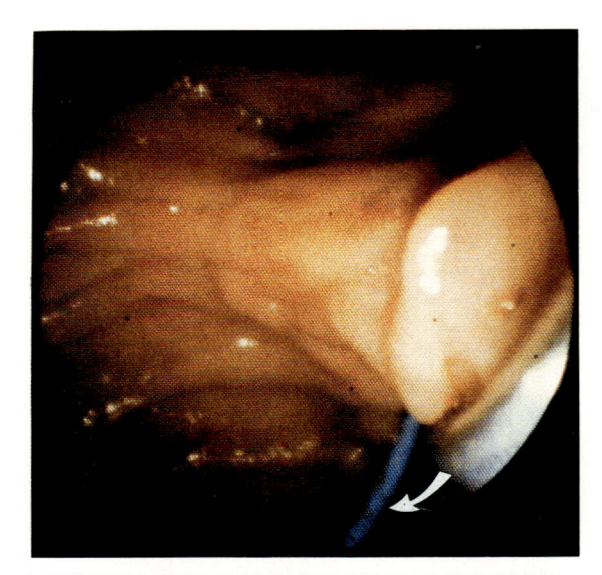

Plate 10 14 Fr miniscope in patient who underwent laser lithotripsy for large CBD stone; arrow shows nasobiliary drain (see Fig. 14-9D).

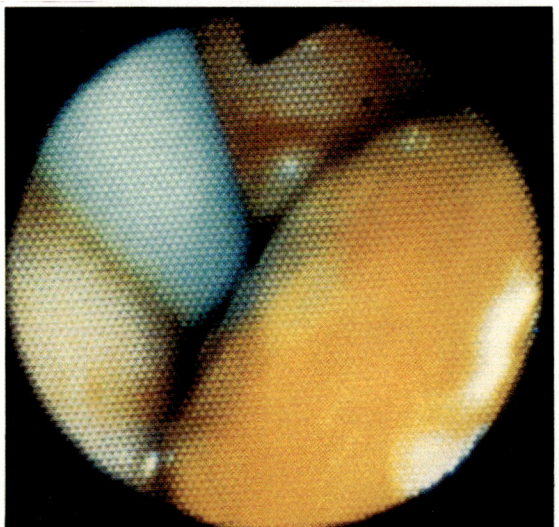

Plate 11 CBD stone in patient depicted in Plate 10; note nasobiliary drain (see Fig. 14-9E).

US with few exceptions. This study indicates the importance of evaluating gallbladder function in patients with indeterminate biliary-pancreatic-type pain and demonstrates that the majority of such patients with poor gallbladder ejection fractions have associated SO dysfunction. It also demonstrates that in noncholecystetomized patients, evaluation of gallbladder contraction is much more likely to detect abnormalities in the biliary tract than evaluation of a possible increase in CBD caliber.

Provocative QHBS and US are noninvasive studies and appear to be important tests to diagnose SO dysfunction in cholecystectomized and noncholecystectomized subjects. When done in noncholecystectomized patients, gallbladder ejection fractions, which are frequently abnormal in patients with suggested SO dysfunction, should always accompany evaluation of CBD diameter. Increases in CBD diameter appear to be more common in cholecystectomized patients with suspected SO dysfunction than in noncholecystectomized patients.

Effects of Drugs on Sphincter of Oddi and Pancreatic Sphincter Function

Several observers indicated that nitrates inhibit the sphincter of Oddi.[4,47–49] In one patient with a dysfunctional sphincter of Oddi and elevated basal sphincter pressures, Bar-Meir et al[47] demonstrated that sublingual nitroglycerin obliterated all phasic wave activity and dropped basal sphincter pressures to 0 mm Hg with relief of obstructive biliary pain while the patient took long-acting nitrites. Staritz et al[48] using glyceryl trinitrate sprayed on the tongue, demonstrated a marked reduction in basal and peak sphincter pressures, but no change in rate of PWA within a few minutes after its application in patients with normal sphincter pressures. In most cases there was also a decrease in CBD pressure. These authors used nitrates to aid in the removal of small common duct stones through the intact sphincter.[49] Other studies by McGowan et al[4] in cholecystectomized subjects demonstrated a decrease in CBD pressure and relief of obstructive pain, induced by morphine, by both amyl nitrite and nitroglycerin.

Morphine was shown by Venu et al[50] to increase phasic wave activity in small doses and basal pressure in larger doses. Similar findings are illustrated in Figures 8-6 and 8-7 from the author's unit. In contrast, diazepam does not appear to affect sphincter of Oddi activity or pressures.[17,51] Accordingly, diazepam is usually given as the sole premedication in patients undergoing sphincter of Oddi manometry.

Atropine appears to have mild effects on the sphincter of Oddi.[52,53] While the existence of an inhibitory effect on phasic wave activity only has been suggested,[52] one study showed a decrease in basal SO pressure, but only in patients with dysfunctional sphincters.[53]

Calcium channel blockers have proven effective in the treatment of esophageal motility disorders such as achalasia and diffuse esophageal spasm. More recently, they have also been used in the treatment of functional disorders of the SO. In one study, using HIDA scans, nifedipine in 20- to 30-mg doses relieved SO spasm induced by morphine.[54] Symptomatically, patients with a hypertonic SO were relieved of their pain by 20–30 mg nifedipine PO. Guelrud et al[55] found that 10 mg nifedipine sublingually did not affect SO pressures in 21 normal

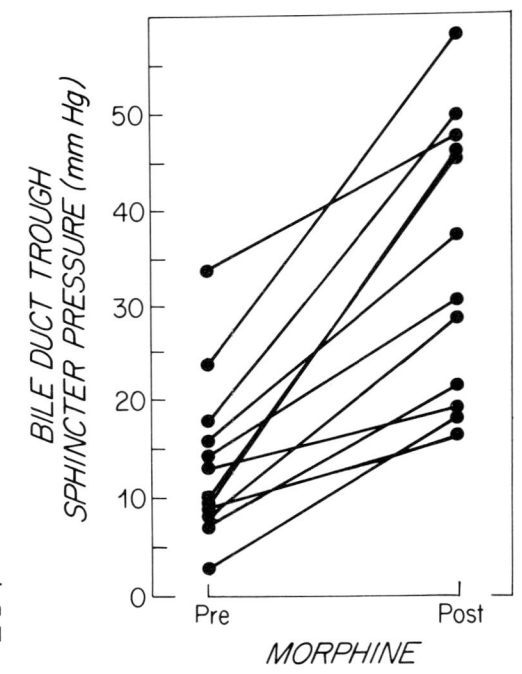

Figure 8-6 Effects of intravenous morphine on trough sphincter pressures in the common bile duct. There is a marked increase in pressures after morphine.

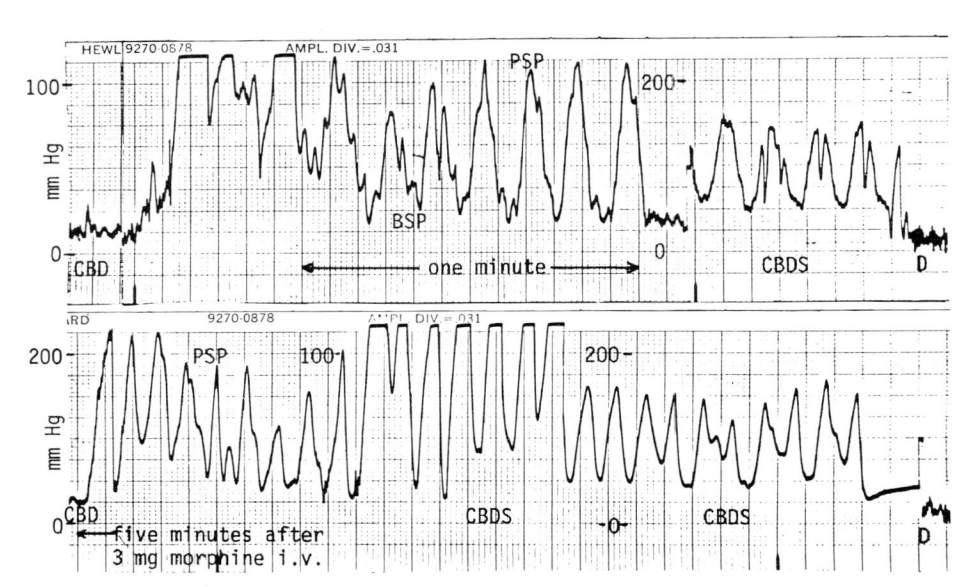

Figure 8-7 Endoscopic manometry study of choledochal sphincter in noncholecystectomized patient before and after morphine showing typical increase in phasic wave activity, trough and peak sphincter pressures, but no change in CBD pressures after morphine. D = duodenum, CBD = common bile duct, CBDS = common bile duct sphincter, PSP = peak sphincter pressure, BSP = basal (trough) sphincter pressure.

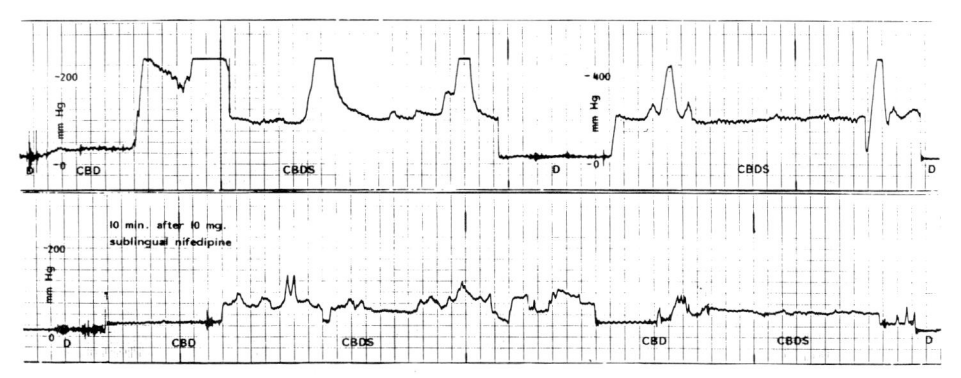

Figure 8-8 Endoscopic biliary manometry study illustrating the effect of sublingual nifedipine on cholecochal sphincter pressures of patient with severely dysfunctional sphincter. There is a marked decrease in elevated peak and basal sphincter pressures and an almost total ablation of phasic wave activity after nifedipine. CBD = common bile duct, D = duodenum, CBDS = common bile duct sphincter.

volunteers or in 9 patients with SO dysfunction, but that 20 mg sublingually produced a significant decrease in basal sphincter pressures in 8/9 volunteers and a marked decrease in basal pressures in the 9 patients with SO dyskinesia. Peak effects were noted between 20 and 30 minutes after administration.

The author studied 25 patients and 8 controls using 10 mg nifedipine sublingually. In normals there was little effect on SO pressures, except for a slowing of phasic wave activity; but in some patients with a severely dysfunctional SO, there was total ablation of all PWA and a marked decrease in BSP, which in one patient decreased from 400 to 29 mm Hg within 10 minutes. Figure 8-8 illustrates the effects of sublingual nifedipine on biliary sphincter pressures in this case. Chronic administration of nifedipine 10–20 mg qid eliminated obstructive biliary pancreatic pain, however, in probably no more than 20% of patients we studied with SO dysfunction. This low response rate may be due to the use of inadequate doses since the sphincter response seems, at least in part, to be dose-related. Future double-blind studies of SO response to calcium channel blockers will prove interesting and this group of compounds will undoubtedly have some place in the treatment of SO disorders.

Clinical Manifestations of Sphincter of Oddi Dysfunction

The majority of patients with sphincter dysfunction are detected after cholecystectomy. In part this is probably because the symptoms of sphincter dysfunction are similar to those of cholecystitis or cholelithiasis. In addition, symptoms related to increased bile duct pressures caused by sphincter dysfunction may be unmasked by the loss of the reservoir function of the gallbladder.

There is also some evidence that cholecystectomy may alter sphincter pressures and sphincter response to hormones. Thune et al[56] demonstrated that the resistance of the feline choledochoduodenal junction to a constant flow of bile is reduced when hydrostatic pressures within the duct are increased within the physiologic range. Administration of tetrodotoxin or infiltration of the junction between the cystic duct and common duct with a local anesthetic eliminated this response. The findings indicate that reflex regulation of the biliary sphincter occurs and is modulated by distending pressures in the biliary tract and that this reflex regulation is in part mediated by inhibitory nerves running along the common bile duct. Damage to such nerves could easily happen during cholecystectomy.

Grace et al[57,58] studied biliary sphincter function in cholecystectomized prairie dogs in response to CCK-OP. There was a blunted response to CCK-OP in the cholecystectomized animals. This also suggests that neural pathways along the common duct mediate the response of the biliary sphincter to hormonal stimulation.

Biliary pain related to SO dysfunction can occur in a variety of locations but, in the author's experience, is generally in the epigastrium and/or right upper quadrant, and usually radiates through to the interscapular area or around to the right scapula. Occasionally the pain is circumferential and in rare instances is experienced principally in the right flank and may initiate an investigation for renal disease. Radiation of pain to the low substernal area is common. In rare instances pain may be entirely in the midanterior chest and occasionally radiate from there to the back and be indistinguisable from coronary or esophageal pain.[59-62]

When the pain is epigastric, it may be indistinguishable from that of pancreatitis, which is frequently associated with SO dysfunction, particularly when there is associated pancreatic sphincter stenosis. The patient may also experience episodic pain in separate areas in the upper abdomen, one from biliary pain and the other from pancreatitis. The author has seen patients in whom removal of a diseased gallbladder relieved the episodes of right upper quadrant pain but did not alleviate the epigastric component due to associated sphincter dysfunction and/or associated pancreatitis. Other clinical conditions which may produce episodes of pain in the same areas include esophageal disorders, large- and small-bowel disease, stomach disorders, and coronary artery disease. Since esophageal motility disorders, gastric emptying disorders, and irritable bowel problems are commonly associated with SO dysfunction as part of a pandysautonomia (see below), diagnosis becomes even more complex.

A few clinical studies document the difficulties in ascribing pain to a specific gastrointestinal etiology on the basis of location alone. Chapman et al[59] showed that during balloon distention of either the esophagus or common bile duct, four of nine patients could not distinguish between the two sites as the origin of pain. Doran[62] found that pain produced by inflating a Foley catheter in the common duct through a T tube was most often noted in the epigastrium and low substernal area, but also occurred in the right upper quadrant and interscapular area. Ravdin et al[61] first noted the association of chest pain with biliary tract disease. In a recent study by Kingham and Dawson,[63] of 22 patients with indeterminate right upper quadrant pain, balloon distention of at least one area of large and small bowel produced a similar pain and further emphasizes that right upper quadrant pain is not always of biliary origin. In the author's experience, pain from an irritable bowel may be experienced entirely in the right upper quadrant and lead to the erroneous diagnosis of biliary tract disease and unnecessary cholecystectomy, with persistent pain after surgery. Such considerations underscore the importance of having accurate diagnostic criteria for SO dysfunction.

Episodes of pain due to SO dysfunction may last from 20–30 minutes to days. They may awaken the patient from sleep or only occur during the daytime, and in some patients they may occur only after meals. Occasionally, pain ultimately becomes constant with superimposed episodes of more severe pain.

In some patients there are definite clues as to etiology. One is the occurrence of biliary-type pain in postcholecystectomy patients after administration of narcotics, principally codeine and morphine. In some this may be a single episode occurring only after ingestion of a teaspoonful of cough medicine containing 6–8 mg of codeine and the patient, recognizing this, no longer uses the medicine. The author has also seen patients given morphine in the postcholecystectomy period who developed severe biliary pain. In such patients there may also be non-narcotic-induced episodes of pain, and such pain may ultimately become constant.

The other clue that the patient may have SO dysfunction is the production of biliary-like pain after the ingestion of a fatty meal. In the author's large experience, this history has been strongly associated with a dysfunctional biliary and/or pancreatic sphincter and the mechanism for this is discussed elsewhere. In some of these patients, pain occurs only after fat ingestion and the patients have no pain if they remain on a low-fat diet. In most patients with fat-induced biliary pain, however, there are also spontaneous, non-fat-related episodes of pain.

Laboratory Abnormalities Associated with SO Dysfunction

Laboratory studies to diagnose SO dysfunction have been disappointing and few. The abnormalities associated with SO dysfunction consist of elevations of liver function tests, usually in association with episodes of pain. These occur in less than 25% of those seen by the author. Occasionally, there may be persistent elevation of the serum alkaline phosphatase, usually in those with chronic pain. Elevated serum amylase may occasionally occur in patients with associated pancreatic sphincter dysfunction and/or associated pancreatitis, which is usually obstructive in etiology. Jaundice is very rare unless there are associated common duct stones.

Association of Sphincter of Oddi Dysfunction with Other Biliary-Pancreatic Disorders

There is a significant relationship between SO dysfunction and several other biliary-pancreatic disorders, most of which have only been appreciated since the development of ERCP and endoscopic manometric techniques.

One of the most common of these is the association of SO disorders with acalculous cholecystitis. In many instances, CCK-OP, fatty meal ultrasonography or radionuclide ejection studies show that these patients have poorly functioning gallbladders. It has been well known for over 50 years that removal of an acalculous gallbladder in a patient with recurrent right upper quadrant biliary-type pain is associated with a significant rate of recurrent biliary-type pain within a period of several years. The principal reason for this is probably SO dysfunction, possibly in association with chronic cholecystitis. The resected gallbladder usually only demonstrates mild chronic cholecystitis. It is the author's feeling that patients with presumed acalculous cholecystitis should have endoscopic biliary manometry prior to cholecystectomy.

SO dysfunction is also common in those patients with so-called postcholecystectomy syndrome who have recurrent biliary-type pain after cholecystectomy for either calculous or acalculous disease. We found that the majority of such patients have SO dysfunction rather than common duct stones or pancreatitis. In most cases, symptoms recurred within 6 months of surgery, but in a small number of patients, symptoms may develop only many years after cholecystectomy.

The other clinical situations associated with a high incidence of SO dysfunction are pancreas divisum and incomplete pancreas divisum, both of which are associated with dorsal duct sphincter stenosis in patients with pancreatitis. The author found, principally by endoscopic manometry, that over 50% of these patients also have elevated trough pressures in their choledochal sphincter. This is important information for the surgeon since dorsal duct sphincteroplasty alone in these cases may not relieve all pain. For this reason, the author recommends that choledochal sphincteroplasty should also be done in all patients with pancreas divisum or incomplete pancreas divisum, unless the surgeon knows preoperatively that the biliary sphincter is normal.

The other two clinical situations associated with SO dysfunction, already briefly discussed, are: (1) patients with narcotic hypersensitive sphincter encountered clinically only postcholecystecotomy, and (2) patients with recurrent biliary pain after fat ingestion, all of whom in the author's large experience have a dysfunctional biliary and/or pancreatic sphincter by manometry. In some of these cases, the abnormality can only be demonstrated by a challenge test with either CCK-OP IV or administration of a fatty meal during endoscopic manometry.

There is also an association of sphincter stenosis or dysfunction of the pancreatic sphincter with idiopathic pancreatitis. The author has found such abnormalities in approximately 30% of such patients. Sphincteroplasty of the biliary and pancreatic sphincters in these patients is usually curative.

The Morphine-Prostigmine Provocative Test of Biliary-Pancreatic Sphincter Dysfunction

The morphine-prostigmine test (MPT) was introduced initially by Nardi and Acosta[16] to select patients with obstructive pancreatitis who would benefit from sphincteroplasty. Subsequently, it was also proposed as a diagnostic test for sphincter dysfunction in postcholecystectomy patients with biliary pain. This test has been controversial. Only a few studies included controls, and they were not always normal subjects. The criteria for abnormality were changed several times. An initial requirement for a fourfold rise in amylase was later changed to a twofold increase and reproduction of pain, or even development of pain alone. Since the test may produce abdominal pain of bowel origin, pain alone is a poor predictor.

Among the studies purporting to show a possible role for the MPT, that of Roberts-Thomson and Toouli[64] showed reproduction of pain in 65 of 80 patients with biliary pain after cholecystectomy and only 2 of 25 controls. Hyperamylasemia and elevations in liver enzymes were significantly higher in patients than in controls. Among 33 patients who had manometry, however, no significant differences in the frequency of elevated liver enzymes could be found between those with normal manometry and those with fixed stenosis or biliary dyskinesia.

Madura et al[65] evaluated the MPT in 50 patients who underwent sphincteroplasty for stenosis or a dysfunctional sphincter. Using a fourfold increase in amylase or SGOT as positive, 43 of 50 had one or more abnormalities. ERCP was abnormal in 55%. Intraoperative bile duct pressures were elevated in 80%, but transsphincteric flow rates were abnormal in only 45%. Abnormal sphincter tissue was seen microscopically in 71%. Relief of pain was achieved in 88%. Persistent or recurrent sphincter stenosis accounted for poor results in some and this was associated with a persistently positive MPT. A group of 34 patients undergoing biliary surgery for a variety of other reasons served as a control group and in this group four had positive MPT.

In a study of normal volunteers, Carr-Locke and Gregg demonstrated that the maximal amylase response in 24 subjects was 3.0 times normal. None developed pain except for occasional cramps and mild nausea. When 70 patients with stenosis by manometry were evaluated, 65% had an abnormal response. On the other hand, in the author's experience at least 25% of patients with a positive MPT will have normal manometry.

Several studies have led to skepticism about the utility of the MPT test. LoGiudice et al[66] found that serum amylase and lipase values exceeded six times normal in three of six subjects and also that three of four patients with sphincter stenosis at operation had less than a twofold rise, while two of four patients found to have anatomically normal sphincters at surgery had greater than a fourfold rise in amylase. Of six patients with a positive MPT and normal ERCP manometry, only one had SO stenosis at operation. Of eight patients with a negative MPT, elevated SO pressure was recorded in three, with SO stenosis confirmed at surgery. Steinberg et al[67] evaluated 10 normal volunteers and five patients with irritable bowel, and four with unspecified chronic abdominal pain. A rise in amylase of five times the upper limits of normal occured in six of 10 normal controls. Several patients with irritable bowel also had a significant but lesser rise. The test also failed to give reproducible results in two of four patients when repeated on separate days. Some patients with irritable bowel developed abdominal pain of unspecified type. Warshaw et al[68] compared the MPT results to evaluation of the sphincter at surgery. Twenty-four to twenty-six percent had a positive test with stenosis, a figure similar to that of their controls. Unfortunately, abdominal pain alone during the test or a rise in serum amylase or lipase greater than two times normal was considered a positive test, rendering the study of limited value.

Although the MPT has limitations and has been abandoned in many centers, in the author's opinion it has occasional value if strict criteria are used for a positive test. A negative study does not exclude the presence of sphincter disease and the study does not differentiate between stenotic and dysfunctional sphincters.

Secretin-Ultrasound Provocation Test to Detect Sphincter Stenosis

Warshaw et al[68] investigated the value of a provocative test using ultrasound and secretin to detect SO stenosis. They evaluated an increase in the caliber of the pancreatic and/or common bile duct after secretin. Ultrasound was done prior to and 5, 15, and 30 min after secretin in 34 controls, 30 symptomatic patients suspected of having sphincter stenosis, and 22 patients with symptomatic pancreas divisum. Diagnosis of sphincter stenosis was made at surgery by sphincter calibration.

A positive test was defined as one in which the common hepatic duct (CHD) increased at least 1–2 mm and the pancreatic duct at least 1 mm in diameter. A grade 3 positive result consisted of an increase in CHD diameter of greater than 5 mm and at least a 2-mm increase in PD diameter in all three parts of the gland. They were able to visualize the pancreatic duct in a surprisingly high 94% of cases. Eighty-three percent of 16 cases with sphincter stenosis documented at surgery demonstrated an increase in diameter of the pancreatic duct by at least 1 mm and 72% of patients with pancreas divisum did likewise, while only 14% of control subjects did so. The response was abolished by sphincteroplasty.

Unfortunately, no patients had sphincter manometry and no patients had an intraductal secretin test of pancreatic function to define flow rates. No mention is made of how many subjects had already had cholecystectomy. Although the statement is made that secretin has no effect on the sphincters, secretin at physiologic and pharmacologic doses has profound effects on the pancreatic sphincter, which consist of a decrease in peak and basal sphincter pressures and a decrease in phasic wave frequency, but no effect on bile duct sphincter pressures. Since pharmacologic doses of secretin have a slight cholecystokinetic effect and an increased hepatic bile flow to approximately 1.3 ml/min (Gregg, unpublished data), an increase in CBD diameter may be solely related to these factors and bear no relationship to presence or absence of stenosis. The author has done similar studies and compared them to sphincter pressures and pancreatic juice flow rates, and not found the test to be useful or discriminatory.

Hepatobiliary Scintigraphy for Diagnosis of Sphincter of Oddi Dysfunction

A few studies have evaluated the use of hepatobiliary scintigraphy (HBS) in the diagnosis of SO disorders and suggest that it may be a useful adjunct. Lee et al,[69] for example, studied 21 patients with typical biliary pain suggestive of SO dysfunction. Duodenal appearance time (DAT) of the nuclide was delayed beyond 60 minutes in eight cases, and the longest delays were principally in those patients with such tight sphincters that the biliary tract could not be entered for manometry. However, several patients with elevated biliary sphincter pressures had rapid DAT. Time-activity dynamics were abnormal in seven patients, including several with rapid DAT. We concluded that a prolonged DAT is probably a reliable indicator of SO dysfunction but that some patients with elevated sphincter pressures may still have normal DAT. This is probably less likely with structural stenosis. Further studies by the author in 20 normal controls and 70 patients with SO dysfunction have confirmed that DAT beyond 60 minutes is abnormal.

Zeman et al[70] studied 30 postcholecystectomy patients with upper abdominal pain suggesting SO dysfunction. Of 10 diagnosed with SO stenosis by intraoperative calibration of the sphincter or by dilated duct and delayed drainage, 9 had abnormal time-density relationships with no decrease in CBD radioactivity between 1–2 hr. DAT was less reliable, with times over 60 minutes being present in only 4 of 10 patients.

Shaffer et al[71] evaluated HBS in 35 symptomatic postcholecystectomy patients, 9 with suspected SO dysfunction (cholestasis, CBD dilation, and delayed drainage) and 18 with intrahepatic cholestasis or extrahepatic obstruction. The parameter that discriminated best between controls and SO dysfunction was the T peak, or time for maximal uptake by the liver. However, T peaks were similar in SO dysfunction and overt cholestatic disorders. Emptying rates were also abnormal in patients with SO dysfunction and in cholestatic disease.

Scintigraphy appears to be a useful adjunct, though it cannot be used as the sole basis for diagnosis or therapy in these patients. It will not distinguish sphincter dysfunction from other causes of duct obstruction or intrahepatic cholestasis. It is important that narcotics not be used within 6–8 hours of HBS since these drugs may delay DAT.

Treatment of Biliary-Pancreatic Sphincter Dysfunction

The initial treatment of patients with biliary-pancreatic sphincter dysfunction should be dietary management. Many of these patients have episodic pain in relation to fat ingestion and should be placed on a strict, 40-g, low-fat diet. This will eliminate or improve pain in some patients. Patients who are postcholecystectomy and have biliary dyskinesia related to morphine, codeine, and other narcotics should be told to avoid these medications and be cautious of cough medications containing codeine.

For those patients who do not respond to dietary treatment alone, nitrates or nitrites taken during an acute episode of pain may provide transient relief. Use of a long-acting nitrate may prevent episodic pain in some patients but these have not been studied in detail. In my experience, calcium channel blockers offer the best relief or prevention of episodic or interruption of constant pain. I prefer to start treatment with nifedipine 10 mg t.i.d. and h.s. and will increase the dose if necessary. I have also found diltiazem 30–60 mg taken at the same time intervals to be helpful.

For patients who do not respond well to diet and drug treatment, either endoscopic or surgical ablation of the biliary sphincter, or of both sphincters, is necessary. Such treatment should be undertaken only when the patient understands the magnitude of the procedure and that the procedure may not relieve pain. Generally, I feel that the biliary sphincter is best treated by endoscopic sphincterotomy and the pancreatic sphincter by balloon dilation; stents offer an interesting but less permanent solution. When only the biliary sphincter is abnormal, biliary sphincterotomy alone should suffice. When both sphincters are abnormal, I have often found that both need to be treated, especially when the patient presents with pancreatitis. Although it is possible to treat both biliary and pancreatic sphincters at the same endoscopy, I prefer to treat them on separate occasions. This may decrease the incidence of complications and affords the opportunity to observe the patient for improvement after biliary sphincterotomy alone. If the procedure is to be done surgically, the surgeon should be prepared to do both biliary and pancreatic sphincters with septectomy.

Evaluation of Adequacy of Sphincterotomy

Evaluation of the adequacy of sphincterotomy is important in the patient with persistent upper abdominal pain similar to that before surgery. Aerobilia or barium reflux into the bile duct and/or pancreatic duct are reliable indicators of complete sphincter ablation. Barium reflux appears somewhat more sensitive in this regard, but its absence does not invariably imply lack of total sphincter ablation. These studies are much less satisfactory in evaluating pancreatic sphincter surgery, after which some residual sphincter usually remains.

If these noninvasive studies cannot determine the adequacy of sphincter surgery, endoscopic manometry of both biliary and pancreatic sphincters may be required. If residual sphincter activity is present but sphincter pressures are normal, it is advisable to do a manometry challenge test with CCK-OP or a challenge with intravenous morphine. Elevated basal pressures in either sphincter, a paradoxical sphincter response to either a fatty meal or CCK-OP, or a persistently positive morphine-neostigmine test for either abnormal elevations of serum amylase or SGOT indicates the need for further sphincter ablation if there is persistent or recurrent biliary pain. Almost all postsphincterotomy manometry studies except those by the author[74] have failed to address the status of the pancreatic sphincter, which is indispensable in postoperative evaluation of the patient with persistent biliary-pancreatic pain.

Complications of Endoscopic Sphincterotomy for Biliary Sphincter Disease

In the author's experience and that of some others, ES for SO dysfunction has a higher complication rate than ES for stones.[75-78] One factor contributing to an increased incidence of duodenal perforation is probably the significant number of these patients with normal caliber bile ducts, lowering the safety margin in doing a complete ES. Hypertrophic or fibrotic sphincters may also increase the risk since extended periods of high-intensity current may be required for sphincter ablation. This increases the risk of deep tissue burns and therefore pancreatitis, perforation, or late fibrosis. The extended time required to attempt a difficult cannulation also increases the risk of pancreatitis. The use of a guide-wire can expedite cannulation in difficult cases. Precut sphincterotomy also increases the risk of pancreatitis in our experience, occurring in 15% of such patients. The author is currently reluctant to perform precuts.

In 51 patients treated by Thatcher et al,[77] there were four perforations, two patients with hemorrhage, and two cases of pancreatitis. Three patients with perforation and one other patient required emergency surgery. Leese et al[78] noted complications in 16.2% of patients with stenosis and 10.3% having ES for stones. Roberts-Thomson and Toouli[79] had few complications in their 50 cases. Only 1 had bleeding and one had pancreatitis. The author also had a low incidence of perforation with only 1 in 120 for stenosis. There were 3 cases of hemorrhage of which 1 required surgery, 2 cases of hemorrhagic pancreatitis, and 11 others with milder pancreatitis, many occurring in our early experience when precuts were used in the more difficult procedures. Seifert et al[76] also noted an increased incidence of complications after ES for stenosis and a twofold increase in mortality.

Because of the relatively high incidence of major complications, a period of medical treatment is desirable to determine if the patients are medically manageable.

Determinants of Success After Endoscopic Sphincterotomy for Benign Biliary Sphincter Disease

Factors affecting outcome after endoscopic sphincterotomy or surgical choledochal sphincteroplasty for benign biliary sphincter disease include (1) the accuracy of the diagnosis; (2) the degree to which stenosis or sphincter dysfunction was relieved by the procedure, (3) the presence of associated pancreatic duct sphincter stenosis, and (4) the presence of associated pancreatitis. Unfortunately, most reports concerning results of ES do not address all these questions, particularly that concerning the presence of associated pancreatic sphincter stenosis, which in the author's experience, occurs in 25–30% of patients with biliary sphincter disease.

Roberts-Thomson and Toouli[79] found pain relief to correlate poorly with a dilated common duct and cholestasis. Pain resolved or improved in 5 of 7 patients with normal sphincter manometry and 10 of 17 with various manometric abnormalities. Five of seven with elevated basal sphincter pressures did not improve. There was no mention of the status of the pancreatic duct sphincter.

In contrast, Carr-Locke et al[80] felt that the best predictors of success in their series were a dilated common duct and delayed drainage of contrast material. The place of endoscopic manometry was unclear, but the majority of their subjects did not have manometry.

Thatcher et al[77] also found that the best results among 51 patients who had had ES were in those with a CBD dilated greater than 12 mm and/or delayed drainage of contrast material greater than 45 min. These amounted to 34 of 51 cases. Of those 17 with a normal caliber CBD, 13 of 17 had associated pancreatitis. The presence of pancreatitis and the increased difficulties and risks of doing a total choledochal sphincterotomy in patients with normal caliber CBD may have contributed to the lesser success of ES in this group. The value of endoscopic manometry in these patients is hard to assess since it was only done in 29 cases, and the authors were not always certain in which duct and sphincter they were measuring pressures.

Tanaka et al[81] studied 17 patients with postcholecystectomy biliary pain by microtransducer manometry before and after administration of morphine. They found that a parallel elevation in CBD pressure and the intensity of pain produced by morphine was the best predictor of pain relief after ESP. This occurred in

13/17 cases. Unfortunately, no mention was made of duct diameter or drainage time by ERCP and no sphincter manometry was performed.

Bar-Meir et al,[26] in a highly selected group of 10 patients who had ES, felt that elevated basal sphincter pressures were the most significant factor for future pain relief since all 10 with elevated BSP were free of pain after sphincter surgery. Of the 10, however, 8 had a markedly dilated CBD with a diameter over 15 mm and delayed drainage of contrast material.

The strongest evidence that manometric findings correlate with therapeutic results comes from the randomized study of Geenen et al.[82] Forty-seven patients had postcholecystectomy pain and one or two of the following: dilated bile duct, delayed drainage beyond 45 min at ERCP, and abnormal liver tests on at least two occasions. Patients were randomized to treatment with sphincterotomy or sham sphincterotomy, and the results at 1 year subsequently correlated with manometric findings prior to treatment. Of the 23 patients who initially had high basal SO pressure, 10 of 11 (91%) who underwent sphincterotomy had improved compared with only 3 of 12 (25%) who had sham sphincterotomy. Of the 24 patients with normal SO pressure initially, 5 of 12 (42%) improved after sphincterotomy but 4 of 12 (33%) did so after the sham procedure as well. In the group of 12 with initial high SO pressure treated by sham ES, 7 subsequently had real ES. At 4-year followup, 17 of the 18 patients who had ES in this study remained improved.[83]

In the author's experience, of 120 ES for either stenosis or sphincter dysfunction, patients with either appeared to benefit equally from ES, and 78% were either pain-free or had marked improvement in follow-up from 12 months to 11 years. The principal reasons for failure of pain relief were associated pancreatitis and/or pancreatic sphincter stenosis, the latter diagnosed by endoscopic manometry in 37 cases. Patients with significant pain due to pancreatic sphincter stenosis underwent either ES or surgical sphincteroplasty of the pancreatic sphincter with resolution or improvement. The least immediate relief was in those with associated pancreatitis, but even in these, pain continued to improve over several months after relief of pancreatic sphincter obstruction. This was so in our early experience and continued to be so through 1989. The great majority of our patients have had prior cholecystectomy. Five of 120 patients restenosed the ES.

Unlike patients in some other studies, the majority of ours had a CBD that was of normal caliber or only slightly dilated from 8–13 mm. There was no significant difference in relief of symptoms in those with or without dilated CBD if patients with associated pancreatitis or pancreatic sphincter dysfunction are excluded. Patients with dysfunctional sphincters for narcotics and those dysfunctional for fats who had normal basal sphincter pressures did as well as those who had elevated basal sphincter pressures in the absence of pancreatitis and pancreatic sphincter dysfunction.

One reason that patients with a dilated common duct do better in some series after ES than others is that complete biliary sphincter ablation may not be as easily and safely achieved in those with a normal caliber duct. Another consideration that affects improvement after ES is whether or not the patient has an associated motility disorder of the GI tract.

It appears that multiple factors may predict results of sphincterotomy for SO dysfunction. The presence or absence of a dilated CBD is not predictive in the absence of pancreatitis or pancreatic sphincter dysfunction. Elevated basal sphincter pressures are a reliable indicator of SO dysfunction and, if the CBD basal sphincter pressures alone are elevated, are a good predictor of excellent response to ES. Rapid phasic wave activity alone is probably a poor predictor of good response to ES since it may be encountered as a normal part of the MMC. Paradoxical sphincter response to CCK-OP or fat is a good predictor of relief from ES. In the author's experience, usually both biliary and pancreatic sphincters respond in this manner in the same patient and ES may fail to relieve pain unless both biliary and pancreatic sphincters are ablated. Associated motility disorders in the GI tract may be present and cause persistent symptoms after satisfactory sphincterotomy or sphincteroplasty. The presence of associated pancreatitis and/or pancreatic sphincter dysfunction will be associated with poor results from biliary ES alone unless the obstructive pancreatitis is also treated. Early or late restenosis of the ES and incomplete ES may account for failure of pain relief in a small number of cases.

Pancreatitis and Pancreatic-Type Pain in Patients with Pancreatic Sphincter Stenosis or Dysfunction

Direct measurements of pancreatic sphincter and duct pressures have become important means of determining the presence or absence of pancreatic sphincter dysfunction. As a corollary, manometry is useful in determining whether or not patients with pancreatic-type pain and/or pancreatitis may benefit from sphincteroplasty or endoscopic sphincterotomy of the pancreatic duct sphincter. It is the author's feeling that pancreatic sphincter manometry should always be done in conjunction with biliary sphincter manometry. Our studies demonstrated the presence of pancreatic sphincter dysfunction in some patients with pancreatitis and/or pain with pancreatitis, and relief of pain after either endoscopic pancreatic duct sphincterotomy or surgical sphincteroplasty. Conventional sphincteroplasty or endoscopic biliary sphincterotomy failed to relieve pain and pancreatitis in some of these patients.

Several groups have investigated the sphincter in patients with pancreatitis.[84-89] Toouli et al[87] studied 28 patients with idiopathic recurrent pancreatitis and either normal or slightly abnormal ($N = 14$) pancreatic duct on ERCP. Although the manometry cannula was positioned to "favor" cannulation of the pancreatic duct, the actual position of the cannula was not determined. An elevated SO basal pressure was recorded in 16 cases, excess retrograde sphincter contractions in 9, a tachyarrythmia in 9, and absence of PWA in 3, 2 of whom had very elevated basal sphincter pressures. Three patients had a paradoxical response to IV CCK-OP. Selecting a rate of PWA of greater than 7/min as abnormal is probably not realistic since PWA may exceed this rate in normal controls and be part of the normal frequency range encountered during parts of the MMC. It is unfortunate that in this and the other studies above a more precise knowledge of which sphincter pressure was actually measured was not determined. However, the study does demonstrate that biliary-pancreatic sphincter dysfunction is present in a significant number of patients with idiopathic pancreatitis.

Guelrud and Siegel[88] described four cases of pancreatitis associated with a hypersensitive pancreatic duct sphincter by endoscopic manometry, and all had a marked delay in duct emptying after ERCP. In another series, Guelrud et al[89] evaluated 42 patients with idiopathic relapsing pancreatitis by manometry and demonstrated that 17 had SO dysfunction with elevated basal sphincter pressures. The 17 were initially treated with ES followed by balloon dilation of the pancreatic sphincter several weeks later but pancreatic sphincter pressures were not measured. There was an alarming 43% incidence of pancreatitis due to the balloon dilation.

Hogan et al[90] noted that conventional biliary sphincter ablation, either endoscopically ($N = 4$) or surgically ($N = 5$), failed to prevent further episodes of pancreatitis in nine patients with idiopathic recurrent pancreatitis. All nine had virtual ablation of CBD–duodenal pressure gradients after ESP but were demonstrated to have elevated peak and basal pancreatic duct sphincter pressures. Pancreatic duct sphincter pressures were normal in another nine patients who underwent endoscopic sphincterotomy for common duct stones who did not have associated pancreatitis. Carr-Locke and Gregg[21] demonstrated that endoscopic sphincterotomy in 12 patients with recurrent pancreatitis associated with ampullary stenosis failed to relieve obstructive pain in all cases. After sphincterotomy, endoscopic evaluation of the pancreatic sphincter demonstrated pancreatic sphincter stenosis in 6 of the 12.

In a recently completed study of 125 patients with idiopathic pancreatitis who did not have pancreas divisum, Gregg (manuscript in progress) found elevated basal pancreatic duct sphincter pressures ranging from 42 to over 400 mm Hg by endoscopic manometry in 38. This study also documented, as have others, that SO dysfunction was also present in a substantial number of these patients. Conversely, we found that 29% of our patients with biliary sphincter dysfunction have similar disorders of their pancreatic duct sphincters. Venu et al[91] studied 116 patients with idiopathic relapsing pancreatitis by manometry and ERCP. Seventeen had elevated basal sphincter of Oddi pressures and 11 pancreas divisum.

The classic example of obstructive pancreatitis and/or obstructive pancreatic pain is the congenital anomaly, pancreas divisum. In this syndrome, the dorsal pancreatic sphincter is always stenotic in those who present with pain and/or pancreatitis. Calibration of the sphincter at surgery or during ERCP has consistently confirmed the sphincter caliber to be 1 mm or less in diameter in virtually all cases. Dorsal pancreatic duct pressures measured with an end-hole cannula by Staritz et al[92] were elevated compared to normals, and dorsal sphincter pressures measured by Gregg (unpublished data) in three patients by endoscopic manometry demonstrated basal sphincter pressures of 104, 136, and 400 mm Hg after dilation just adequate to permit manometry with a standard 1.7-mm-OD manometry cannula. Pressures measured by the same manometry system preoperatively, after minimal sphincter dilation at surgery just sufficient to permit manometry, ranged from 84 to 196 mm in six cases. It is likely that the basal sphincter pressures would have been even higher if one did not have to dilate the sphincter prior to manometry. Phasic wave activity was demonstrated in the dorsal sphincter. We also found that at least 50% of patients with pancreas divisum have coexistent choledochal sphincter dysfunction, as do many patients with incomplete pancreas divisum. In this condition, there is a minute connection between dorsal and ventral pancreatic ducts but the dorsal duct is the dominant drainage system. Clinically, it behaves similarly to pancreas divisum.

Thus it appears that pancreatic sphincter dysfunction is a cause of idiopathic pancreatitis. The etiology of the pain is probably elevated pancreatic duct pressures. Unfortunately, elevated pancreatic duct pressures in patients with pancreatitis do not always indicate sphincter dysfunction and may be a reflection solely of a high-viscosity juice due to chronic pancreatitis.[84] Pressures in the duct may also not be elevated during the nonsecretory period due to decompression of the duct through a patent dorsal ampulla. Since endoscopic measurement of pancreatic duct pressures alone is not adequate to determine the presence of sphincter dysfunction, endoscopic pancreatic sphincter manometry is important to determine the presence of pancreatic sphincter dysfunction. A small subset of patients have normal basal sphincter pressures and have a paradoxical CCK response as discussed elsewhere in the text.

Endoscopic Treatment of Pancreatic Sphincter Dysfunction and/or Stenosis

Relatively few reports appeared until recently concerning endoscopic treatment of disorders of the pancreatic sphincter. Endoscopic treatment of pancreatic disease is discussed in detail in Chapter 10 and will be reviewed only briefly here with regard to pancreatic sphincter disease.

A small number of investigators reported improvement in pancreatitis after sphincterotomy of the dorsal duct sphincter in patients with pancreas divisum[93-95]; the author treated three such patients endoscopically with good results. Poor results have also been reported.[96] ES may have a place in the treatment of pancreas divisum, but the technique is difficult and the safety of the procedure has not been established. There has been a trend in favor of stents for these patients rather than sphincterotomy.[97-100] We have had good results in 7 of 10 patients treated with hydrostatic balloon dilation. Ultimately, these techniques must be compared to surgical sphincteroplasty. If the gallbladder is in situ and there is coexistent SO dysfunction, these patients are better treated by surgery, which should include cholecystectomy.

The treatment of stenosis or dysfunction of the ventral pancreatic sphincter is similar but easier than that of dorsal sphincter disorders because of greater accessibility. Similar modalities have been used, including sphincterotomy of the pancreatic sphincter,[101] balloon dilation,[103-105] and stents.[99,106] The author performed sphincterotomy in 33 patients from 1978 to 1981 with normalization of sphincter pressures in most and resolution of pain in all but two. Pancreatitis occurred in three patients, one severe. More recently, hydrostatic dilatation with a 4-mm balloon was performed in 12 patients, again with normalization of pressures and improvement or resolution of pain in all, but with two instances of pancreatitis, one severe. Guelrud et al[105] had good results with a 4- or 6-mm balloon, but a 43% incidence of pancreatitis which probably was related to the use of the larger, 6-mm balloon which we prefer to avoid. Subsequently, Guelrud et al[107] reported that somatostatin infusion begun prior to the procedure significantly decreases the frequency and severity of pancreatitis. This concept requires further evaluation.

Endoscopic treatment of pancreatic sphincter dysfunction has a place in the treatment of both sphincter stenosis and dysfunction, particularly those in whom medical therapy has been ineffective. However, endoscopic sphincterotomy and hydrostatic balloon dilation of the ventral and dorsal sphincters carry more risk than the same procedures when used to relieve biliary sphincter dysfunction. The risks must be compared to those of transabdominal sphincter surgery. The long-term relief of pancreatic sphincter dysfunction appears to be satisfactory with the endoscopic procedures. The place of endoscopic stents to relieve sphincter obstruction appears to be less apparent, and to be a temporary rather than permanent solution to the problem of pancreatic sphincter disorders.

Gastrointestinal Smooth Muscle Disorders Associated with Biliary-Pancreatic Sphincter Dysfunction

Although the majority of patients with biliary-pancreatic sphincter disorders are either pain-free or markedly improved after sphincterotomy or sphincteroplasty, some are not. This may be related to associated pancreatitis or inadequate sphincteroplasty, or restenosis of the sphincter, especially the pancreatic sphincter. There may be persistent upper abdominal and/or low chest pain which is different from the patient's biliary-pancreatic pain, or persistent nausea and/or vomiting. The author observed that some of these patients had esophageal motility disorders or functional bowel disorders. This association has been noted by others as well.[108–110] For example, of 43 postcholecystectomy patients with right upper quadrant pain, 18 had elevated bile duct basal sphincter pressures greater than 35 mm Hg and 9 had an esophageal motility disorder consisting of high-amplitude contractions. Esophageal dysmotility occurred priniciplly in those with elevated basal pressures in either the biliary or pancreatic duct sphincters.[108]

In 47 consecutive patients with biliary-pancreatic sphincter dysfunction we did gastric emptying studies and esophageal manometry. Most of the patients had elevated biliary basal sphincter pressures, and both biliary and pancreatic sphincters were dysfunctional or stenotic in 19. Delayed gastric emptying was documented in 12 cases using an egg white meal labeled with [^{99}Tc]sulfur colloid with 55–90% retention at 60 min with an average of 76% (normal less than 50%). Two of these patients had pyloric stenosis. Neither had a history of peptic ulcer disease and both required hydrostatic balloon dilation of the pylorus for relief of pyloric stenosis. Metoclopramide relieved symptoms of gastric retention in the remaining subjects. Seven patients in this group had esophageal motility disorders. These were achalasia (2), diffuse esophageal spasm (2), hypertensive LES (2), and a variant of nutcracker esophagus (1). Other problems were migraine headaches (6) and functional bowel disorders (7).

It appears that biliary-pancreatic sphincter dysfunction probably represents part of a spectrum of smooth muscle disorders which affect many areas of the digestive tract and may also involve the cerebral arteries.

Conclusions

Dysfunction of the biliary and pancreatic sphincters has long been recognized as a cause of recurrent or constant upper abdominal pain. These disorders are recognized principally in the postcholecystomized patient and are the principle cause of postcholecystectomy biliary-pancreatic pain. They comprise a diverse group of disorders including hypersensitivity to narcotics, paradoxical response to CCK or fat similar to that of the lower esophageal sphincter in achalasia, and other as yet undefined neuromuscular abnormalities of the sphincter which probably will ultimately compose the major portion of these disorders. They occur frequently as part of a pandysautonomia of the upper gastrointestinal tract and may be associated with poor gallbladder function, esophageal motility disorders, gastric emptying disorders, and functional bowel problems. They also occur frequently in association with pancreas divisum and pancreas divisum variant.

Diagnosis has been facilitated by endoscopic biliary-pancreatic sphincter manometry, but challenge studies with fatty meals or CCK-OP may be needed to detect sphincter dysfunction in some patients during manometry. A number of other studies, including ERCP with demonstration of a dilated bile duct and delayed drainage, hepatobiliary scintigraphy, fatty meal ultrasonography, particularly in the postcholecystectomized patient, evaluation of gallbladder function with CCK-OP or a fatty meal, or provocative tests with morphine-neostigmine, are also helpful diagnostic tests. No one test alone will detect sphincter dysfunction in all patients.

Treatment with a low-fat diet and elimination of drugs which precipitate episodes of pain will be helpful in less than 50% of cases. Treatment with calcium channel blockers appears promising. Persistent or severe recurrent pain can be relieved by either endoscopic or surgical sphincteroplasty in the majority of patients. Treatment failures are either due to coexistent pancreatic sphincter dysfunction, pancreatitis, or associated functional disorders of the upper GI tract.

References

1. Meltzer SJ: The disturbance of the law of contrary innervation as a pathogenic factor in the diseases of the bile ducts and gallbladder. *Am J Med Sci* 1917;153:469–472.
2. Berg J: Studies on function of biliary ducts. *Acta Chir Scand* 1922:suppl. 2,1–185.
3. Del Valle D, and Donovan R: Coledoco-Odditis retractil cronica concepto clinico y quirurgico. *Arch Argnt Enerm Ap Diges* 1926;4:1–6.
4. McGowan JM, Butsch WL, Walters W: Pressure in the common bile duct of man: its relation to pain following cholecystectomy. *J Am Med Assoc* 1936;106:2227–2230.
5. Ivy AC, Voegtlin WI, and Greengard H: Physiology of common bile duct. *J Am Med Assoc* 1933:100:1319–1320.
6. Best RR, and Hicken NF: Cholangiographic demonstration of biliary dyssenergia. *J Am Med Assoc* 1936;107:1615–1620.
7. Boyden EA: Hypertrophy of the sphincter choledochus, a cause of internal biliary fistula. *Surgery* 1941;10:567–571.
8. Ivy AC: Motor dysfunction of the biliary tract. *Am J Roentegerol Rad Tor* 1947;57:1–11.
9. Trommald JF, and Seabrook DB: Benign fibrosis of the sphincter of Oddi. Report of 8 cases. *World J Surg* 1950;58:84–88.
10. Colp R: Treatment of postoperative biliary dyskinesia; Report of 8 cases of endocoledochal sphincterotomy. *Gastroenterology* 1946;7:414–417.
11. Cattell RB, Colcock BP, and Pollack JL: Stenosis of the sphincter of Oddi. *N Engl J Med* 1957;256:429–435.
12. Grage TB, Lober PH, Imamoglu K, and Wangensteen OH: Stenosis of sphincter of Oddi. A clinicopathological review of 50 cases. *Surgery* 1960;48:304–317.

13. Partington PP: Sphincterotomy for stenosis of the Sphincter of Oddi. *Surg Gynec Obstet* 1966;143:2282–2288.
14. Wise RE, and O'Brien RG: Interpretation of the intravenous cholangiogram. *J Am Med Assoc* 1956;160:819–827.
15. Rose JD: Serial cholecystography: A means of preoperative diagnosis of biliary dyskinesia. *Arch Surg* 1959;78:56–58.
16. Nardi GL, and Acosta JM: Papillitis as a cause of pancreatitis and abdominal pain: Role of evocative test, operative pancreatography and histologic evaluation. *Ann Surg* 1966;164:611–621.
17. Nebel OT: Manometric evaluation of the papilla of Vater. Gastrointest Endosc. *Gastroint Endosc* 1975;21:126–128.
18. Funch-Jensen P, Csendes A, Kruse A, Oster MJ, and Amdrup E: Common bile duct and Oddi sphincter pressure before and after endoscopic papillotomy in patients with common duct stones. *Ann Surg* 1979;190:176–178.
19. Geenen JE, Hogan WJ, Schaffer RD, Stewart ET, Dodds WJ, and Arndorfer RC: Endocscopic electrosurgical papillotomy and manometry in biliary tract disease. *J Am Med Assoc* 1977;237:2075–2078.
20. Hagenmueller F, Ossenberg FW, and Classen M: Duodenoscopic manometry of the common bile duct. The sphincter of Oddi *Proceedings of the 3rd Gastrointestinal Symposium*. Nice, 1976. Basel, Karger, 1977, pp 72–76.
21. Carr-Locke DL, and Gregg JA: Endoscopic manometry of pancreatic and biliary sphincters; Findings in biliary and pancreatic disease and after sphincter surgery. *Am J Gastroenterol* 1979;72:333 (abstract).
22. Csendes A, Kruse A, Funch-Jensen P, Oster MJ, Ornsholt J, and Amdrup E: Pressure measurements in the biliary and pancreatic duct system in controls and in patients with gallstones, previous cholecystectomy or common bile duct stones. *Gastroenterology* 1979;77:1203–1210.
23. Geenen JE, Hogan WJ, Dodds WJ, Stewart ET, and Arndorfer RC: Intraluminal pressure recordings from the human sphincter of Oddi. *Gastroenterology* 1980;78:317–328.
24. Rosch W, Koch H, Demling L: Manometric studies during ERCP and endoscopic papillotomy. *Endoscopy* 1976;8:30–33.
25. Carr-Locke DL, and Gregg JA: Endoscopic manometry of pancreatic and biliary sphincter zones in man. *Dig Dis Sci* 1981;26:7–15.
26. Bar-Meir S, Geenen JE, Hogan WJ, Dodds WJ, Stewart ET, and Arndorfer RC: Biliary and pancreatic duct pressures measured by ERCP manometry in patients with suspected papillary stenosis. *Dig Dis Sci* 1979;24:209–213.
27. Toouli J, Roberts-Thomson C, Dent J, and Lee J: Manometric disorders in patients with suspected sphincter of Oddi dysfunction. *Gastroenterology* 1985;88:1243–1250.
28. Tanaka M, Ikeda S, and Nakayama F: Nonoperative measurement of pancreatic and common bile duct pressures with a microtransducer catheter and effects of duodenoscopic sphincterotomy. *Dig Dis Sci* 1981;26:545–552.
29. von Vondrasek P, and Eberhardt G: Endoskopische Druckmessungen mittels Halbleitertechnik. *Z. Gastroenterol* 1974;12:453–458.
30. Guelrud M, Mendoza S, Rossiter G, and Villegas M: Sphincter of Oddi manometry in healthy volunteers. *Gastroenterology* 1988;94:(abstract).
31. Funch-Jensen P, Kruse A, and Ravnsbaek J: Endoscopic sphincter of Oddi manometry in healthy volunteers. *Scand J Gastroenterol* 1987;22:243–249.
32. Torsoli A, Corazziara E, Habib FI, De Masi E, Biliotti D, Mazzarella R, Giubilei D, and Fegiz G: Frequencies and cyclical pattern of the human sphincter of Oddi phasic activity. *Gut* 1986;27:363–369.
33. Hogan WJ, Geenen JE, Venu RP, Dodds WJ, Helm JF, and Toouli J: Abnormally rapid phasic contractions of the human sphincter of Oddi: (tachyoddia). *Gastroenterology* 1983;84:1189 (abstract).

34. Toouli J, Geenen JE, Hogan WJ, Dodds WJ, and Arndorfer RC: Sphincter of Oddi motor activity: a comparison between patients with common bile duct stones and controls. *Gastroenterology* 1982;82:111–117.
35. Boyden EA: The sphincter of Oddi in man and certain representative mammals. *Surgery* 1937;1:25–37.
36. King CE, Kalvaria I, and Sninsky CA: Pancreatitis due to endoscopic biliary manometry. Proceed with caution. *Gastroenterology* 1988;94:A227.
37. Toouli J, Hogan WJ, Geenen JE, Dodds WJ, and Arndorfer RC: Action of cholecystokinin-octapeptide on sphincter of Oddi basal pressure and phasic wave activity in humans. *Surgery* 1982;92:497–503.
38. Carr-Locke DL, and Bentley S: Endoscopic manometry evaluation of exogenous cholecystokinin octapeptide on the pancreatic and biliary sphincters of man. *Gut* 1984;25:A1328.
39. Carr-Locke DL, Gregg JA, and Chey WY: Effect of exogenous secretin on pancreatic and biliary ductal and sphincteric pressures in man demonstrated by endoscopic manometry and correlated with plasma secretin levels. *Am J Gastroenterol* 1979;72:333.
40. Venu RP, and Geenen JE: Diagnosis and treatment of diseases of the papilla. *Clin Gastroenterol* 1986;15:439–456.
41. Carr-Locke D, Gregg JA, and Aoki T: Effects of exogenous glucagon on pancreatic and biliary ductal and sphincteric pressures in man demonstrated by endoscopic manometry and correlation with plasma glucagon. *Dig Dis Sci* 1983;28:312–320.
42. Corraziari E, De Masi E, Gatti V, Battistini A, Habib FI, Pellegrini M, Fegiz GF, and Torsoli A: Effect of somatostatin (SRIF) on the sphincter of Oddi (SO) motor activity. *Gastroenterology* 1986;84:1130.
43. Hogan WJ, Geenen JE, Dodds WJ, Toouli J, Venu R, and Helm J: Paradoxical motor response to cholecystokinin (CCK-OP) in patients with suspected sphincter of Oddi dysfunction. *Gastroenterology* 1983;82:1085 (abstract).
44. Rolny P, Arlebäck A, Funch-Jensen P, Kruse A, Ravnsbaeck J, and Järnest G: Paradoxical response of sphincter of Oddi to intravenous injection of cholecystokinin or ceruletide. Manometric findings and results of treatment in biliary dyskinesia. *Gut* 1986;27:1507–1511.
45. Behar J, and Biancani P: Effect of cholecystokinin and the octapeptide of cholecystokinin on the feline sphincter of Oddi and gallbladder. *Am Soc Clin Invest* 1980;66:1231–1239.
46. Behar J, and Biancani P: Pharmacologic characterization of excitatory and inhibitory cholecystokinin receptors of the cat gallbladder and sphincter of Oddi. *Gastroenterology* 1987;92:764–770.
47. Bar-Meir S, Halpern Z, and Bardan E: Nitrate therapy in a patient with papillary dysfunction. *Am J Gastroenterol* 1983;78:94–95.
48. Staritz M, Poralla T, Ewe K, and Meyer zum Buschenfelde KH: Effect of glyceryl trinitrate on the sphincter of Oddi motility and baseline pressure. *Gut* 1985;26:194–197.
49. Staritz M, Poralla, T. Dormeyer H-H, Meyer zum Büschenfelde KH: Endoscopic removal of common bile duct stones through the intact papilla following medical sphincter dilatation. *Gastroenterology* 1988;88:1807–1811.
50. Venu R, Toouli J, Geenen JE, Hogan WJ, Helm J, Dodds WJ, and Arndorfer RC: Effect of morphine on motor activity of the human sphincter of Oddi. *Gastroenterology* 1983;84:1342 (abstract).
51. Staritz M, and Meyer zum Buschenfelde KH: Investigation of the effect of diazepam and other drugs on the sphincter of Oddi motility. *Ital J Gastroenterol* 1986;18:41.
52. Garrigues V, Ponce J, Perejo V, Sala T, Berenguer J: Effects of atropine and pirenzipine on sphincter motility. A manometric study. *J Hepatol* 1986;3:247–250.
53. Meshkinpour H, Mullot M, Eckerling GB, and Bookman L: Bile duct dyskinesia. Clinical and manometric study. *Gastroenterology* 1984;87:759–762.

54. Laszlo S, and Sandor EK: A hipertonias Oddi-szfinkter diszkinezis kezelese Kalcium-antagonista szerekkel. *Orv Hetil* 1983;124:2805–2809.
55. Guelrud M, Mendoza S, Rossiter G, Ramirez L, and Barkin J: Effect of nifedipine on sphincter of Oddi motor activity: Studies in healthy volunteers and patients with biliary dyskinesia. *Gastroenterology* 1988;95:1050–1055.
56. Thune A, Thornell E, and Svanvik J: Reflex regulation of flow resistance in the feline sphincter of Oddi by hydrostatic pressure in the biliary tract. *Gastroenterology* 1986;91:1364–1369.
57. Grace PA, Muller EL, Conter RL, Roslyn JJ, Taylor IA, and Pitt HA: Peptide YY inhibits sphincter of Oddi phasic wave activity in the prairie dog. *Gastroenterology* 1985;88:1402 (abstract).
58. Grace PA, Couse NF, and Pitt HA: Peptide YY inhibits cholecystokinin (CCK) stimulated sphincter of Oddi activity in the prairie dog. *Gastroenterology* 1986;90:1435 (abstract).
59. Chapman WP, Herrera R, and Jones CM: Comparison of pain produced experimentally inlower esophagis, common bile duct and upper intestine with pain experienced by patients with diseases of the biliary tract and pancreas. *Surg Gynec Obstet* 1949;89:573–582.
60. Ravdin IS, Fitzhugh T, Jr, Wolferth CC, Barbieri EA, Ravdin RG: Relation of gallstone disease to angina pectoris. *Arch Surg* 1955;70:333–342.
61. Ravdin IS, Royster HP, and Sanders GP: Reflexes originating in the common duct giving rise to pain simulating angina pectoris. *Ann Surg* 1942;115:1055.
62. Doran F: Sites of pain referred from the common bile duct. *Br J Surg* 1967;54:599–606.
63. Kingham JCG, and Dawson AM: Origin of chronic right upper quadrant pain. *Gut* 1985;26:783–788.
64. Roberts-Thomson IC, and Toouli J: Abnormal responses to morphine-neostigmine in patients with undefined biliary type pain. *Gut* 1985;26:1367–1372.
65. Madura JA, McCammon RL, Paris JM, Jesseph JE: The Nordi test and biliary manometry in the diagnosis of pancreatobiliary sphincter dysfunction. *Surgery* 1981;90:588–595.
66. LoGiudice JA, Geenen JE, Hogan WJ, and Dodds WJ: Efficacy of the morphine-prostigmine test for evaluating patients with suspected papillary stenosis. *Dig Dis Sci* 1979;24:455–458.
67. Steinberg WM, Salvato RF, and Toskes PP: The morphine-Prostigmin provocative test: is it useful for making clinical decisions? *Gastroenterology* 1980;78:728–731.
68. Warshaw AL, Simeone J, Schapiro RH, Hedberg SE, Mueller PE, Ferrucci JT, Jr: Objective evaluation of ampullary stenosis with ultrasonography and pancreatic stimulation. *Am J Surg* 1985;149:65–72.
69. Lee RG, Gregg JA, Koroshetz, AM, Hill TC, Clouse ME: Sphincter of Oddi stenosis: diagnosis using hepatobiliary scintigraphy and endoscopic manometry. *Radiology* 1985;156:793–796.
70. Zeman RK, Burrell MI, and Dobbins J, et al: Postcholecystectomy syndrome: Evaluation using biliary scintigraphy and endoscopic retrograde cholangiopancreatography. *Radiology* 1985;156:787–792.
71. Shaffer EA, Hershfield NB, Logan K, and Kloiber R: Cholescintigraphic detection of functional obstruction of the sphincter of Oddi: Effect of papillotomy. *Gastroenterology* 1986;90:728–733.
72. Aronchick CA, Ritchie W, Kaplan S, Wright SH, Retig JN, and Lipschutz WH: Bile duct pathology, defined by ERCP and sphincter of Oddi (SO) manometry, correlates with sincalide (S) aided ultrasonography of the common bile duct (CBD). *Gastroint Endosc* 1986;32:153A.
73. Darweesh R, Dodds WJ, Hogan WJ, Geenen JE, Collier BD, Shaker R, and Kishk S: Efficacy of quantitative hepatibiliary scintigraphy and fatty-meal sonography for detecting partial common duct obstruction. *Gastroenterology* 1987;92:1363A.

74. Gregg JA, Carr-Locke DL: Endoscopic pancreatic and biliary manometry in pancreatic, biliary and papillary disease, and after endoscopic sphincterotomy and surgical sphincteroplasty. *Gut* 1984;25:1247–1254.
75. Mustard R, Jr, Mackenzie R, Jamieson C, Haber GB: Surgical complications of endoscopic sphincterotomy. *Can J Surg* 1984;27:215–217.
76. Seifert E, Gail K, Weismuller J: Langzeitresultate nach endoskopischer sphinkterotomie. *Dtsch Med Wschr* 1982;107:610–614.
77. Thatcher BS, Sivak MV, Tedesco FJ, Vennes JA, Hutton SW, and Achkari EA: Endoscopic sphincterotomy for suspected dysfunction of the sphincter of Oddi. *Gastroint Endosc* 1987;33:91–95.
78. Leese T, Neoptolemos JP, Carr-Locke DL: Successes, failures, early complications and their management following endoscopic sphincterotomy: Results in 394 consecutive patients from a single center. *Br J Surg* 1985;72:215–219.
79. Roberts-Thomson IC, and Toouli J: Is endoscopic sphincterotomy for disabling biliary-type pain after cholecystectomy effective? *Gastroint Endosc* 1985;31:370–373.
80. Carr-Locke DL, Bailey I, Neoptolemos JP, Leese T, and Heath D: Outcome of endoscopic sphincterotomy for papillary stenosis. *Gut* 1986;27:A1280.
81. Tanaka M, Ikeda S, Matsumato S, Yoshimato H, and Nakayama F: Manometric diagnosis of sphincter of Oddi spasm as a cause of post-cholecystectomy pain and its treatment by endoscopic sphincterotomy. *Ann Surg* 1985;202:712–719.
82. Geenen JE, Hogan WJ, Toouli J, Dodds WJ, and Venu RP: A prospective randomized study of the efficacy of endoscopic sphincterotomy for patients with presumptive sphincter of Oddi dysfunction. *Gastroenterology* 1984;86:(abstract).
83. Geenen JE, Hogan WJ, Dodds WJ, Toouli J, and Venu RP: The efficacy of endoscopic sphincterotomy in patients with sphincter-of-oddi dysfunction. *N Engl J Med* 1989;320:82–87.
84. Okazaki K, Yamamoto Y, Nishimori I, and Nishioka T: Motility of the sphincter of Oddi and pancreatic main ductal pressure in patients with alcholic, gallstone-associated, and idiopathic chronic pancreatitis. *Am J Gastroenterol* 1988;83:820–826.
85. Novis BH, Bornman PC, Girdwood AW, and Marks IN: Endoscopic manometry of the pancreatic duct and sphincter zone in patients with chronic pancreatitis. *Dig Dis Sci* 1985;30:225–228.
86. Rolny P, Arleback A, Jarnerot G, and Andersson T: Endoscopic manometry of the sphincter of Oddi and pancreatic duct in chronic pancreatitis. *Scand J Gastroenterol* 1986;21:415–420.
87. Toouli J, Roberts-Thomson IC, Dent J, and Lee J: Sphincter of Oddi motility disorders in patients with idiopathic recurrent pancreatitis. *Br J Surg* 1985;72:18–63.
88. Guelrud M, and Siegel JH: Hypertensive pancreatic duct sphincter as a cause of pancreatitis. Successful treatment with hydrostatic balloon dilatation. *Dig Dis Sci* 1984;29:225–231.
89. Guelrud M, Mendoza S, and Viera L: Idiopathic recurrent pancreatitis and hypercontractile sphincter of Oddi. Treatment with endoscopic sphincterotomy and pancreatic duct dilation. *Gastroenterology* 1986;90:1443 (abstract).
90. Hogan WJ, Geenen JE, Kruidenier J, Venu RP, Helm J, Dodds WJ, and Wilson SD: Ineffectiveness of conventional sphincteroplasty in relieving pancreatic duct sphincter pressure in patients with idiopathic recurrent pancreatitis. *Gastroenterology* 1983;84:1189 (abstract).
91. Venu RP, Geenen JE, and Hogan WJ: Idiopathic recurrent pancreatitis (IRP): diagnostic role of ERCP and sphincter of Oddi manometry. *Gastroint Endosc* 1985;31:141 (abstract).
92. Staritz M, Hutteroth T, Manns M, and Meyer zum Buschenfelde KH: Pancreas divisum: praedisposition zur chronischen pankratitis durch chronischen sekretstau. *Deutsch Med Wochen* 1986;111:421–423.
93. Sahel J, Boustiere C, Sarles J-C, Chevillote G, Sarles H: Traitment du pancreas divisum. Resultats preliminaires. *Gastroenterol Clin Biol* 1983;7:293–298.

94. Liguory C, Lefebvre JF, Canard TM, Bonnel D, and Etienne JP: Pancreas divisum: therapeutic results in 12 patients. *Dig Dis Sci* 1986;31(suppl):530S (abstract).
95. Gregg JA, Monaco AP, and McDermott WV: Pancreas divisum. Results of surgical intervention. *Am J Surg* 1983;145:488–492.
96. Russell RCG, Wong NW, and Cotton PB: Accessory sphincterotomy (endoscopic and surgical) in patients with pancreas divisum. *Br J Surg* 1984;71:954–957.
97. Pullano W, Siegel JH, Ramsey WH, and Cooperman A: Pancreas divisum: The camps are divided—to decompress preoperatively is the answer. *Gastroenterology* 1986;32:153 A58.
98. Pullano W, Siegel JH, Ramsey WH, and Cooperman A: Effectiveness of endoscopic drainage in patients with pancreas divisum: Endoscopic and surgical results in 31 patients. *Gastroint Endosc* 1986;81:887 (Abstract).
99. McCarthy J, Geenen JE, and Hogan WJ: Preliminary experience with endoscopic stent placement in benign pancreatic diseases. *Gastroint Endosc* 1988;34:16–18.
100. Grimm H, de Heer K, and Sohendra N: Endoscopic transpapillary drainage in chronic pancreatitis. *Dig Dis Sci* 1986;31suppl:530S (abstract).
101. Fuji T, Amano H, Aibe T, Asagami F, Kinukawa K, Ariyama S, and Takemoto T: Pancreatic sphincterotomy and pancreatic endoprosthesis. *Endoscopy* 1985;17:69–72.
102. Cotton PB: Pancreatic orifice sphincterotomy; experience from 15 centres. *Gut* 1983;24:A967.
103. Siegel JH, and Guelrud M: Endoscopic cholangiopancreatoplasty: hydrostatic balloon dilation in the bile duct and pancreas. *Gastroint Endosc* 1983;29:99–103.
104. Guelrud M, and Siegel JH: Hypertensive pancreatic duct sphincter as a cause of pancreatitis. Successful treatment with hydrostatic balloon dilation. *Dig Dis Sci* 1984;29:225–231.
105. Guelrud M, Mendoza S, and Viera L. Idiopathic recurrent pancreatitis and hypercontractile sphincter of Oddi. Treatment with endoscopic sphincterotomy and pancreatic duct dilation. *Gastroenterology* 1986;90:1443 (abstract).
106. Huibregste MD, Schneider B, Vrij AA, and Tytgat GNJ: Endoscopic pancreatic drainage in chronic pancreatitis. *Gastroint Endosc* 1988;34:9–15.
107. Guelrud M, Mendoza S, and Viera L: Does somatostatin prevent acute pancreatitis after pancreatic duct sphincter balloon dilatation? *Gastroint Endosc* 1987;33:148.
108. Sunshine A, Long WB, Marcus R, Smith H, and Ouyang A: Esophageal and biliary manometry in post-cholecystectomy patients with right upper quadrant pain. *Gastroenterology* 1986;90:1652A.
109. Burton FR, Knight WA, Jr: Esophageal motility patterns in patients with sphincter of Oddi dysfunction. *Am J Gastroenterol* 1986;81:882–A148.
110. Johnson DA, Cattau EL, and Winters C, Jr: Biliary dyskinesia with associated high amplitude esophageal peristaltic contractions. *Am J Gastroenterol* 1986;81:254–256.

Chapter 9

Endoscopic Management of Benign Biliary Strictures, Biliary Tract Fistulae, and Sclerosing Cholangitis

Jerome H. Siegel, M.D.

Introduction

Prior to the introduction of percutaneous and endoscopic techniques for the management of biliary tract strictures, the only methods available for their treatment were surgical.[1-3] These surgical techniques have generally been successful, but recurrences of strictures or complications subsequent to surgery occur as frequently as 25%. The most serious of the long-term complications of surgery are the formation of recurrent strictures, which most often occurs at the anastomotic site. This can lead to the development of jaundice, recurrent cholangitis, and, utimately, secondary biliary cirrhosis.

Biliary strictures are acquired, frequently resulting from injury to the bile duct during cholecystectomy and common duct exploration. A less frequent cause is recurrent inflammatory disease due to stones and consequent intermittent biliary tract infection. An inflammatory reaction induced by foreign material introduced at surgery, i.e., staples and clips, results in fibrosis and scar formation (Figure 9-1). Primary repair of bile duct strictures can be attempted initially, although a bypass procedure is preferred by most surgeons. Primary repair requires an experienced surgeon and a suitable length of common hepatic duct which can be mobilized for an anastomosis. If a stricture should develop as a sequela to primary repair, it can be successfully managed nonsurgically using either the percutaneous (radiologic) or endoscopic approach.[4-8]

The radiologic approach to biliary tract disorders will only be alluded to in this chapter; the major emphasis will be on the endoscopic techniques currently in use or in evolution. The management of malignant strictures, although similar in many ways to the handling of benign strictures, is also beyond the scope of this chapter.[9-15]

The use of endoscopically placed biliary stents in patients with bile duct fistulae is an exciting new treatment method which prevents bile from exiting through the fistula, thus avoiding a whole series of problems for the patient, and at the same time allowing the fistula to heal and close.

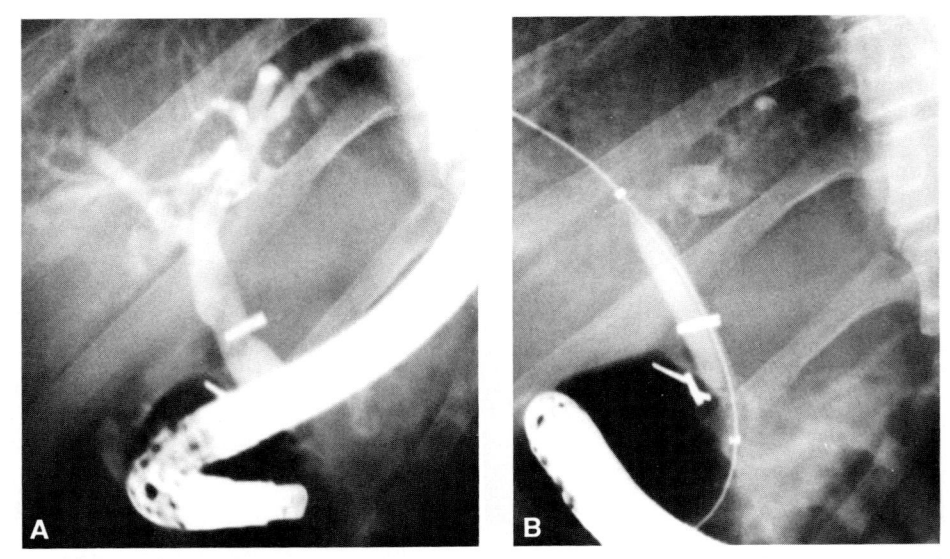

Figure 9-1 (A) Cholangiogram demonstrating stricture of common hepatic duct at site of surgical clip. **(B)** Dilating balloon inflated in stricture.

Sclerosing cholangitis, a disease that had formerly resisted all attempts at therapy and in which the patient ultimately succumbed to liver failure, is now definitively managed by liver transplantation. Endoscopic retrograde cholangiography plays a major role in the diagnosis of this entity, and we have shown that for patients awaiting transplant, or for those whose disease is relatively early, relief of cholestasis may be achieved by defining the strictures in the common bile duct and in the common hepatic duct and its major branches and dilating them with endoscopically placed balloon dilators.

ERCP as a Therapeutic Tool

As increased experience with endoscopic retrograde cholangiopancreatography (ERCP) accrues,[16–22] we have begun to appreciate the important contribution to the diagnosis and management of pancreatobiliary disorders that this technique makes. Although the diagnostic capabilities of ERCP are well accepted and have been available for some time, the evolution of therapeutic ERCP was relatively slow because it was dependent on the development of instrumentation, accessories, and, most importantly, experienced endoscopists. As experience with ERCP developed, a new appreciation of ductular morphology evolved, but when a lesion was identified, the patient was automatically referred to a surgeon for definitive care. A similar sequence had occurred at an earlier time with other endoscopic therapeutic techniques, i.e., polypectomy. As biliary and pancreatic accessories were introduced, aggressive endoscopists applied the experience gained in animal models and at necropsy to living patients. Many therapeutic techniques were developed at the outset on patients to whom a careful explanation of risks and alternatives was presented after consultation with their referring primary physicians.

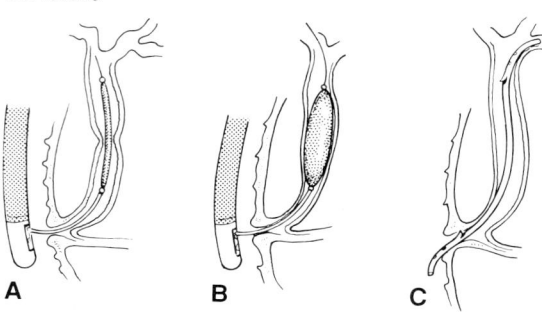

Figure 9-2 **(A)** Balloon catheter advanced over guidewire in stricture. **(B)** Balloon inflated to maximum diameter dilating stricture. **(C)** Prosthesis placed proximal to stricture to maintain lumen integrity.

Treatment of Benign Strictures

Benign, acquired biliary strictures are approached endoscopically by passing a catheter and guidewire through the stricture and, with the guidewire in place, advancing a dilating catheter over it. A balloon catheter is then passed over the guidewire so that the balloon engages the stricture and the balloon is then inflated to dilate the stricture[23-25] (Figure 9-2), resulting in the stretching and disruption of the collagen fibrils. The area that is dilated may slowly return to the predilation caliber over an indeterminate period of time; to prevent stricture reformation, insertion of a large-diameter prosthesis is performed immediately upon completion of the dilation (Figure 9-2).[28-31]

The initial step in endoscopic dilation of benign biliary strictures is the performance of ERCP in the usual manner with a standard 2.8-mm channel instrument (outer diameter of the insertion tube is 11 mm). After identifying the papilla, a cannula is inserted selectively into the bile duct and contrast is injected. Once the stricture is identified, my preference at this juncture is to perform a sphincterotomy to facilitate access to the bile duct. This approach avoids unnecessary trauma to the pancreas, especially when subsequent procedures or manipulation become necessary, such as when prostheses need to be changed. The sphincterotomy is tailored to permit insertion of a large-caliber prosthesis and should be approximately 1 cm in length. After the sphincterotomy is performed, the standard duodenoscope is removed and a large-channel instrument introduced. Currently, the largest production model therapeutic duodenoscope has a channel size of 4.2 mm and an insertion tube diameter of 13 mm. The sphincterotomy is cannulated, and a catheter-guidewire assembly is introduced into the bile duct distal to the stricture.[32] My preference for the dilating catheter is a Van Andel tapered catheter, 7-Fr, 180 cm long, or a 6-Fr guiding catheter. The guidewire, 0.035 in. × 350 cm long, is Teflon-coated and has an atraumatic or flexible tip. Under fluoroscopic control, the guidewire is passed into the stricture and manipulated until the stricture is traversed by the catheter-guidewire assembly. Once the guidewire is in the proximal biliary tree, the guiding catheter is removed leaving the wire in place. A 7-Fr dilating balloon catheter containing a polyethylene balloon which, when inflated, distends to a diameter of 6 mm and is 2 cm long, is then advanced over the wire through the sphincterotomy and into the stricture. If the stricture is tight and difficult to negotiate with the standard balloon catheter, a smaller balloon catheter containing a 4-mm balloon, 2 cm long, is used for initial dilation. Progressive dilation

174   J. H. SIEGEL

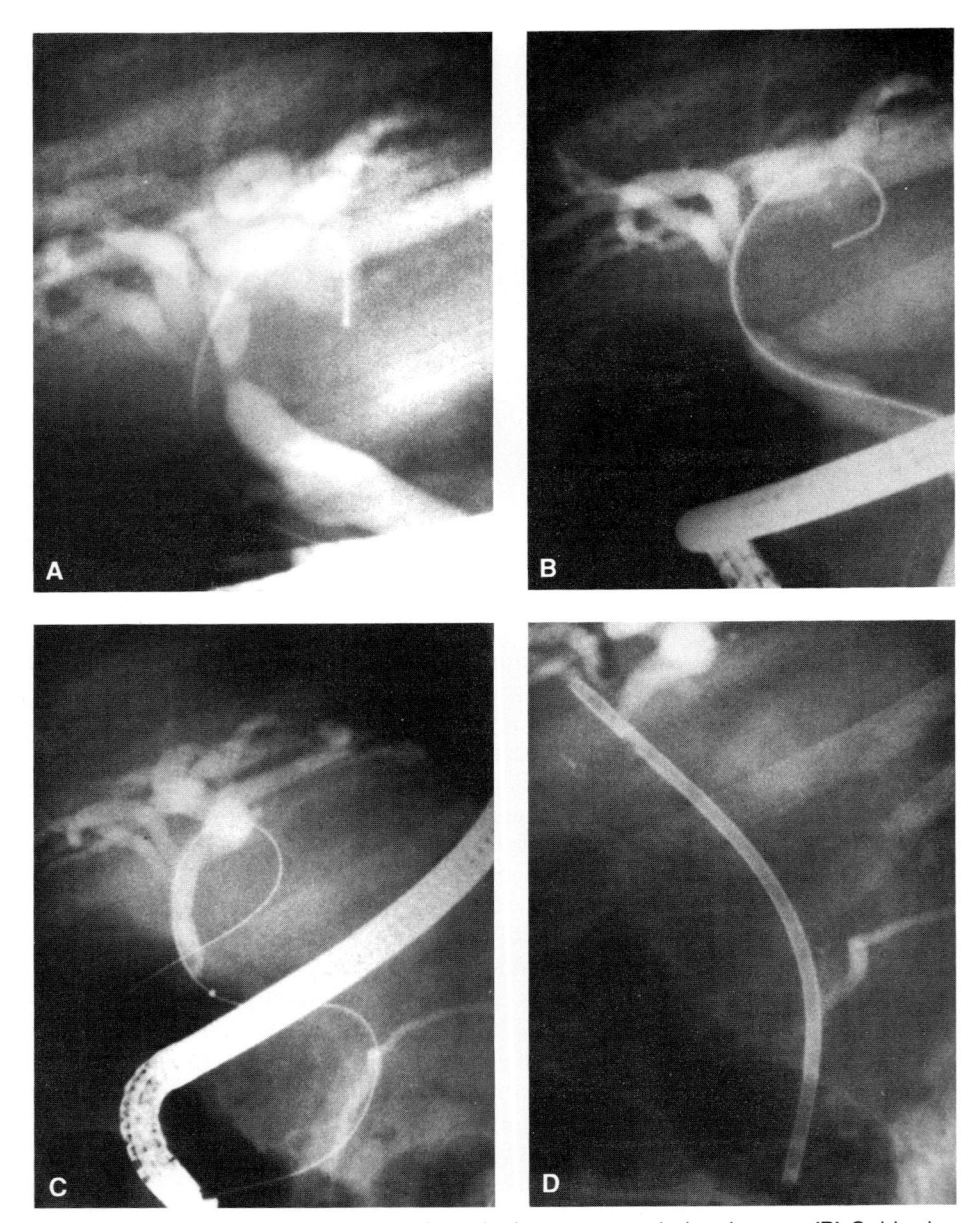

Figure 9-3 (A) Tight-stricture common hepatic duct seen on cholangiogram. **(B)** Guidewire advanced through stricture into left hepatic duct. **(C)** Balloon dilation of stricture carried out. **(D)** Large-caliber prosthesis placed through stricture.

of the stricture is then accomplished using 6-mm and 8-mm balloons sequentially. We inflate to 5 atm for 2 periods of 30 sec each. After adequately dilating the stricture, the guidewire is left in place and a large-caliber prosthesis advanced through the stricture, separated from the guidewire and left in position (Figure 9-3). If a stricture is present in the common hepatic duct and encroaches

ENDOSCOPIC MANAGEMENT OF BENIGN BILIARY STRICTURES 175

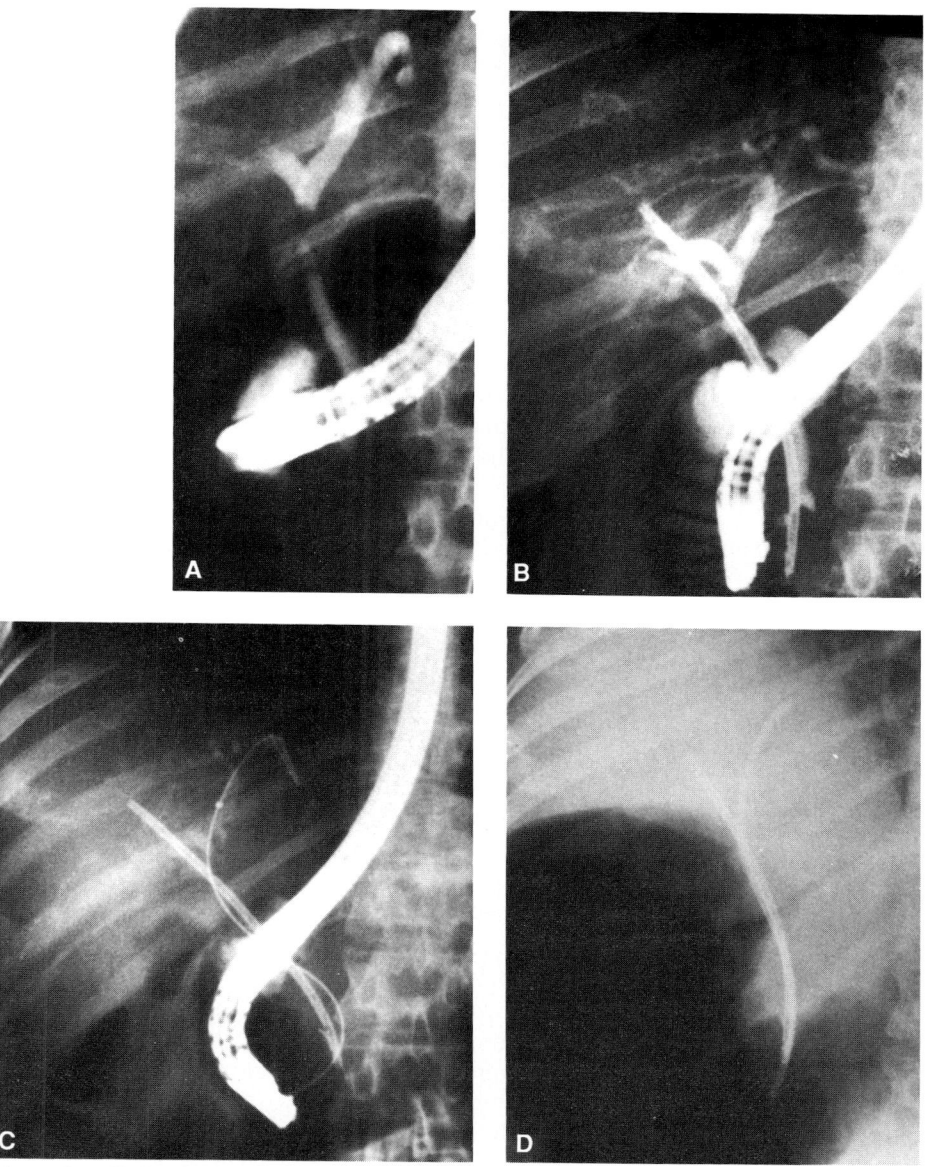

Figure 9-4 **(A)** Cholangiogram demonstrating postoperative stricture of common hepatic duct at bifurcation. **(B)** Large-caliber prosthesis placed into right hepatic duct. **(C)** Guidewire and balloon catheter passed through stricture into left hepatic duct. **(D)** Radiograph showing prostheses in both right and left hepatic ducts; patient asymptomatic 3 years.

on the bifurcation, an additional stent should be placed into the branch which has not already been decompressed (Figure 9-4).

In my experience, 33 consecutive patients with biliary strictures have been successfully treated in the above fashion (Tables 9-1 to 9-3). The major complications of balloon dilation, prior to the use of preprocedure antibiotics, were

Table 9-1 Distribution of Benign Biliary Strictures (*N* = 33)

Upper third	13
Middle third	12
Lower third	8

fever and chills (Table 9-4); this has been minimized by administering prophylactic antibiotics before the procedure.

All patients were successfully decompressed and improvement in cholestatic biochemical indices was noted: reduction of bilirubin, alkaline phosphatase, γ-glutamyl transpepsidase to normal or near-normal values. Patients reported subjective improvement of their symptoms in all cases as well.

No evidence of biliary cirrhosis or deteriorating liver function has been noted in this group.

Long-term results include a voluntary follow-up by either the patients or their referring physicians for the past 7 years. None of these patients has required surgical intervention.

Acceptance of the procedure by the patient includes a commitment to return for periodic stent change within a specified period (4–6 months). Some patients have opted to wait until symptoms occur, ie, pruritis, fever, or cholestasis, before returning for exchange of a prosthesis. None have experienced sepsis or were seriously ill on return for stent exchange. Compliance has been excellent with a patient return rate exceeding 90%. Hospital stay for stent exchange has been less than 2 days with a range of 1–5 days. Some authors recommend early stent exchange; my advice to the patient has been to return when symptoms recur. I arrived at this conclusion after realizing that none of my patients became seriously ill when the prosthesis was failing. I have only removed the prosthesis without replacing it in seven patients whose strictures I felt were no longer significant. These seven patients have all done well after removal of the stent with a mean follow-up time of 3.7 years (range 0.5–6 years). In the majority of patients the prosthesis is replaced when cholangiography performed after the removal of the old stent still demonstrates a significant stricture. Ultimately, the goal is for all prostheses to be removed when the strictures appear to have been permanently dilated on cholangiography.

The duration of stent patency in benign disease exceeds that of malignant disease by at least 50%. In malignant disease, the mean patency of an 11.5- or 12-Fr prosthesis is 195 days (range 3–450 days)[29] whereas in benign disease the mean patency exceeds 300 days. The mechanisms for occlusion of prostheses in both benign and malignant diseases is thought to be the same: formation of

Table 9-2 Patients with Benign Biliary Strictures

Females	21
Males	12
Age range	31–72 yrs
Mean age	53.4 yrs

Table 9-3 Results of Treatment of Benign Biliary Strictures ($N = 33$)

Successful dilations	33
Insertion of prostheses	26
Exchange of prostheses	19
Removal of prostheses	7

a biofilm containing bacteria and amorphous material on the inner walls of the stent, with further deposition of the products of bacterial enzyme action on bile, such as calcium bilirubinate formed by the action of β-glucuronidase on bilirubin diglucuronide.[32,33]

The longer duration of patency in benign disease may be explained by the fact that a benign stricture is static in contrast to the continuous growth and encroachment of a malignancy. It has also been suggested that the constant movement of the prosthesis in the bile duct might be responsible for perpetual dilation of the stricture.[34] It is thought that once a stricture is forcefully dilated and a large prosthesis placed to maintain the integrity of the lumen of the duct, the inert, nonreactive polyethylene tube functions as a continuous dilator, especially if the tubing moves freely in the strictured area.

The choice of material for the prosthesis is polyethylene due to its inert nature, and its construction is preferably that of a straight tube with side flaps to prevent migration. It has been shown[29,34,35] that the larger the prosthesis and the straighter its configuration, the greater the volume of flow will be through it, and the longer the prosthesis remains patent. We have also found that the larger the prosthesis placed, the more rapidly the patient improves clinically and biochemically and the longer the prosthesis will remain patent and functional.

In another relatively large series, Huibregtse et al[27] reported successful endoscopic therapy in 27 of 29 patients with benign postoperative biliary strictures. Their approach varied somewhat in that they inserted one or two 10-Fr endoprostheses in all their patients but reserved balloon dilation, or dilation with metal-tipped dilating catheters, for those patients (12 of 27) in whom the tightness or firmness of the stenosis prevented passage of a guidewire-containing catheter. Of 21 patients followed for over 6 months, 16 had excellent long-term results, with complete clearance of jaundice and/or no recurrence of cholangitis. The stents were removed in 6 patients after a mean of 20 months without adverse sequelae up to 15 months later. Radiographically, the strictures appeared adequately dilated in these patients. The authors noted that the stents were occasionally clogged even when the patient was well, leading them to speculate that intermittent movement of the stent may cause adjacent enlargement of the

Table 9-4 Complications

Fever	5 (15%)
Septicemia	1 (3%)
Surgery	0
Deaths	0

stricture, thus facilitating some flow around as well as through the tube. Nevertheless, they recommended stent exchange every 3 months and consideration of stent removal at 6 months if the patient is well and the stricture appears to be adequately dilated.

Whether all strictures that have been treated by balloon dilation require stenting has not been established conclusively. In a study of 73 patients who underwent percutaneous transphepatic balloon dilation with or without stenting by one of three interventional radiology groups, the data were insufficient to provide definite answers on the efficacy of long-term stenting.[36] Theoretical concerns raised about stenting include the possibility that stents will incite an inflammatory reaction with recurrence of the stricture soon after the tube is removed.[36] On the other hand, some radiologists feel strongly that stents are needed to ensure long-term patency.[37]

Although the available data are uncontrolled and nonrandomized, the experience to date suggests that endoscopic management of biliary strictures is a valid and exciting new approach to treatment. Further trials are needed to confirm this and to resolve issues related to variations in technique.

Biliary Fistulae

Biliary-cutaneous or biliary-peritoneal fistulae may develop following injury to the bile duct during cholecystectomy, or after surgical exploration of the common bile duct and placement of catheters and/or T tubes. If these tubes are removed or dislodged, and if there is obstruction of the distal common bile duct caused by a stone, stricture, or tumor, a fistula will develop[38] as bile flows antegrade through the path of least resistance: the catheter or catheter tract. In patients with T tubes in place, obstruction of the distal duct should be suspected when bile is seen leaking around the T tube, rapidly soiling the dressings. A T-tube cholangiogram is used to confirm this, and the obstruction can then be effectively relieved either by attempting to remove the stone through the T-tube tract percutaneously after maturation of the tract or endoscopically via the duodenoscope. Some patients may present with bile drainage through a T-tube tract/fistula following removal of their T tube. Before removing a T tube, the surgeon usually requests a cholangiogram which, if negative for retained stones or other obstructions to flow like spasm or strictures, is followed by removal of the T tube. If a residual stone is missed on the cholangiogram, it may migrate toward the papilla, subsequently producing obstruction to bile flow through the papilla, making the T-tube fistula the next best alternative path for the bile to take (Figure 9-5). This occurs more commonly than the development of a spontaneous fistula from the cystic duct stump, which can occur in cases of distal duct obstruction as well. The increased pressure in the bile duct that results can cause leakage through the cystic duct remnant especially if dislodgement of a ligature or staple occurs,[39] and a percutaneous fistula or peritoneal fistula may then develop.

Recognition of a percutaneous fistula is made by direct observation; a peritoneal fistula presents as a combination of abdominal signs and symptoms and physical findings of guarding or rebound tenderness. Confirmation of a percutaneous fistula can be easily accomplished by performing a radiologic examination, ie, sinogram or fistulogram. Confirmation of a peritoneal fistula requires endoscopic examination and retrograde cholangiography.

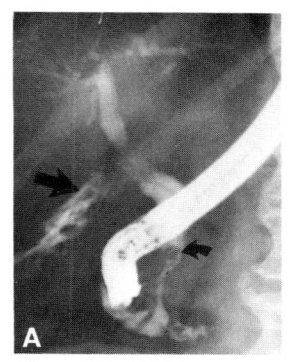

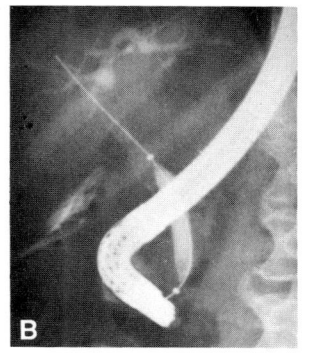

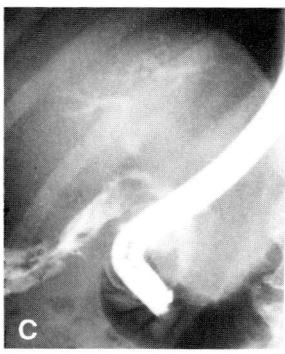

Figure 9-5 (A) Cholangiogram revealing stricture of distal common bile duct with stone (small arrow) seen proximal to stricture. Note percutaneous fistula (large arrow). **(B)** After sphincterotomy, balloon catheter placed into stricture and dilation accomplished. **(C)** Cholangiogram showing disappearance of stone and stricture.

My approach to the treatment of biliary fistulae is as follows: after performing an ERCP confirming the fistula and its location, I routinely perform a sphincterotomy in the usual manner. If an obstructing stone is present in the distal common bile duct, I remove it using a standard basket or occlusion balloon. A cholangiogram is repeated confirming that no other obstructing stones are present. After the repeat cholangiogram, I usually place a prosthesis which allows bile to flow from the proximal bile ducts to the duodenum allowing the fistula to heal spontaneously (Figure 9-6). The prosthesis is usually removed in 4–6 weeks and can be removed during an outpatient visit. A nasobiliary tube can also be used for this purpose but obviously for a shorter period of time. However, I prefer placing a large-caliber endoprosthesis which allows the patient more freedom of movement and an earlier discharge from hospital.

In my experience, successful treatment of 18 patients with biliary fistulae was accomplished incorporating either endoscopic sphincterotomy and/or insertion of prostheses as part of the standard regimen. Fourteen of the fistulae were percutaneous (Table 9-5), 11 closed spontaneously after sphincterotomy, and 7 (3 percutaneous, 4 peritoneal) closed after insertion of a prosthesis[7] (Table 9-6). The rationale for placing a prosthesis in the bile duct of a patient presenting with a bile fistula is as follows: if antegrade flow of bile is reestablished by opening the sphincter (sphincterotomy), bile will flow through the path of least resistance, thus reducing the flow through the fistulous tract allowing formation of granulation tissue and closure of the fistula. Following sphincterotomy, however, edema of the distal common bile duct may occur, paradoxically *increasing* flow through the fistulous tract. This problem is easily remedied by inserting a prosthesis, either of the nasobiliary or transduodenal type, within 48–72 hours.

Table 9-5 Biliary Fistulae

Type of fistulae	
Cutaneous	14
Intraperitoneal	4

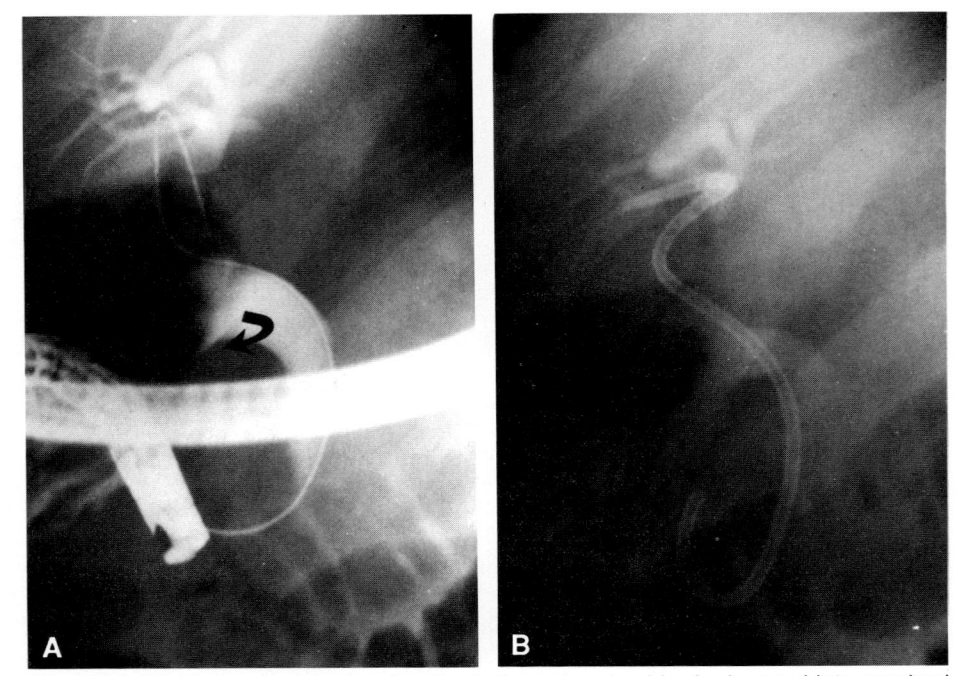

Figure 9-6 (A) Cholangiogram showing fistula (arrow) and guidewire inserted into proximal bile duct. **(B)** Stent (prosthesis) seen in proximal biliary tree allowing bile to drain into duodenum.

Preferential flow of bile through a prosthesis which has been placed proximal to the fistulous tract and extending into the duodenum promotes granulation tissue formation and closure of the tract. Using this technique, I have seen rapid closure of even large-caliber fistulous tracts.

Four patients with intraperitoneal fistulae were referred to me and responded to identical therapy. Two of these patients developed fistulae due to rupture of the cystic duct stump, and two patients developed them due to bile duct injury; in both cases peritonitis resulted. Early documentation of the fistula by ERCP and prompt therapeutic intervention by sphincterotomy and stent placement resulted in rapid improvement and recovery in these patients. This is remarkable when one considers that up until recently the only management for these cases was urgent surgical intervention.

Among other authors who have utilized ERCP for the treatment of biliary fistulas,[38–44] Smith et al[38] treated five patients with biliary-cutaneous fistulas by inserting 7–10 French internal stents endoscopically in four and percutaneously

Table 9-6 Treatment Modalities for Biliary Cutaneous or Peritoneal Fistulae

Sphincterotomy	*Sphincterotomy-Protheses*
Cutaneous, 11	Cutaneous, 3
	Peritoneal, 4

in one. In only one patient treated endoscopically was a sphincterotomy performed at the time of stent placement. Drainage from the fistulaes ceased within 3–7 days in all patients, although the stents were kept in place for 4 or more weeks. Prompt cessation of drainage from biliary-cutaneous fistulaes was also reported in four patients by Sauerbruch et al,[39] two of whom received 7-French endoprostheses and two others nasobiliary tubes. None were reported to have had a sphincterotomy. Percutaneous stent placement can also be effective in closing fistulae, as shown by Kaufman et al.[45] Of 12 patients with biliary leaks, drainage ceased permanently in six.

It has been argued that endoscopic sphinterotomy alone provides effective treatment for postoperative external biliary fistulaes, as it was within 3–5 days in all seven patients in a recent series.[44] This series was somewhat atypical in that four of the patients had fistulaes after operations for hydatid cysts of the liver. Although sphincterotomy alone may be successful in selected patients, it is not appropriate when the fistula is proximal to any sort of obstructing process in the bile duct.

In summary, biliary fistulae, both percutaneous and peritoneal, can be effectively evaluated and treated by endoscopic means, reducing the morbidity of what formerly was considered a major complication. Prolonged periods of hospitalization for these problems have been considerably reduced since endoscopic management has been implemented, and physicians should be made aware of these improved techniques so that the appropriate referrals can be made.

Sclerosing Cholangitis

The etiology and treatment of primary sclerosing cholangitis has been an enigma for clinicians for many years. Many medical and surgical approaches to this disorder have been described with few sustained remissions or cures.[46–48]

The different medical and surgical treatment modalities historically employed in the treatment of this serious entity are seen in Table 9-7. Endoscopic intervention in this disease has been a relatively new development and preliminary results have been promising.[49–52] We previously described our preliminary results[49] in the management of sclerosing cholangitis using several endoscopic

Table 9-7 Therapy for Sclerosing Cholangitis

Medical	*Surgical*
Cholestyramine	Colectomy
Steroids	Cholecystectomy
Azathioprine	Choledochostomy
Penicillamine	T-tube/tube insertion
Colchicine	Sphincteplasty
Methotrexate	Biliary-enteric bypass and/or Roux limb placed subcutaneously
Endoscopic	
Sphincterotomy	
Cholangioplasty	
Endoprosthesis	
Nasobiliary tube	

Table 9-8 Patients with Sclerosing Cholangitis, Demographics

Males	25
Females	11
Age range	17–63 yr
Mean age	31.4 yr

treatment modalities including sphincterotomy, nasobiliary tube perfusion, catheter and/or balloon dilation of dominant strictures, and insertion of prostheses to maintain duct patency. From this initial series, our work has expanded to include a total of 36 patients who have all benefited from a combination of these treatment modalities[52] (Table 9-8). We found that in about 10% of patients with extrahepatic duct strictures in sclerosing cholangitis, balloons and/or prostheses cannot be placed.

Our initial approach to the treatment of patients with sclerosing cholangitis included balloon dilation of the dominant stricture and insertion of a nasobiliary catheter (Figure 9-7) for perfusion of steroids, antibiotics, and saline. Four patients were treated in this fashion with improvement in both their cholestatic biochemical parameters and in their constitutional symptoms. The nasobiliary catheter remained in place for a minimum of 3 months. Initial hospital management made use of an I-Med infuser pump, which was connected to the nasobiliary catheter and used to administer the agents desired. Patients were later taught to irrigate and perfuse the catheter with antibiotics and saline alternately four times a day using a 30-cm^3 syringe. They continued this regimen for 3–4 months and cholangiography performed at specific intervals during this time revealed some improvement in the morphology of the affected ducts paralleling the improvement of their cholestatic biochemical picture. Initial work in this area from Amsterdam[50] utilizing lavage with saline and prednisolone via a nasobiliary tube in eight patients suggested even more significant morphologic improvement than we found in our series. Geenen's group[51] also reported significant improvement in patients with sclerosing cholangitis who had been treated endoscopically. Following endoscopic sphincterotomy, Gruntzig-type balloons were used to dilate strictures in 10 patients with prior attacks of cholangitis. Stents were placed in three because of persistent high-grade strictures after balloon dilation. In an unspecified number of these patients, biliary sludge and stones were removed after sphincterotomy. Following these procedures, the authors observed a significant decrease in the frequency of hospitalizations for cholangitis and significant improvement in liver tests.

Currently, our approach in preparing to treat the strictures of sclerosing cholangitis is to first perform ERCP in the usual manner. Once the bile duct is cannulated and a cholangiogram has been obtained, a sphincterotomy is performed. Again here, my rationale for performing a sphincterotomy is to access the bile duct more easily, thus preventing manipulation and injury to the pancreas. After performing a sphincterotomy, a catheter and guidewire[52] are inserted through the opening and manipulated through the dominant stricture toward the proximal bile ducts. The catheter is then removed and a dilating balloon catheter advanced over the guidewire into the stricture. Under fluoroscopic control, the balloon is inflated to its maximum diameter (Figure 9-8).

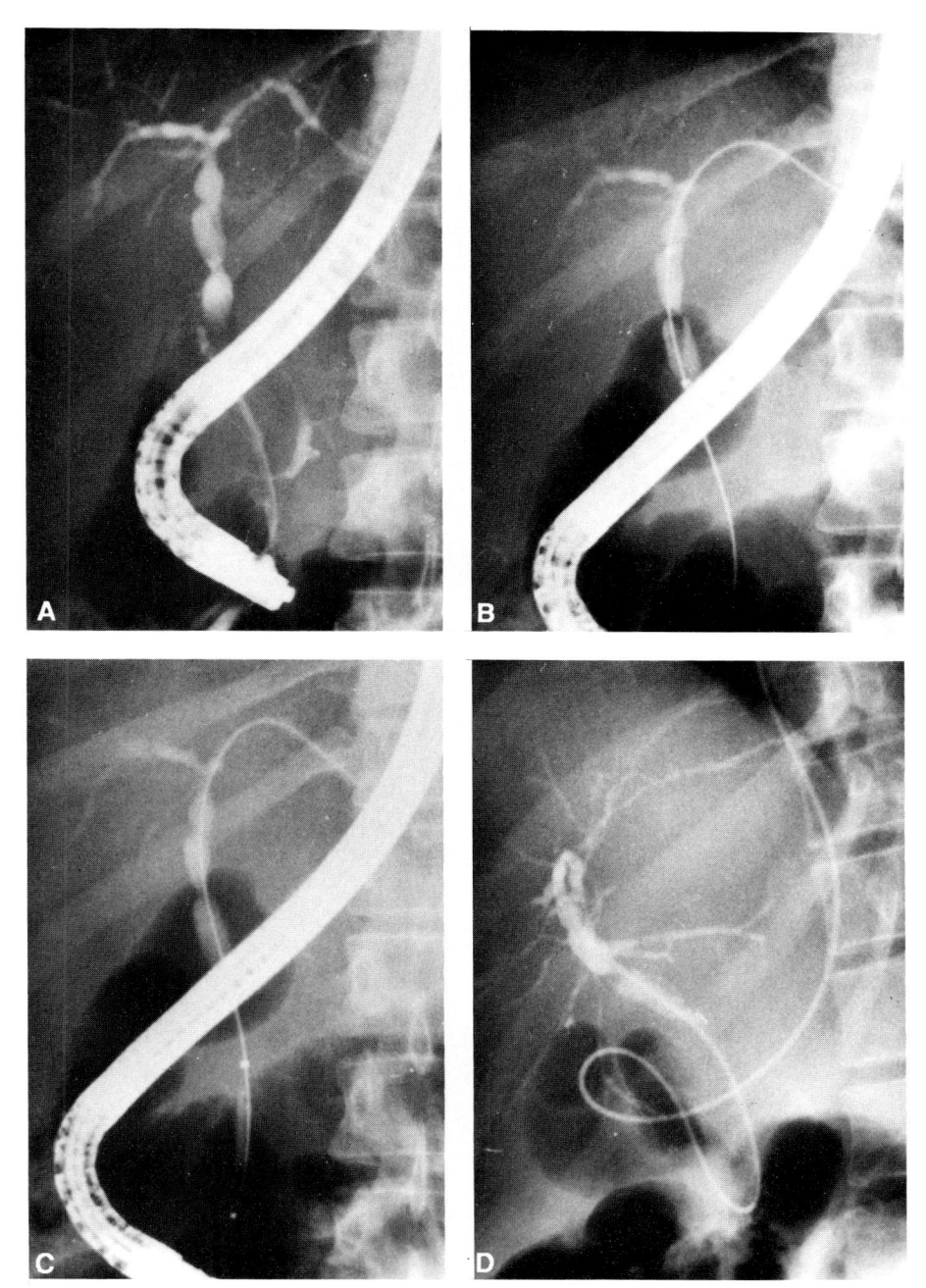

Figure 9-7 (A) Cholangiogram compatible with sclerosing cholangitis. **(B)** Balloon dilator inflated in common hepatic duct to dilate dominant stricture. **(C)** Balloon dilator inflated in ampulla dilating stricture facilitating entry into bile duct. **(D)** Cholangiogram obtained through nasobiliary tube.

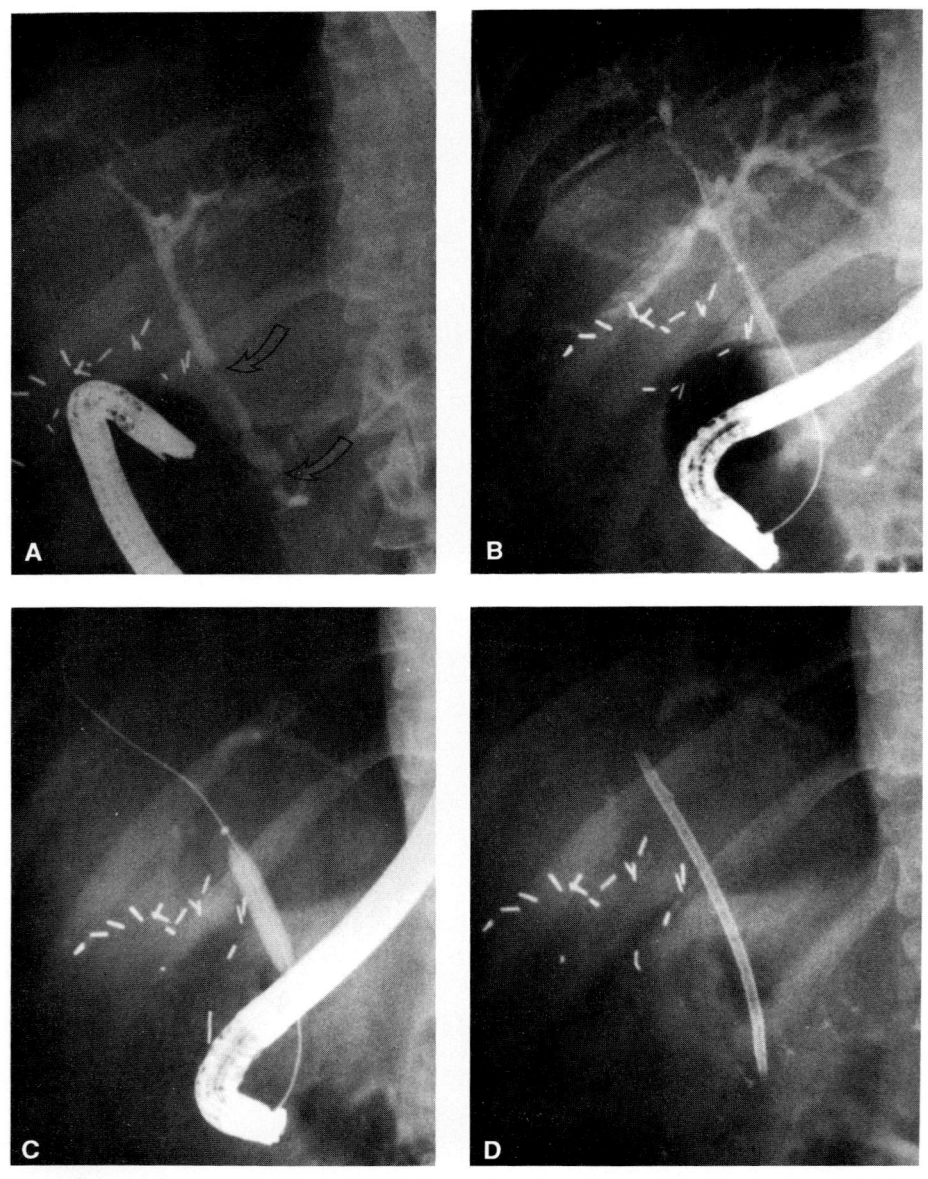

Figure 9-8 (A) Cholangiogram demonstrating sclerosing cholangitis with dominant stricture of distal common bile duct (arrows). **(B)** Small balloon dilating stricture. **(C)** Larger balloon dilating stricture. **(D)** Large-caliber prosthesis placed into extrahepatic bile duct.

In some cases a 4-mm balloon was used initially and in others a balloon as large as 8 mm was inflated. In our experience, edema is a frequent consequence of the dilation. To prevent this from causing even more obstruction after the procedure, a prosthesis is placed to promote drainage. Antibiotics are given prophylactically before and after the procedure. The mean hospital stay for our patients was 3 days with a range of 1–7 days. No serious complications have

Table 9-9 Sclerosing Cholangitis: Treatment Results

Bilirubin	80% decrease
Alkaline phosphatase and γ-glutamyl transpepsidase	60% decrease
Mean follow-up	3.5 yr
Follow-up range	0.5–5 yr

resulted to date from the manipulation, ie, perforation. Most patients experienced transient discomfort during the dilation procedure but few required additional analgesics. Biochemical parameters improved in all cases. A decrease in serum bilirubin of approximately 80% was noted, and a decrease in alkaline phosphatase and γ-glutamyl transpepsidase of approximately 60% has persisted in most patients who have been followed during the past 5 years (Table 9-9).

Prior to the endoscopic management of sclerosing cholangitis, patients followed in our series required hospitalization an average of 2.5 times annually. After endoscopic therapy, hospitalization was only necessary once in 2 years primarily for stent exchange. Our results suggest that with endoscopic management patients may enjoy long periods of remission with less time lost from their jobs or usual activities. Savings to the health care delivery system are made as well—an important consideration in this era of cost-conscious health care. Another advantage of endoscopic over surgical intervention is in the consideration and acceptance of a patient for liver transplantation. If previous surgery of the biliary tract can be avoided before transplantation, the technical peformance of the transplantation surgery is thought to be less complicated, since fewer adhesions are present to obscure the field or delay the surgical dissection necessary in the areas being excised.

Unfortunately, two patients in our series had a cholangiocarcinoma, and initially their lack of improvement following our endoscopic intervention caused us to doubt the effectiveness of our endoscopic efforts. To date, there is no reliable way one can determine or predict which patient may have a neoplasm associated with sclerosing cholangitis, and no serologic markers or biochemical tests are available which can be used as predictors. It is interesting to note, then, that in this large experience, the two patients who did not improve with endoscopic biliary drainage were the same two who had associated cholangiocarcinoma.

The fluctuations in the natural history of sclerosing cholangitis confound our ability to draw definitive conclusions from uncontrolled studies of treatment for this disease, and ideally a multicenter, randomized trial would be required.[51] However, at the present time our data and those of others suggest that sclerosing cholangitis is best evaluated and treated preliminarily with ERCP, sphincterotomy, balloon dilation, and placement of prostheses. Results indicate that the use of these therapeutic options improves liver functions while reducing exacerbations, doctor visits, frequency of hospitalizations, and duration of acute illness. The clinical improvement obtained permits affected patients to continue a near-normal life-style until deteriorating liver function becomes the determinate for liver transplantation.

References

1. Warren KW, and Jefferson MF: Prevention and repair of strictures of the intrahepatic ducts. *Surg Clin N A* 1973;53:1169–1190.
2. Way LW, Bernhoft RA, and Thomas MJ: Biliary strictures. *Surg Clin N A* 1981;61:963–972.
3. Pellegrini CA, Thomas MJ, and Way LW: Recurrent biliary stricture. Patterns of recurrence and outcome of surgical therapy. *Am J Surg* 1984;147:175–180.
4. Vogel SB, Howard RJ, Caridi J, and Hawkins EF: Evaluation of percutaneous transhepatic balloon dilatation of benign biliary strictures in high-risk patients. *Am J Surg* 1985;149:73–78.
5. Gallacher DJ, Kadir S, Kaufman SL, et al: Nonoperative management of benign postoperative biliary strictures. *Radiology* 1985;156:625–629.
6. Siegel JH, and Guelrud M: Endoscopic cholangiopancreatoplasty: hydrostatic balloon dilation in the bile duct and pancreas. *Gastroint Endosc* 1983;29:99–103.
7. Geenen JE: Balloon dilatation of bile duct strictures. pp. 105–108. In: *Nonsurgical Biliary Drainage.* Classsen M, Geenen J, Kawai K, eds. Springer-Verlag, New York, 1984.
8. Foutch PG, and Sivak MV Jr: Therapeutic endoscopic balloon dilatation of the extrahepatic biliary ducts. *Am J Gastroenterol* 1985;80:575–580.
9. Ring EJ, Oleaga JA, Freiman DB, et al: Therapeutic applications of catheter cholangiography. *Radiology* 1978;128:333–338.
10. Smale BF, Ring EJ, Frieman DB, et al: Successful long-term percutaneous decompression of the biliary tract. *Am J Surg* 1981;141:73–76.
11. Dooley JS, Dick R, George P, et al: Percutaneous transhepatic endoprosthesis for bile duct obstruction: complications and results. *Gastroenterology* 1984;86:905–909.
12. Soehendra N, and Reynders-Frederix V: Palliative gallengangsdrainage: Eine neue Methode zur endoskopischen Einfuerhrung eines inneren Drains. *Dtsch Med Wochenschr* 1979;104:206–207.
13. Huibregtse K., and Tytgat GN: Palliative treatment of obstructive jaundice by transpapillary introduction of large bore bile duct endoprosthesis. *Gut* 1982;23:371–375.
14. Siegel JH, Harding GT, and Chateau F: Endoscopic decompression and drainage of benign and malignant biliary obstruction. *Gastroint Endosc* 1982;28:79–82.
15. Siegel JH: Improved biliary decompression using large caliber endoscopic prostheses. *Gastroint Endosc* 1984;30:21–23.
16. Oi I: Fiberduodenoscopy and endoscopic pancreatocholangiography. *Gastroint Endosc* 1970;17:59–62.
17. Cotton PB: Cannulation of the papilla of Vater by endoscopy and retrograde cholangiopancreatography (ERCP). *Gut* 1972;13:1014–1025.
18. Kasugai T, et al: Endoscopic pancreatocholangiography. II. Pathologic endoscopic pancreatocholangiogram. *Gastroenteroloy* 1972;63:227–234.
19. Dickinson PB, Belsito AA, and Cramer GG: Diagnostic value of endoscopic cholangiopancreatography. *J Am Med Assoc* 1973;225:944–948.
20. Zimmon DS, Breslaw J, and Kessler RE: Endoscopy with endoscopic cholangiopancretography. The combination as a primary diagnostic procedure. *J Am Med Assoc* 1975;233:447–449.
21. Cotton PB: ERCP, *Gut* 1977;18:316–341.
22. Siegel JH: ERCP update: diagnostic and therapeutic applications. *Gastroint Radiol* 1978;31:311–318.
23. Siegel JH: Combined endoscopic dilatation and insertion of large diameter endoprostheses for bile duct obstruction. *Gastroint Endosc* 1984;30:91–92.
24. Siegel JH, and Yatto RP: Hydrostatic balloon catheters: A new dimension of therapeutic endoscopy. *Endoscopy* 1984;16:231–236.
25. Foutch PG, and Sivak MV, Jr: Therapeutic endoscopic balloon dilatation of the extrahepatic biliary ducts. *Am J Gastroenterol* 1985;80:575–580.

26. Siegel JH: Interventional endoscopy in diseases of the biliary tree and pancreas. *Mt Sinai J Med* 1984;51:535–547.
27. Huibregtse K, Katon RM, and Tytgat GN: Endoscopic treatment of postoperative biliary strictures. *Endoscopy* 1986;18:133–137.
28. Siegel JH: Improved biliary decompression using large caliber endoscopic prosthesis. *Gastroint Endosc* 1984;30:21–23.
29. Siegel JH, Pullano WE, Kodsi B, Cooperman A, and Ramsey W: Optimal palliation of malignant bile duct obstruction: Experience with endoscopic 12 French prostheses. *Endoscopy* 1988;20:137–141.
30. Huibregtse K, Katon RM, Coeve PP, and Tytgat GNJ: Endoscopic palliative treatment in pancreatic cancer. *Gastroint Endosc* 1986;32:334–338.
31. Siegel JH, and Snady H: The significance of endoscopically placed prostheses in the management of biliary obstruction due to carcinoma of the pancreas: Results of nonoperative decompression in 277 patients. *Am J Gastroenterol* 1986;81:634–641.
32. Leung JWC, Ling TKW, Kung JLS, and Vallance-Owen J: The role of bacteria in the blockage of biliary stents. *Gastroint Endosc* 1988;34:19–22.
33. Speer AG, Cotton PB, Rode J, Seddon AM, Neal CR, Holton J, and Costerton JW: Biliary stent blockage with bacterial biofilm. *Ann Intern Med* 1988;108:546–553.
34. Speer AG, Cotton PB, and MacRae KD: Endoscopic management of malignant biliary obstruction: Stents of 10 French gauge are preferable to stents of 8 French gauge. *Gastroint Endosc* 1988;34:412–417.
35. Leung JWC, DelFavero G, and Cotton PB: Endoscopic biliary prostheses: A comparison of materials. *Gastroint Endosc* 1985;31:93–95.
36. Mueller PR, van Sonnenberg E, Ferrucci JT Jr, et al: Biliary stricture dilatation: Multicenter review of clinical management in 73 patients. *Radiology* 1986;160:17–22.
37. Salomonowitz E, Castaneda-Zuniga WR, Lund G, Cragg AH, Hunter DW, Coleman CC, and Amplatz K: Balloon dilatation of benign biliary strictures. *Radiology* 1984; 151:613–616.
38. Smith AC, Schapiro RJ, Kelsey PB, and Warshaw AL: Successful treatment of non-healing biliary-cutaneous fistulas with biliary stents. *Gastroenterology* 1986;90:764–769.
39. Sauerbruch T, Weinzierl M, Holl J, and Pratschke E: Treatment of nonhealing biliary-cutaneous fistulas by internal endoscopic biliary drainage. *Gastroenterology* 1986; 90:1993–2003.
40. Burmeister W, Koppen MO, and Wurbs D: Treatment of a biliocutaneous fistula by endoscopic insertion of a nasobiliary tube. *Gastroint Endosc* 1985;31:279–281.
41. Janardhanan R, Brodmerkel GJ Jr, Turowski P, Gregory DH, and Agrawal RM: Endoscopic retrograde cholangiopancreatography in the diagnosis and management of postcholecystectomy cystic duct leaks. *Am J Gastroenterol* 1986;81:474–476.
42. Deviere J, von Gunsbeke D, Ansay J et al: Endoscopic management of a post-traumatic biliary fistula. *Endoscopy* 1987;19:136–139.
43. O'Rahilly S, Duignan JP, Lennon JR, and O'Malley E: Successful treatment of a postoperative biliary fistula by endoscopic papillotomy. *Endoscopy* 1983;15:60–68.
44. Del Olmo L, Meroño E, Moreira VF, Garcia T, and Garcia-Plaza A: Successful treatment of postoperative external biliary fistulas by endoscopic sphincterotomy. *Gastroint Endosc* 1988;34:307–309.
45. Kaufman SL, Kadir S, Mitchell SE, Chang R, Kinnison ML, Cameron JL, and White RI, Jr: Percutaneous transhepatic biliary drainage for bile leaks and fistulas. *Am J Roentgenol* 1985;144:1055–1058.
46. Siegel JH, Pullano W, and Ramsey WH: Sclerosing cholangitis, benign bile duct strictures and biliary cutaneous/peritoneal fistulas: Room at the top for endoscopic management. *Gastroint Endosc* 32:166 (abstract).
47. Schwartz SI: Primary sclerosing cholangitis: A disease revisited. *Surg Clin N A* 1973;53:1161–1168.

48. LaRusso NF, Wiesner RH, Ludwig J, et al: Primary sclerosing cholangitis. *N Engl J Med* 1984;310:899–903.
49. Siegel JH, and Halpern G: Endoscopic therapy in the treatment of sclerosing cholangitis: Effective use of sphincterotomy, dilatation and prostheses. *Am J Gastroenterol* 1985;80:831 (abstract).
50. Grijm R, Huibregtse K, Bartelsman J, et al: Therapeutic problems in primary sclerosing cholangitis. *Dig Dis Sci* 1986;31:792–798.
51. Johnson GK, Geenen JE, Venu RP, and Hogan WJ: Endoscopic treatment of biliary duct strictures in sclerosing cholangitis: Follow-up assessment of a new therapeutic approach. *Gastroint Endosc* 1987;33:9–12.
52. Siegel JH, and Ben-Zvi JS: Endoscopic management of sclerosing cholangitis: Results in 36 patients (in prep.).

Chapter **10**

Endoscopic Treatment in Nonmalignant Pancreatic Disease

Justin H. McCarthy, M.D., Joseph E. Geenen, M.D., and Walter J. Hogan, M.D.

Introduction

Endoscopic retrograde cholangiopancreatography (ERCP) and the use of biliary endoprostheses in the treatment of benign and malignant biliary strictures is now a well-established and acceptable alternative to surgical therapy. Although diagnostic ERCP is a routine investigation in the assessment of pancreatic disease, the use of endoscopic therapy in acute and chronic pancreatitis is experimental. The reports discussed in this chapter are preliminary and their role in the treatment of pancreatic diseases remains to be determined. Because alternative methods for the treatment of pancreatic disorders are so unsatisfactory and because early results of endoscopic therapy are sufficiently encouraging, further studies are warranted.

In the past, acute pancreatitis was a contraindication to ERCP. Recently diagnostic and therapeutic ERCP have been performed in patients with acute pancreatitis thought to be secondary to choledocholithiasis. Many reports now attest to the safety of these procedures in acute biliary pancreatitis.

In a recent study, Escourrou et al[1] reviewed their experience with ERCP and acute pancreatitis in 118 patients. ERCP showed choledocholithiasis in 78% of cases and endoscopic sphincterotomy was possible, during initial endoscopy, in 95% of patients. Two patients died from postsphincterotomy hemorrhage; however, no other complications were reported.

These results correspond with earlier reports by Cotton[2] and Classen[3] and indicate that ERCP and sphincterotomy can be safely performed during an acute attack of pancreatitis without greater risk than is usually entailed by the procedure. These studies draw attention to the difficulty in diagnosing choledocholithiasis using conventional techniques. Noninvasive techniques for detecting

---

The authors wish to thank Mrs. Karen Nielsen for her patience and typing, without which this manuscript would not have been completed. They also acknowledge the artistic skills of Ms. Joyce Levandowski and thank her for her help with the illustrations.

common bile duct stones are generally unpredictable. In a recent report comparing ultrasound and ERCP in patients presenting with acute pancreatitis, ultrasound detected common bile duct stones in 18% of patients compared with a 78% detection rate by ERCP.[4,5] An attempt has been made to use a multivariate analysis to determine which biochemical values would most appropriately predict the presence of common bile duct stones. Common bile duct stones were predictable in 85% of the cases where the patient had severe pancreatitis. [Blamey's criteria[1] and a bilirubin greater than 40 μmol/L (2.35 mg/dL)]. In these cases the diagnosis was confirmed by ERCP. However, the accuracy of prediction was less in cases of mild pancreatitis.

Problems have included the absence of good criteria as to the best time to intervene with ERCP, and the lack of critical appraisal as to whether instrumentation of the papilla and injection of contrast into the pancreatic duct makes a serious case of pancreatitis worse. Some European investigators circumvented these concerns and advocated ERCP in all patients. The earlier reports of Cremer et al[6] and Gelin et al[7] have not been substantiated by others. Both investigators advocated routine ERCP in all patients with acute pancreatitis. There was no reported increase in the overall incidence of complications following these procedures. Nonetheless, in most medical institutions there is limited experience in the routine use of urgent ERCP in all patients presenting with acute pancreatitis.

An important argument against such a universal approach is that most patients with biliary pancreatitis have self-limited episodes that permit elective intervention after the acute illness has subsided. This feature of the disease has also contributed to the absence of a clear consensus among surgeons as to the timing of operation in biliary pancreatitis, despite extensive discussion in the surgical literature that predates endoscopists' concerns with this issue.

Recently, the first randomized controlled trial of emergency ERCP and sphincterotomy versus conservative treatment, by Neoptolemos et al,[8] was reported. In patients with predicted severe attacks according to a multifactorial prognostic system, morbidity, and hospital stay were significantly reduced and there was a trend toward reduced mortality. In contrast, in patients with mild attacks, the outcome was not significantly altered.*

Acute Recurrent Pancreatitis

An etiology for acute pancreatitis can be identified in 60–88% of patients with acute recurrent pancreatitis.[11-15] Small gallstones, minimal pancreatic duct abnormalities, and sphincter of Oddi dysfunction have been suggested as causes of pancreatitis in the remaining 12–40% of patients.[16,17]

In a recent study extending the findings of Katon et al[18] and Cotton,[19] Venu et al[20] reviewed 116 patients who had acute recurrent pancreatitis, normal hepatobiliary ultrasound, and normal oral cholecystogram studies. Forty-five patients were found to have a possible cause for their pancreatitis at ERCP (Table 10-1). Twenty-seven patients were found to have a structural abnormality at diagnostic ERCP and 17 patients were found to have significantly elevated sphincter of Oddi basal pressure (50 ± 4.5 mm Hg versus 15 ± 4.5) at ERCP manometry.

---

*This subject is treated in further detail in Chapter 6.

Table 10-1 ERCP Findings in 116 Patients with Idiopathic Recurrent Pancreatitis (N = 116)

Sphincter of Oddi dysfunction	17
Pancreas divisum	11
Choledochocele	4
Cholelithiasis	8
Papillary tumor	3
Malignant stricture/pancreatic duct	1

Source: From Venu RP et al[20]

Cremer et al[6] and Gelin et al[7] suggested that pancreatography was useful in defining those patients with "chronic" pancreatitis who were having an "acute" attack of pancreatitis. The significance of this information is questionable. It has also been claimed that this technique combined with CT and ultrasound gives a precise definition of pancreatitic necrosis should surgery be necessary. This line of reasoning has been reinforced by a published small series which advocates ERCP in acute hemorrhagic necrotizing pancreatitis as a preoperative guide.[9] It was suggested that this aids surgical dissection and may help overcome the problem of assessing the extent of pancreatic necrosis at laparotomy. Further studies in this area are anticipated.

Acute pancreatitis can occur following diagnostic ERCP and there have been few advances in the prevention of post-ERCP pancreatitis. A recent study by Guelrud et al[10] suggested that the incidence of pancreatitis following balloon dilation of the pancreatitic sphincter could be reduced by the intravenous infusion of somatostatin during and after the procedure. This study found that 25% of patients developed pancreatitis following a 12-hr infusion of somatostatin; 37% developed pancreatitis following a 36-hr somatostatin infusion compared with 62% incidence of post-ERCP pancreatitis in the patient controls who received normal saline infusion for 12 hr. There have been no reports of the use of somatostatin in diagnostic ERCP to prevent postprocedure pancreatitis. Preliminary observations at our center suggest that insertion of a temporary nasopancreatic tube after ERCP in which postprocedure pancreatitis is thought to be a major possibility can reduce the likelihood of this complication.

Chronic Pancreatitis

There are preliminary reports indicating that pancreatic endoprostheses may be beneficial in patients with ductal abnormalities who are having recurrent episodes of pancreatitis or chronic pain. Huibregtse et al[21] inserted pancreatic stents in patients with chronic pancreatitis of varying etiologies (Tables 10-2 and 10-3). These patients had either recurrent episodes of pancreatitis or chronic pain. In 22 of the 32 patients referred with the diagnosis of chronic pancreatitis, a sphincterotomy of the pancreatic sphincter was performed to facilitate deep cannulation. A guidewire was placed prior to insertion of a nasopancreatic drain or endoprosthesis. Stents were successfully placed in 8 out of 11 patients with pancreatic strictures, 6 of 7 patients with pseudocysts, and 6 of 11 patients with pancreatic duct stones. Of 3 patients with papillary stenosis and ductal dilation,

Table 10-2 Pancreatic Endoprosthesis Treatment (N = 32)

Abnormalities	Recurrent pancreatitis (N = 21)	Chronic pain (N = 11)
Dominant strictures	9	2
Stricture + stones	1	5
Pancreatic stones	4	1
Papillary stones	3	0
Pseudocyst	4	3

Source: From Huibregtse et al: Endoscopic pancreatic drainage in chronic pancreatitis. *Gastroint Endosc* 1988;34:9–15.

a pancreatic sphincterotomy was performed in 3 and a stent placed in 1. Among the patients receiving long-term endoscopic treatment, all 17 with recurrent episodes of acute pancreatitis improved, while 7 of the 10 patients with chronic pain due to pancreatitis also improved. These results suggest the provision of a conduit to improve pancreatic drainage may be an important factor in treating certain cases of pancreatitis. The overall complication rate in this study was 22%. There was 1 death from perforation and 2 patients required surgery for infectious complications subsequent to endoscopic therapy.

In a similar study carried out by the authors,[22] pancreatic stents were successfully inserted in a small group of 14 patients with benign pancreatic disorders (Figure 10-1). There was symptomatic improvement in approximately 50% of patients (Table 10-4). Soehendra et al[23] also reported encouraging results following endoscopic papillotomy of the sphincter of Oddi and the pancreatic duct component in patients with chronic obstructive pancreatitis. No serious complications were reported following this procedure and it appeared to be very effective in relieving pancreatic pain. Fuji et al[24] also reported that pancreatic sphincterotomy is safe in chronic pancreatitis and that it can be combined with pancreatoscopy and endoprosthesis insertion. In this study a pancreatic sphincterotomy was successfully performed in 10 out of 13 patients with chronic pancreatitis; pancreatoscopy was performed in 3 cases to exclude calculi and pancreatic stents were placed in 3 cases. Clinical symptoms improved in 9 out of 10 patients following sphincterotomy and in 1 case after stent placement. In 1

Table 10-3 Pancreatic Endoprostheses Treatment: Etiology of Chronic Pancreatitis

Etiologic factor	Patients
Alcohol	18
Gallstones	2
Pancreas divisum	3
Benign papillary tumor	1
Congenital ductal anomaly	1
Idiopathic	7

Source: From Huibregtse et al: Endoscopic pancreatic drainage in chronic pancreatitis. *Gastroint Endosc* 1988;34:9–15.

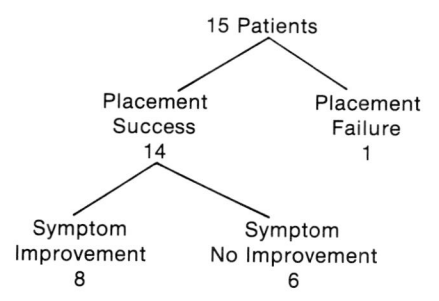

```
                    15 Patients
                   /          \
         Placement              Placement
         Success                Failure
            14                     1
         /       \
   Symptom       Symptom
   Improvement   No Improvement
       8              6
```

Figure 10-1 Stent Placement in Benign Pancreatic Disease.

case the stent had to be removed following the development of severe abdominal pain and 1 patient did not benefit at all from stent placement.

The accumulated experience to date involves only small numbers of patients. Problems to be resolved involve the optimal time for stent insertions, the duration of treatment of stent placement, and the interval between stent removal and replacement. It has been the authors' policy to routinely exchange pancreatic stents at 6-month intervals. In a total of 30 stent placements during 2 years, five stents were found to be occluded at the time of removal, two stents had dislodged and passed spontaneously through the gut, and two stents had to be removed following insertion because of an exacerbation of the patients' pain. (Table 10-5).

There have been preliminary reports indicating that the removal of pancreatic debris is helpful for pain relief in chronic pancreatitis.[25,26] Several endoscopists[21,27–29] also proposed endoscopic drainage of pancreatic cysts as an alternative to the usual internal or external operative drainage techniques.

Liguory[27] attempted endoscopic drainage in four patients outside the pancreas proper. Two patients had chronic alcoholic pancreatitis and two patients had acute pancreatitis, both complicated by pseudocyst formation. The cysts were localized with ultrasound and/or abdominal computed tomography, and they were found to be bulging into the stomach or duodenum at the time of endoscopy. Two endoscopic cystogastrostomies and two cystoduodenostomies were performed using a straight-wire sphincterotome and nasocystic drainage. The two patients with chronic pancreatitis benefited from this form of therapy but the two patients with acute pancreatitis subsequently underwent an operation because of complications.

Sahel et al[28] attempted to perform endoscopic cystoduodenostomy in 19 patients with chronic calcific pancreatitis with a success rate of 90%. The only two failures, as well as two perforations, occurred in patients without a visible

Table 10-4 Stent Placement in Benign Pancreatic Disease

Indications for stents	No. of patients with stents	No. of patients with symptomatic improvement
ETOH and stricture	5	4
Acute recurrent with papillary stenosis	7	3
Idiopathic chronic	2	1

Table 10-5 Endoscopic Stent Failure in Pancreatic Diseases*

Occluded stents	5
Spontaneous passage	2
Early pain	2

* Stents changed at 6-month intervals. Total stent placements, 30.

bulge created by the cyst on the duodenum, and the authors recommended avoidance of this approach in such patients.

Cremer et al[29] performed endoscopic cystoduodenostomy, using diathermy, on 22 patients and cystogastrostomy on 11, all of whom had cysts bulging into the wall of the appropriate adjacent structure. The success rate for the two groups were 95–100% with only a 10–20% long-term recurrence rate. Of the 33 patients, one with attempted cystoduodenostomy developed retroperitonitis treated with antibiotics followed by surgical cystojejunostomy. Two others undergoing cystogastrostomy developed infected pseudocysts treated nonsurgically. One of these had self-limited arterial bleeding at the time of the initial endoscopic excision.

It remains to be seen how many patients with pseudocysts will have the appropriate anatomy for endoscopic treatment. More data from additional centers are needed to establish the efficacy and safety of this approach compared with surgery before this approach can be considered beyond the investigational stage.

In contrast to the above studies, Huibregtse et al[21] worked within the pancreas, positioning endoprostheses into the pseudocysts in five patients with chronic pancreatitis via the main pancreatic duct. Four patients experienced relief of their complaints and resolution of their cysts. In one patient, a cystoduodenal fistula was created with an excellent result. Again, it is yet to be determined whether these techniques are superior to CT or ultrasound-directed needle aspiration or operative drainage.

Pancreas Divisum

There is still controversy over the role of pancreas divisum as a cause of acute pancreatitis and/or obscure abdominal pain.

However, there have been continuing reports[26] that dilation and stent placement in the minor papilla of patients with pancreas divisum relieves their symptoms. In an attempt to determine if pancreatic stent therapy is beneficial in patients with pancreas divisum, 22 of our patients underwent stent insertion either for pancreas divisum and acute recurrent pancreatitis or for pancreas divisum and severe abdominal pain.[22] Six of these patients had a previous operation on the minor papilla before being referred to us. A stent was successfully placed endoscopically in 19 of these 22 patients (Figure 10-2). Stents were changed at 6-month intervals.

Of these 19 patients, 17 had symptomatic improvement with marked decrease in pain, decrease in number of attacks of pancreatitis, and fewer visits to the emergency room. The two patients who did not have symptomatic improvement had their stents replaced twice before this treatment was abandoned.

```
                    22 Patients
                   /          \
          Placement            Placement
           Success              Failure
             19                    3
           /      \
    Symptom       Symptom
  Improvement   No Improvement
       17             2
```

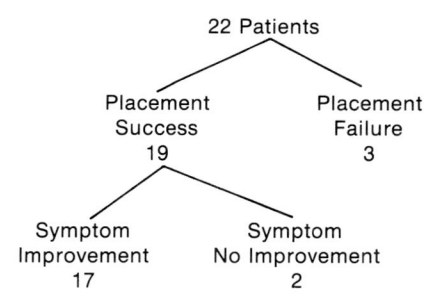

Figure 10-2 Stent Placement in Pancreas Divisum.

Paradoxically, serial pancreatograms showed the development of dorsal ductal changes consistent with chronic pancreatitis in two patients during stent therapy despite their symptomatic improvement (Figure 10-3). These patients have been followed for 6 months to 3 years. Over this period, a total of 48 stents have been placed in the dorsal duct. At the time of the 6-month stent exchange, it was noted that 10 stents had become occluded and four stents had passed spontaneously out of the GI tract. Two stents had migrated into the body of the pancreas. Attempts to remove them with a minisnare retriever were successful in one patient. The other patient with the stent retained inside the pancreas has had no problems to date (Table 10-6).

Following endoscopic stenting, there were five episodes of pancreatitis, three of which responded spontaneously to conservative management, and two in which the stents had to be removed. One stent was removed 24 hr after insertion and the other 5 days after insertion.

This preliminary experience with the endoscopic insertion of transpapillary

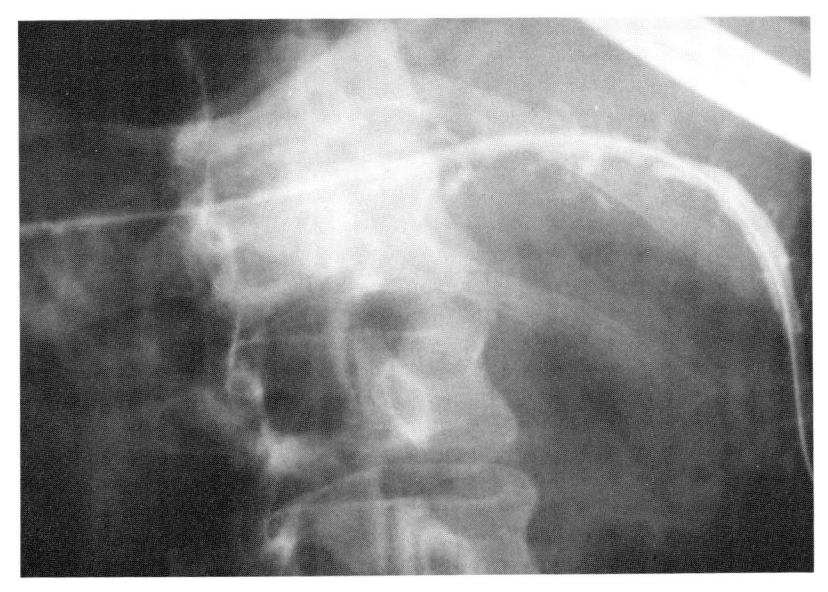

Figure 10-3 Radiograph illustrating ductal changes of chronic pancreatitis which have developed despite stent insertion.

Table 10-6 Problems Associated with Stent Placement in Patients with Pancreas Divisum*

Total stent placements	48
Occluded stents	10
Spontaneous passage	4
Migration into pancreas	2
Early pain	2

* Stents routinely changed every 6 months in 17 patients.

stents in pancreatic diseases corroborates the report of Soehendra et al.[30] Furthermore, it demonstrates that manipulation of the dorsal pancreatic duct is comparatively safe and less hazardous than formerly believed. Symptomatic improvement in the patients treated by transpapillary stent placement is encouraging but a careful prospective clinical trial is needed. Endoscopic therapy may provide an effective way of obtaining symptomatic relief in a select group of patients with benign pancreatic problems.

Techniques

The technique for placing a stent in the pancreatic duct is similar to that used for inserting nasobiliary stents and drainage tubes. A diagnostic pancreatogram is performed. Following this a 0.025-in. guidewire is inserted into the pancreatic duct and advanced midway toward the tail of the pancreas (Figure 10-4). A 5-Fr or 7-Fr barbed stent is then introduced over the guidewire into the pancreatic duct and positioned so that its distal end protrudes into the duodenal lumen. The stents are 5–7 cm in length (Figure 10-5).

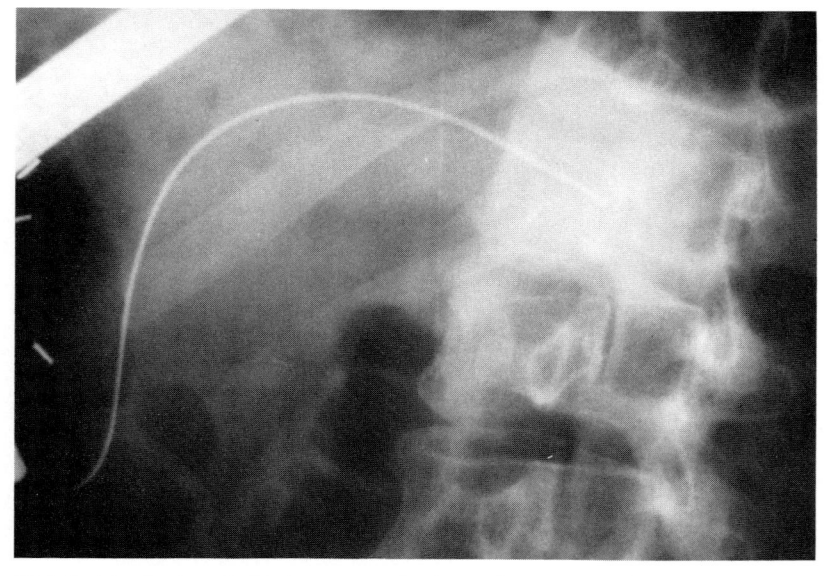

Figure 10-4 Guidewire inserted into pancreatic duct prior to stent placement.

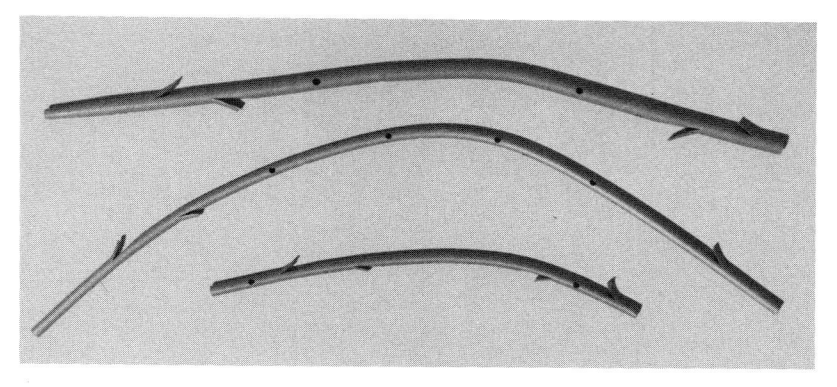

Figure 10-5 Straight-barbed stents, 5 and 7 Fr, 5–7 cm in length used for insertion into the pancreatic duct.

In patients with suspected pancreas divisum, a dorsal duct pancreatogram can be obtained by cannulating the minor papilla with either a tapered-tip catheter, a needle-tip catheter, or a 3-Fr angiocatheter which may or may not require prior insertion of a 0.018-in. guidewire (Figure 10-6). The identification of the minor papilla is assisted by the long endoscopic approach and/or the injection of secretin which stimulates pancreatic juice outpouring and demarcation of the orifice (1 unit/kg). When a stent is to be placed into the dorsal pancreatic duct via the minor papilla, it is preferable to cannulate the papilla with a 3-Fr angiographic catheter through which a 0.018-in. guidewire is inserted. The guidewire is then advanced toward the tail of the pancreas and the stent positioned over the guidewire in the usual method (Figures 10-7, 10-8, 10-9).

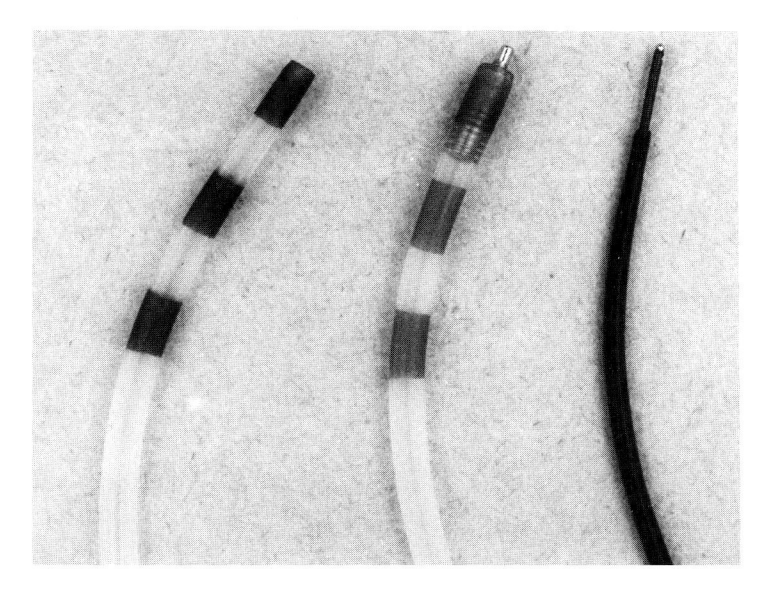

Figure 10-6 Three types of catheters used for cannulating the minor papilla (left to right): tapered-tip catheter, needle-point catheter, 3-Fr angiographic catheter over a 0.018-in. guidewire.

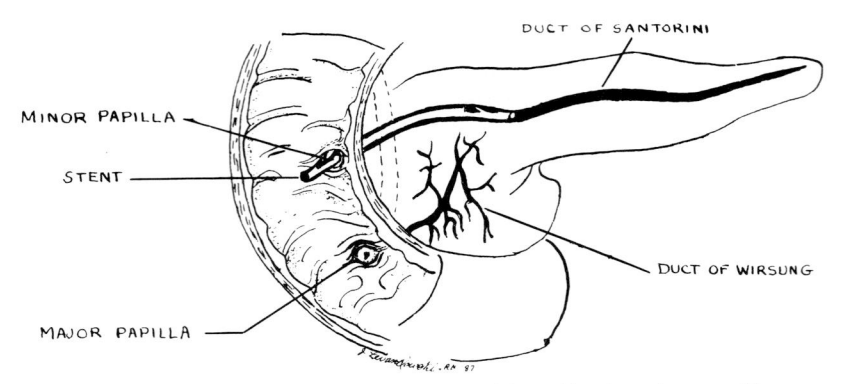

Figure 10-7 Schematic representation of a stent positioned in the minor papilla.

In those cases where the stent has migrated into the body of the pancreas, a minisnare can be inserted into the pancreatic duct and used to retrieve the stent (Figure 10-10). Using this technique, the authors managed to retrieve all but one of the stents that migrated into the body of the pancreas (Figure 10-11).

Dilation of the major and minor papilla is not routinely undertaken prior to stent placement. In the authors' experience, approximately 50% of cases required dilation prior to stent insertion. Dilation appears to be associated with an increased risk of pancreatitis as compared to a diagnostic ERCP study. In some patients with acute recurrent pancreatitis and papillary stenosis who have not benefitted from conventional sphincterotomy, dilation of the pancreatic sphincter with angiographic catheters has been undertaken with some improvement in symptoms. A larger controlled study is required to elucidate the value of dilation at the pancreatic sphincter in patients with papillary stenosis.

Pancreatic sphincterotomy is not routinely practiced by the authors. In a preliminary study, four patients with papillary stenosis and acute recurrent pan-

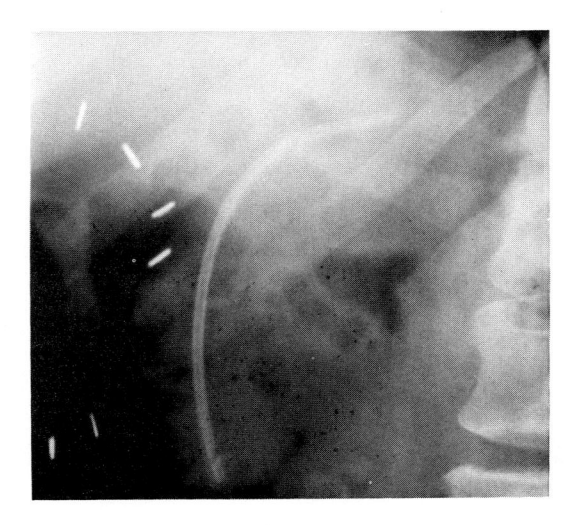

Figure 10-8 Oblique abdominal radiograph depicting a barbed stent positioned through the minor papilla into the dorsal pancreatic duct.

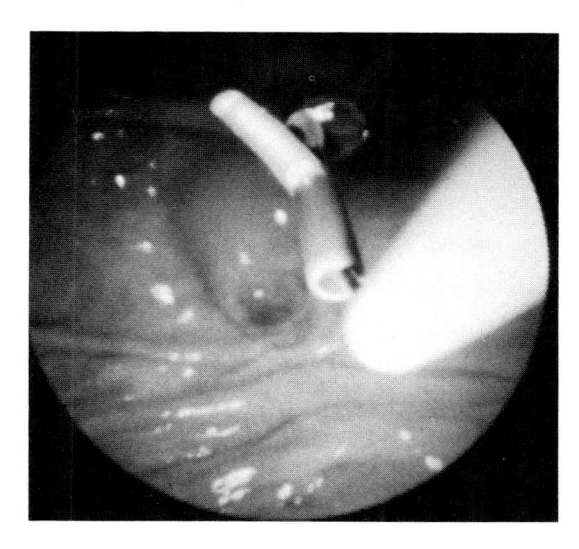

Figure 10-9 Endoscopic view of a stent positioned in the minor papilla. The major papilla can be seen to the immediate left of the stent.

creatitis and two patients with papillary stenosis and chronic pancreatitis underwent pancreatic sphincterotomy. All patients had failed to improve following sphincterotomy on the common bile duct. Of this group of six patients, two developed pancreatitis and one bled following the procedure. None of this group of patients had lasting benefit following endoscopic pancreatic sphincterotomy. One patient with idiopathic pancreatitis benefitted from sphincterotomy. The significant incidence of complications has made us cautious about embarking on a larger study of endoscopic pancreatic sphincterotomy.

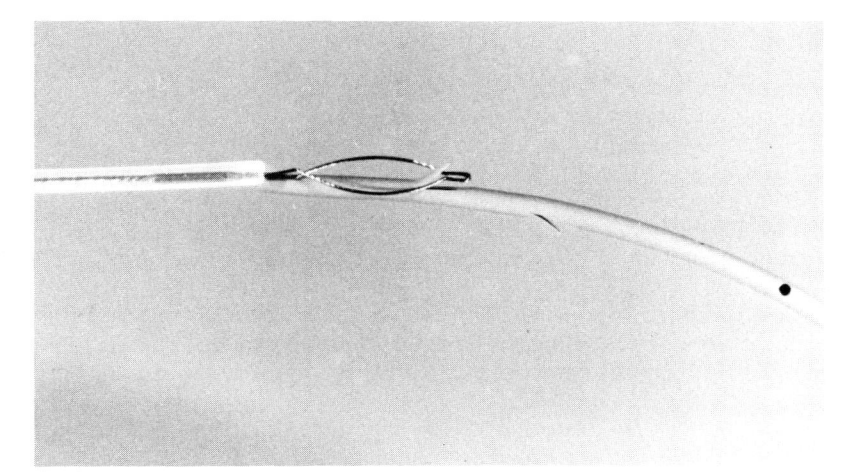

Figure 10-10 Endoscopic minisnare used to remove wandering pancreatic stents. (Prototype manufactured by Wilson Cook Co., North Carolina.)

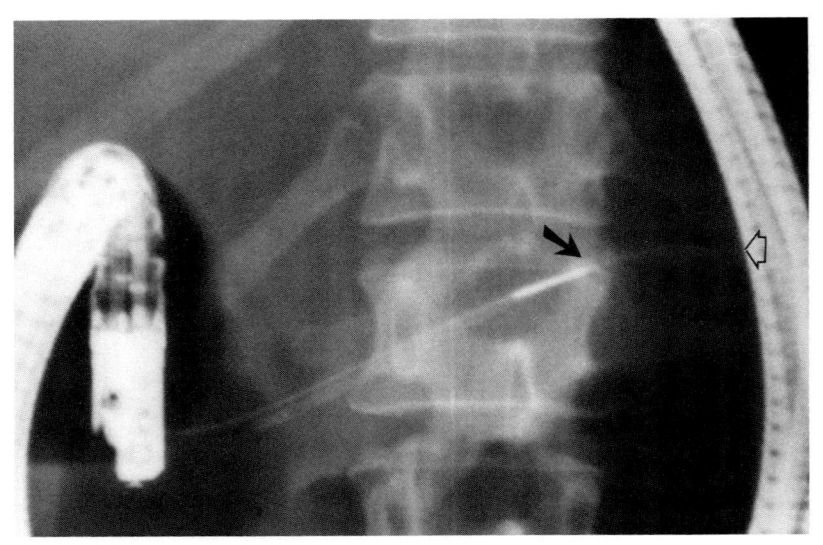

Figure 10-11 Radiograph illustrating snare positioned around the proximal end of a pancreatic stent immediately prior to its removal. Solid arrow points to the edge of the metal shaft and open arrow points to the end of the snare wire.

References

1. Escourrou J, Liguory C, Boyer J, and Sahel J: Emergency endoscopic sphincterotomy in acute biliary pancreatitis; results of a multicenter study (abstract). *Gastroint Endosc* 1987;33:2:187.
2. Cotton PB, and Saffrany L: Urgent duodenoscopic sphincterotomy for acute gallstone pancreatitis (abstract). *Gastroint Endosc* 1980;26:2:65.
3. Classen M, and Phillip J: Endoscopic retrograde cholangiopancreatography (ERCP) and endoscopic therapy in pancreatic disease. *Clin Gastroenterol* 1984;13;3:819–843.
4. Neoptolemos JP, Hall AW, Finaly DF, et al: The urgent diagnosis of gallstones in acute pancreatitis: A prospective study of these methods. *Br J Surg* 1984;71:230–233.
5. Neoptolemos JP, London N, Slater ND, Carr-Locke DL, Fossard DP, and Moosa R: A prospective study of ERCP and endoscopic sphincterotomy in the diagnosis and treatment of gallstone acute pancreatitis. *Arch Surg* 1986;121:697–702.
6. Dunham F, DeToeut J, Jeanty P, Bourgeois N, and Cremer M: Complementary and limits of the different techniques of pancreatic morphologic investigation for the diagnosis of acute pancreatitis and complications. *Acta Chir Belg* 1981;Nov–Dec 80;6:323–629.
7. Gelin M, Dunham F, Engelholm L, Cremer M, and Lambilliotte JP. Interest of biliopancreatic morphologic study in management of acute pancreatitis. *Acta Chir Belg* 1981;Nov–Dec 80(6):357–362.
8. Neoptolemos JP, Carr-Locke DL, London NJ, et al: Controlled trial of urgent endoscopic retrograde cholangiopancreatography and endoscopic sphincterotomy versus conservative treatment for acute pancreatitis due to gallstones. *Lancet* 1988;2:979–983.
9. Gebhardt CH, Rieman JF, and Lux G: The importance of ERCP for the surgical tactic in hemorrhagic necrotizing pancreatitis (preliminary report). *Endoscopy* 1983;15:55–58.
10. Guelrud M, Mendoza S, and Viera L: Does somatostatin prevent acute pancreatitis

after pancreatic duct sphincter hydrostatic balloon dilatation? [abstract]. *Gastroint Endosc* 1987;33:148 (Abstract).
11. Ranson JM: Etiological and prognostic factors in human acute pancreatitis: A review. *Am J Gastroenterol* 1983;77:683–688.
12. Soergel KH: Acute pancreatitis. In: Sleisenger and Fordtran, eds. *Gastrointestinal Disease*, 2nd Ed. Philadelphia, W.B. Saunders, 1983; pp 1463–1485.
13. Howard JM: Pancreatitis associated with gallstones. In: Howard JM, Jordan GL, eds. *Surgical Diseases of the Pancreas*. Philadelphia, J.B. Lippincott, 1960; pp. 169–189.
14. Svensson JO, Norbach B, Bokey EL, and Edlung Y: Changing patterns in etiology of pancreatitis. *Br J Surg* 1979;66:159–161.
15. Trapnell JE, and Duncan EHL: Patterns of incidence in acute pancreatitis. *Br Med J* 1975;2:179–182.
16. O'Sullivan JN, Nobrega FT, Morlock CG, et al: Acute and chronic pancreatitis. *Gastroenterology* 1972;3:373–379.
17. Bar-Meir S, Geenen JE, Hogan WJ, Dodds WJ, Stewart ET, and Arndorfer RC: Biliary and pancreatic duct pressures measured by ERCP manometry in patients with suspected papillary stenosis. *Dig Dis Sci* 1979;24:209–213.
18. Katon RM, Bilbao MR, Eidemiller LR, et al: Endoscopic retrograde cholangiopancreatography in the diagnosis and management of nonalcoholic pancreatitis. *Surg Gynecol Obstet* 1978;147;3:333–338.
19. Cotton PB, and Beales JSM: Endoscopic pancreatography in the diagnosis and management of relapsing acute pancreatitis. *Br Med J* 1974;1:608–612.
20. Venu RP, Geenen JE, Hogan WJ, Johnson GK, and Soergel K: Idiopathic recurrent pancreatitis: An approach to diagnosis and treatment, *Dig Dis Sci* 1989;34:56–60.
21. Huibregtse K, Schneider B, Vrij AA, and Tytgat GNJ: Endoscopic pancreatic drainage in chronic pancreatitis. *Gastroint Endosc* 1988;34:9–15.
22. McCarthy JH, Geenen JE, and Hogan WJ: Preliminary experience with endoscopic stent placement in pancreatic diseases. *Gastroint Endosc* 1988;34:16–18.
23. Grimm H, de Herr K, and Soehendra N: Endoscopic transpapillary drainage in chronic pancreatitis (abstract). *Dig Dis Sci* 1986;131(supp 10):31.
24. Fuji T, Amano H, Hanima K, Aibe T, Asagami F, Kinukawa K, Ariyama S, and Takemoto T: Pancreatic sphincterotomy and pancreatic endoprosthesis. *Endoscopy* 1985;17:69–72.
25. Tsurumi T, Fujii Y, Takeda M, Tanaka J, Harada H, and Oka H: A case of chronic pancreatitis successfully treated by endoscopic removal of protein plugs. *Acta Med Okayama* 1984;38(2):169–174.
26. Schneider MV, and Lux G: Floating pancreatic duct concrements in chronic pancreatitis. Pain relief by endoscopic removal. *Endoscopy* 1985;17:8–10.
27. Liguory C, Letebure JF, Canard JM, Bonnel, and Lemaire A: Endoscopic drainage of four pancreatic cysts (abstract). *Dig Dis Sci* 1986;31(suppl 10):531S.
28. Sahel J, Bastid C, Pellat B, Schurgers P, and Sarles H: Endoscopic cystoduodenostomy of cysts of chronic calcifying pancreatitis: A report of 20 cases. *Pancreas* 1987;2:447–453.
29. Cremer M, Deviere J, and Engelhom L: Endoscopic management of cysts of pseudocysts: long-term follow-up after years of experience. *Gastrointest Endosc* 1989;35:1–9.
30. Soehendra N, Kempeneers I, Nam VCH, and Grimm H: Endoscopic dilatation and papillotomy of the accessory papilla and internal drainage in pancreas divisum. *Gastroint Endosc* 1986;18:129–132.

Chapter **11**

Endoscopic Stents for Biliary Obstruction Due to Malignancy

Anthony G. Speer, B.E., M.B.B.S., F.R.A.C.P., and Peter B. Cotton, M.D., F.R.C.P.

Malignant Obstructive Jaundice: The Problem

Endoscopic stenting needs to be considered against the background of the epidemiology of malignant obstructive jaundice. Carcinoma of the pancreas is the most common tumor causing biliary obstruction. In the United States more than 20,000 persons present with this problem each year.[1] Approximately one-fifth of this number will present with carcinoma of the gallbladder or cholangiocarcinoma. These cancers are diseases of the elderly. The age-specific incidence increases rapidly with increasing age for both males and females.[1] The median age at onset for carcinoma of the pancreas in the United Kingdom in 1982 was over 70 years (Figure 11-1). The age distribution for carcinoma of the gallbladder and cholangiocarcinoma is similar.[2] The age distribution for these lesions is similar in the United States.

Ideally, we would like to resect the tumor and cure the patients. However, this is not possible in the majority of patients. Carcinoma of the pancreas presents late, and 90% have extended beyond the pancreas or metastasized at presentation.[3] Carcinoma of the gallbladder and cholangiocarcinoma spreads to adjacent liver and blood vessels, and the detergent properties of bile allow it to pass through a very narrow lumen without producing signs of obstruction.[4] The tumors are usually far advanced when symptoms appear.[5] Thus, most patients require palliation rather than resection. This will involve a variety of treatments including analgesics or celiac plexus block for pain, counseling about the nature of the disease, and perhaps surgery for duodenal obstruction. Biliary obstruction causes intractable pruritus, malabsorption, and progressive hepatocellular and renal dysfunction. Many patients will benefit from relief of biliary obstruction.

Surgical bypass is the established method for relieving biliary obstruction. However, surgery has a substantial morbidity and mortality. The risk of surgery increases with increasing age and in the presence of extensive metastatic dis-

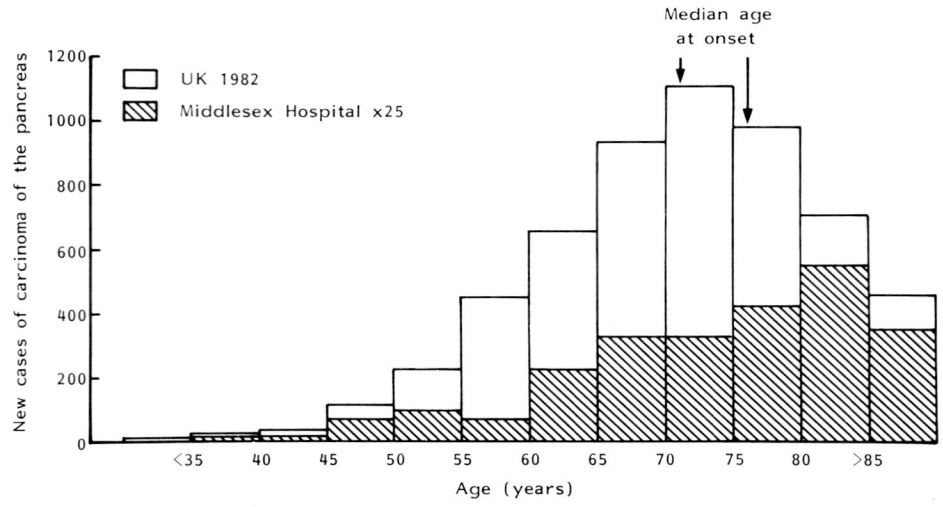

Figure 11-1 Age at first diagnosis of carcinoma of the pancreas in the United Kingdom in 1982 and in the group of patients referred to the Middlesex Hospital for endoscopic stenting. In order to fit the scale, the number presenting to the Middlesex hospital has been multiplied by 25.

ease. Age greater than 60 years has been reported as a risk factor in biliary surgery,[6] and Ransohoff found that the mortality for cholecystectomy and exploration of the common bile duct increases rapidly over 70 years of age.[7] The operative mortality for pancreatic resection over 65 and 70 years of age has been reported as 41 and 58%, respectively.[8,9] The risk of surgery also increases in the presence of extensive metastatic disease. Blievernich reports a mortality for bypass surgery for carcinoma of the pancreas of 12.3% for patients with local extension of the disease, rising to 20% with liver metastases and 43% for patients with peritoneal metastases and ascites.[10] Operative mortalities of 28% in the presence of liver metastases and 59% with extensive metastatic disease have also been reported.[11,12] Many patients presenting with malignant obstructive jaundice are elderly with extensive metastatic disease, and thus are at high risk with bypass surgery. In the hope of reducing the morbidity, mortality, and hospitalization time associated with surgery in these patients, several nonsurgical techniques to establish biliary drainage were developed.

Nonsurgical Palliation

Initially, nonsurgical palliation was accomplished through external drainage by percutaneous transhepatic insertion of a catheter.[13] Later a guidewire and drainage catheter were manipulated through the stricture allowing both internal and external bile flow.[14] However, external biliary drainage has several disadvantages including pain at the catheter site, the risk of spontaneous catheter dislodgement, and leaks of ascitic fluid and bile around the catheter.[15] The use of nonsurgical techniques was advanced by the description of the transhepatic insertion of an indwelling stent without an external catheter.[16] Endoscopic insertion of a biliary stent through the papilla was described more recently.[17] At

Table 11-1 Results of Prospective Randomized Trial Comparing Endoscopic and Percutaneous Stenting for Malignant Obstructive Jaundice in Patients Judged Not Fit for Surgery

	Endoscopic stents ($N = 39$) (%)	Percutaneous stents ($N = 36$) (%)
Successful stent insertion	89	76
Successful relief of jaundice	81	61*
Early complications	19	67
30-Day mortality	15	33**

* $P = 0.017$ Mantel-Haenszel analysis.
** $P = 0.016$ Log-rank analysis.

first it was not obvious which would be the best technique. The endoscopic approach seems technically more difficult than the percutaneous transhepatic method, but is less traumatic for the patient and has the advantage that blocked stents can be removed and easily changed. Variations in technique and patient selection make it difficult to compare these methods from published retrospective series.

We recently published results of the first prospective randomized trial comparing the two methods.[18] Between February 1983 and March 1985, 75 patients with biliary obstruction due to malignancy were randomized to receive either an endoscopic or a percutaneous transhepatic stent. A total of 29 patients had hilar strictures due to cholangiocarcinoma or carcinoma of the gallbladder, and the remainder had low biliary strictures due to carcinoma of the pancreas. The lesions were not resectable and the patients were considered to be unsuitable for bypass surgery because of their age, the extent of the disease, or associated medical conditions. The patients were elderly (median age 73), deeply jaundiced, and 20% had renal impairment due to prolonged biliary obstruction. The two groups were well matched apart from a higher incidence of hilar strictures in the endoscopic group. This was allowed for by stratifying the statistical analysis for the site of the obstruction. The stenting procedures were performed at the London or Middlesex Hospital by experienced gastroenterologists and radiologists.

Endoscopic stents were significantly more successful in relieving jaundice and had a significantly lower 30-day mortality (Table 11-1). The higher mortality with percutaneous stents was due to the high incidence of complications, mainly those of puncturing the liver with large-bore tubes, causing hemorrhage and bile leak. This study convinced us that the endoscopic approach should be attempted first when there are clinical indications for a biliary stent. The percutaneous method should be reserved for those patients in whom the endoscopic approach fails. The main question is whether our results can be applied to other centers or, indeed, to other groups of patients. Some may say that the results reflect greater endoscopic skills and that the complication rate for percutaneous stents is unreasonably high. We do not believe that such criticisms are valid.

We reviewed the published series of percutaneous and endoscopic stents and found that our results are comparable with those of other groups[18-28] (Table 11-2). Other series cite 30-day mortality and survival data of only those patients

Table 11-2 Summary of Results in Published Series of Endoscopic and Percutaneous Stents

Ref.	Patients with malignancy	Successful insertion (%)	Successful drainage (%)	30-Day mortality (%)	Early complications (%)	Median survival (days)
Endoscopic Stents						
Trial[18]	39	89	81	6	18	159
Hagenmuller[19]	454	84	NA	8	26	47–81*
Huibregtse[20]	297	89	86	15	17	162**
Leung[21]	64	89	NA	16	NA	154
Percutaneous Stents						
Mueller[22]	109	92	NA	10	17	NA
Leung[21]	48	88	NA	17	NA	190
Trial[18]	36	76	61	24	61	113
Dooley[23]	40	86	70	25	29	92
Hoevels[24]	13	NA	57	29	38	NA
Burcharth[25]	94	82	66	30	15	62
Coons[26]	62	NA	60	27	13	NA
Burcharth[27]	455	88	73	NA	6	98
Pereiras[28]	12	100	83	NA	58	NA

* Median survival reported from three centers varied between 47 and 81 days.
** Mean survival.
NA = data not available.

in whom stenting was successful; our corresponding figures are given. Our results with endoscopic stents are similar to several other series.

Our success rate for percutaneous route insertion is lower than in other series but the success rate for the relief of jaundice is similar. Our incidence of complications with percutaneous stents is the highest in the literature. However, the reported incidence of complications depends on how these events are defined and how carefully they are sought. We feel that our high complication rate is due to strict definitions and careful clinical follow-up in a prospective trial.

Interestingly, the published percutaneous stent complication rates vary widely while the 30-day mortality rates are remarkably similar. Our trial has one of the lowest reported 30-day mortality figures. Indeed a 30-day mortality is an unambiguous clinical event, not subject to observer bias, and was used for the definitive statistical analysis in this trial. For similar groups of patients we would expect that the 30-day mortality is proportional to the incidence of complications. These considerations lead us to conclude that our results reflect real differences in the potential of the two techniques.

Endoscopic Stenting Technique

Patients are assessed in detail with full consideration given to alternative methods, including the possibility of surgical resection and the apparent risk of duodenal obstruction. Coagulation is checked and corrected with vitamin K when necessary. Most patients, particularly those who are deeply jaundiced and elderly, are given fluids intravenously while fasting to maintain hydration. Approximately a quarter of our patients with malignant obstructive jaundice have renal impairment due to prolonged biliary obstruction. It is important to maintain urinary output and prevent further deterioration of renal function. Antibiotics are given prophylactically 2 hr before the procedure so that tissue levels are adequate at the time of the procedure. We use broad-spectrum antibiotics that are secreted in the bile.[29]

The endoscopic procedure is performed under sedation with diazepam and meperidine. As obstructive jaundice may adversely affect myocardial function,[30] sedation is carefully titrated to prevent hypotension or respiratory depression. High-risk patients can be monitored with automatic pulse- and blood pressure-recording machines.

Stenting procedures require an endoscope with a large channel. A prototype Olympus JFIT with a 3.7-mm channel became available in 1983 and other endoscopes (Pentax, Fujinon) with similar sized channels have since been produced. An endoscope with a 4.2-mm channel (Olympus TJF) was recently introduced. An 11.5-French guage (FG) stent can be inserted through this endoscope.

We use a 4.2-mm channel endoscope for the initial cholangiogram, sphincterotomy (where indicated), and stent insertion. Others prefer to use a smaller, 2.8-mm diameter channel endoscope for the initial cholangiogram and sphincterotomy and then change to the large-channel endoscope for the remainder of the procedure. The smaller endoscope is more maneuverable; however, the procedure may be prolonged due to the change in endoscope. The stent is

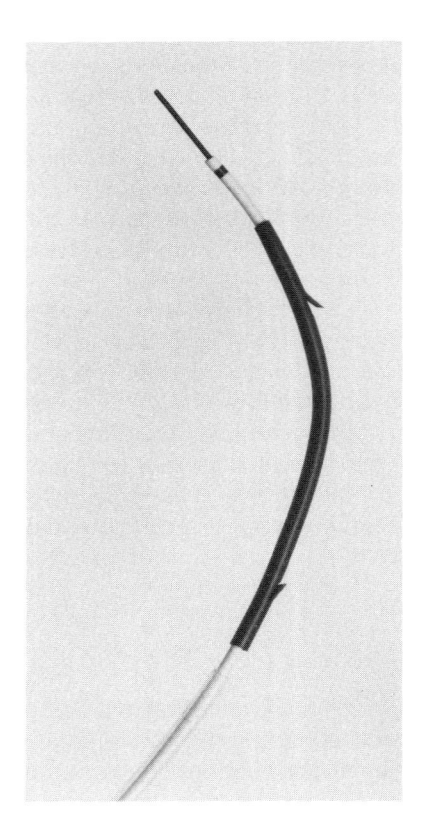

Figure 11-2 The three-layer coaxial system used for stent insertion consists of, from the top down, an 0.035-in. guidewire, a 6-FG Teflon inner catheter with a metal ring, a 10-FG polyethylene stent, and a 10-FG clear Teflon pusher.

inserted using a three-layer coaxial system (Figure 11-2). This consists of a 300-cm-long, 0.035-in.-diameter, 3-cm floppy-tip safety guidewire, 6-FG Teflon inner tube, and a 10-FG dilating and pusher tube. A metal ring on the inner catheter makes the tip clearly visible on the X-ray screen. We prefer stents made from 11.5-FG polyethylene with flaps at both ends to prevent migration and a slight bend in the middle to conform with the shape of the bile duct.

A diagnostic cholangiogram is performed with the inner catheter and this is then maneuvered deep into the bile duct (Figure 11-3). A small sphincterotomy is performed when stents greater than 10 FG are used. This facilitates stent placement (and exchange). Once selective biliary cannulation is achieved, the inner catheter is advanced up the bile duct until it is 1–2 cm below the stricture. The guidewire is inserted through the catheter and then maneuvered through the stricture (Figure 11-4). Once the guidewire is through the stricture, it is advanced until the floppy tip is beyond the stricture, and the inner catheter is then pushed through the stricture over the wire. The bile duct above the stricture can now be outlined more completely by a further injection of dilute contrast through the catheter after the wire is removed. Bile can be aspirated for culture and cytology. A coaxial 10-FG dilator is used to stretch the stricture (Figure 11-5), and the dilator is then removed leaving the inner catheter and guidewire in place. A stent of suitable length is selected after examination of the X rays. The length of the stent must be such that the top flap is above the stricture while the bottom flap is in the duodenum. The distance from 1 cm above the stricture

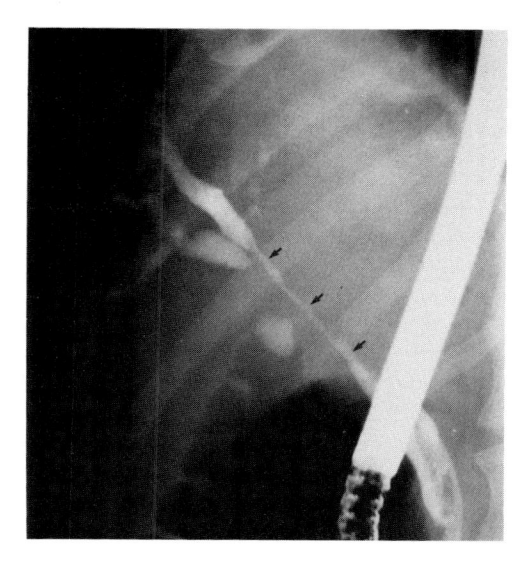

Figure 11-3 Cholangiogram shows a long hilar stricture (arrows) extending up into the right intrahepatic ducts. The top of the inner catheter is behind the endoscope.

to 1 cm below the point where the duct enters the duodenum is measured on the X ray. This is adjusted for magnification (usually about 30%) and this is the length required between the flaps of the stent. The magnification factor can be calculated by comparing the known diameter of the endoscope with that on the X-ray film. Stents with a distance of 5–7 cm between flaps are usually suitable for pancreatic carcinoma while 10–13 cm between the flaps may be needed for hilar strictures.

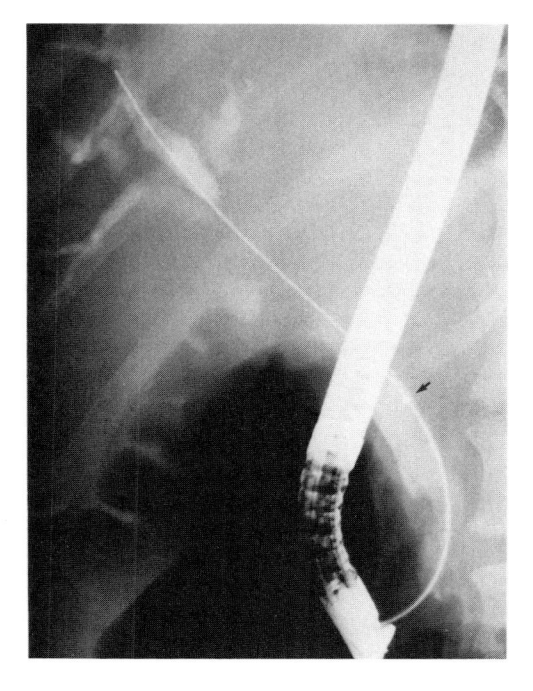

Figure 11-4 The metal ring near the top of the catheter (arrow) is just below the stricture. A guidewire has been maneuvered through the stricture and the floppy tip is well above the stricture.

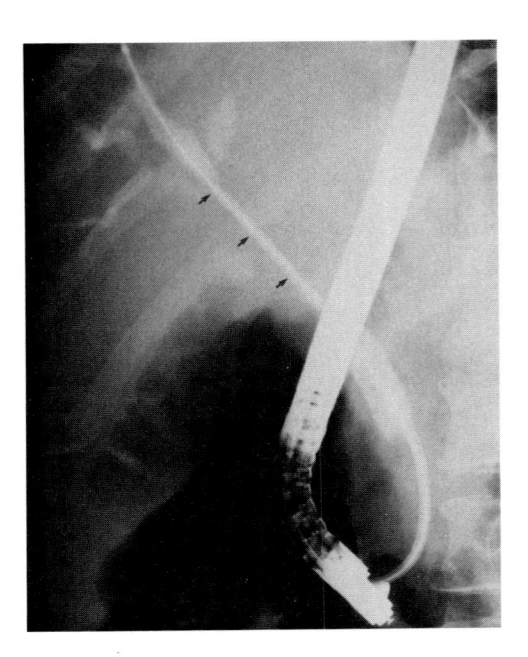

Figure 11-5 The 10-FG dilator (arrows) has been pushed through the stricture. The "short-scope" position is being used and the tip of the endoscope is kept close to the papilla.

The stent is then pushed down over the inner catheter, into the duct, and through the stricture by a combination of pushing on the push catheter and upward movement of the elevator and tension by the nurse on the inner tube. The endoscope must be kept close to the papilla to avoid the formation of a loop in the inner catheter and pusher. When the top flap is above the stricture, the inner catheter and guidewire are removed while the stent is held in place with the pusher (Figure 11-6). About 1 cm of the stent is left protruding from the papilla into the duodenum, so that it can be easily removed if it blocks. Endoscopic stenting can often be performed in less than 30 minutes but difficult cases may take longer. The procedure is usually well tolerated and most patients are able to eat within a few hours.

Technical Problems

Selective Cannulation

Selective cannulation of the bile duct is the first step in endoscopic stenting. This is most easily achieved with the endoscope in the "short-scope" position. In some elderly patients a floppy duodenum makes positioning the endoscope difficult. Rolling these patients onto their left side may help.

We first attempt cannulation with the inner catheter. If this is unsuccessful we then try a sphincterotome. We prefer a sphincterotome with a short tip (2–3 mm) distal to the wire. The variable bow can then be used to adjust position in the papilla and help select the bile duct. A biliary cannulation sleeve can be used together with the sphincterotome.[31] This 10-FG sleeve fits over the sphincterotome and steadies it in the large channel of the endoscope. During difficult sphincterotomies part of the diathermy wire can be covered with the sleeve to

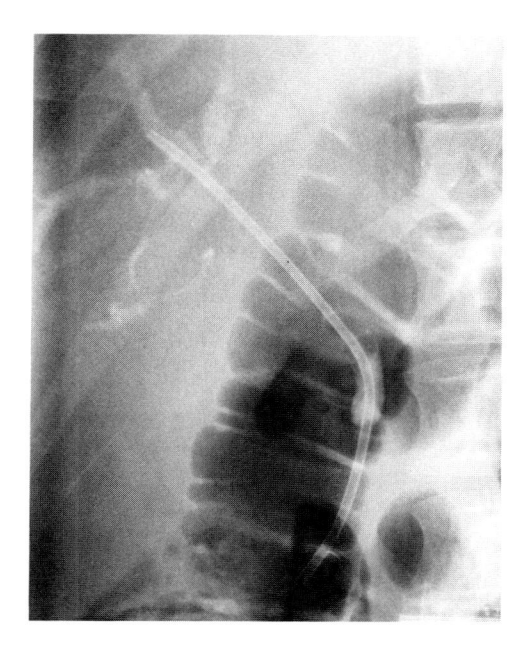

Figure 11-6 10-FG stent in place across the long hilar stricture.

prevent shorting out on the endoscope. Once the sphincterotomy has been performed the sphincterotome and sleeve are placed deep in the duct. The sphincterotome is removed leaving the sleeve in place. The guidewire and inner tube are then inserted through the sleeve directly into the duct. This avoids the problem of having to recannulate the fresh sphincterotomy, which is often oozing and edematous.

In some patients with low bile duct obstruction the tumor extends down close to the papilla and distorts the normal anatomy. This makes selective cannulation with a standard sphincterotome particularly difficult. One approach to this problem is to perform a precut sphincterotomy with a needle knife.[32] This technique has a theoretical risk of an increased incidence of pancreatitis; however, it seems safe when used by experienced endoscopists. We have used a combined percutaneous/endoscopic procedure as another solution to this difficult problem. A radiologist inserts a 5-FG catheter and guidewire into the bile duct percutaneously. The guidewire is maneuvered through the stricture and into the duodenum. The endoscopist, can then insert a catheter (or sphincterotome) over the radiologists guidewire into the duct and through the stricture. A stent is then inserted endoscopically in the usual manner. This approach may have fewer complications than percutaneous stenting as the tract through the liver needs only to be dilated to 5 FG rather than 10–12 FG.

Stricture Intubation and Dilation

Some strictures, particularly those due to cholangiocarcinoma, are irregular and sharply angulated. If passing the guidewire is difficult, a variety of angles and positions in the bile duct below the stricture should be tried. If still unsuccessful, X rays taken while injecting contrast may help to define the position and direction the stricture comes off uninvolved duct. Care should be taken to avoid creating false passages, particularly with strictures at the hilum. Always lead with the floppy tip of a guidewire rather than the stiffer catheter and avoid excessive force. Occasionally a J-tip guidewire may assist in negotiating acutely angled strictures. Prototype torque stable and steerable guidewires have also been tried. These have not been as successful as hoped for because of the long lengths and sharp turns required for endoscopy.

Low biliary strictures are usually easily dilated. Compression is often extrinsic and the distance from the endoscope tip to the stricture is short, and considerable force can be applied to the dilator. However, hilar strictures can be more difficult. If the coaxial 10-FG dilator cannot be passed, a dilator with a long tapered tip or a graduated metal tip dilator can be tried. Balloon dilators have been suggested; however, we have found it difficult to introduce the balloon into tight angulated strictures.

It may be helpful to take bile specimens from above the lesion for cytology (as well as culture); brushing cytology results have so far proved disappointing. If it is not possible to dilate the stricture to 10 FG, then one option is to insert a smaller stent, 7 or 8 FG, with a higher risk of early cholangitis. Alternatively, a nasobiliary drain can be placed above the stricture to provide temporary drainage and prevent cholangitis. We found that strictures are usually much easier to dilate after the biliary tree has been decompressed by several days of nasobiliary drainage.

A combined percutaneous/endoscopic approach can also be used for these difficult strictures. Strictures may be more easily negotiated from above, particularly if the biliary tree has been decompressed by several days of external drainage. If the percutaneous guidewire is held at either end by the radiologist and the endoscopist, considerable force can be applied for endoscopic dilation and stent insertion.

Complications

The most important early complication is cholangitis. This is more common with hilar strictures, the exact incidence depending on the definitions used and how carefully patients are reviewed. Endoscopes must be carefully cleaned and disinfected[33] and accessory equipment should be sterilized. The incidence of cholangitis was high with the 7- and 8-FG stents used initially and decreased when larger stents were introduced. We recommend that stents of at least 10 FG diameter should be used. Occasionally, stenting in a patient with multiple intrahepatic strictures will be complicated by cholangitis in an undrained segment of liver. It is difficult to selectively cannulate and drain the infected segments endoscopically. These patients are best managed by percutaneous drainage of these ducts.

Hemorrhage and pancreatitis have been reported following sphincterotomy for stent insertion. The incidence of these can be reduced by performing a small sphincterotomy or, if possible, by inserting the stent without a sphincterotomy. Perforation complicating stenting may be due to the sphincterotomy or may occur in the bile duct at or below the stricture. Strictures should be gently negotiated with the floppy tip of the guidewire. The wire usually passes easily once the correct position and angle are located. Perforations can usually be managed conservatively by obtaining adequate drainage of the bile duct with an endoscopic stent or percutaneously if this is not possible.

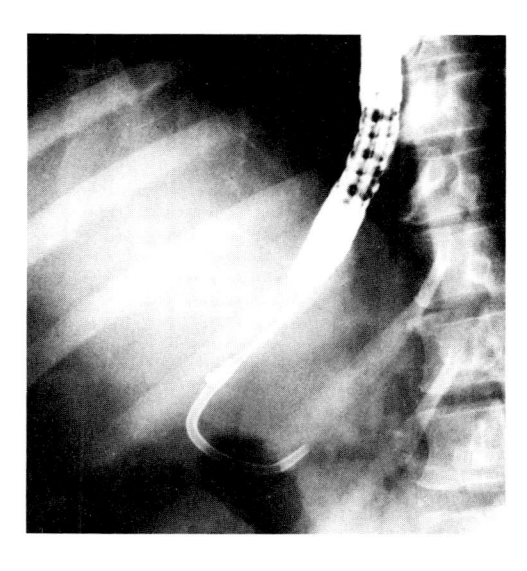

Figure 11-7 A blocked stent is removed by grasping the tip with a basket and pulling the endoscope, basket, and stent out through the mouth.

Poststent Management

Antibiotics are continued until it is clear that the stent is draining adequately, which is usually 24–48 hours. Bilirubin levels are performed daily; a falling bilirubin indicates adequate stent function. Abdominal ultrasound is usually performed 24–48 hours to assess stent function. Decompression of the biliary tree and the presence of air in the ducts indicates successful drainage.[34] The histological diagnosis of malignancy can be confirmed by ultrasound- or CT-guided fine-needle aspiration biopsy at the time.[35] The patients need only be hospitalized for a few days after the procedure; however, the stay may be prolonged due to their poor general condition or the need for further investigations. After a successful stent insertion, pruritus is usually relieved in 2–3 days and jaundice will resolve over 2–3 weeks depending on initial bilirubin levels and hepatocellular function. In the absence of liver metastases or advanced cirrhosis, we would expect the liver function tests to return to normal. On discharge, patients are advised that a recurrence of the jaundice or cholangitis would suggest a blocked stent and should prompt an immediate return for further management. Consideration should be given to exchanging stents prophylactically at about 4 months in patients who remain vital (and in any patient with benign disease). Stent blockage is diagnosed on ultrasound examination by finding a dilated biliary tree that does not contain gas. The blocked stent is removed endoscopically by grasping the tip with a basket or snare and pulling the stent, snare, and endoscope out through the mouth (Figure 11-7). Insertion of a new stent is usually much easier than the initial procedure. Stent migration upward or downward is extremely rare if the initial position is correct.

Carcinoma of the Pancreas
Results in High-Risk Patients

Since its introduction in 1979, endoscopic stenting has been used mainly for patients considered unfit for palliative bypass surgery. There was an initial learn-

Table 11-3 Results of Endoscopic Stenting for Carcinoma of the Pancreas in Patients Who Are High Risks for Surgery

	The Middlesex Hospital ($N = 99$)	University of Amsterdam ($N = 221$)
Relief of jaundice	88%	87%
30-Day mortality	9%	10%
Mean survival	25 weeks	26 weeks
Late duodenal stenosis	6%	7.5%

ing phase where endoscopists developed the technique and equipment. The results of endoscopic stenting have been published in several series. At the Middlesex Hospital between March 1983 and March 1986, 102 patients with carcinoma of the pancreas were assessed for endoscopic stenting. The diagnosis was made by finding a mass in the pancreas on abdominal ultrasound and obstruction of the bile duct and pancreatic duct at ERCP. If there was doubt about the diagnosis, computed axial tomography and endoscopic ultrasound were also used. The lesions were judged to be not resectable because of the size of the tumor or spread of the tumor beyond the pancreas. The patients were considered to be unfit for bypass surgery because of their age, associated medical conditions, or extent of disease. Histologic confirmation of adenocarcinoma was obtained in 76 (76%) of the patients, usually by ultrasound-guided fine-needle aspiration biopsy.

The patients were elderly (median age 76 years). The age distribution at the Middlesex Hospital has been superimposed on that of the United Kingdom in 1982 in Figure 11-1. Our age distribution is skewed to the right, and the biggest group of patients is that aged 80–85 years. The patients were deeply jaundiced; a quarter had renal impairment due to prolonged biliary obstruction. Seventeen patients (17%) had had previous unsuccessful surgical or percutaneous attempts at biliary drainage. Four of these patients had a biliary fistula. Three patients were so sick that further intervention was considered meddlesome and all three died within one week. Stenting was attempted in 99 patients and a stent was successfully inserted in 88 (89%). Jaundice was relieved in all but one of the patients (Table 11-3). The stents used were 10 FG ($N = 71$) with some 11.5 FG ($N = 9$) recently and 8 FG ($N = 8$) double-pigtail stents in our early experience. Eight patients with successfully inserted stents died within 30 days of the procedure. Three died with complications of the procedure: one cholangitis, one pancreatitis, and one patient died during the procedure, probably from oversedation. Three patients died with disseminated disease between days 6 and 26 following the procedure. One patient died with a bleeding gastric ulcer and another with bleeding gastric erosions. Those patients with failed procedures were managed by percutaneous intervention ($N = 4$), bypass surgery ($N = 4$), and no further treatment ($N = 3$). Five of these patients died within 30 days.

The median survival of patients with successfully inserted stents was 21 weeks (mean 25 weeks). Late complications were stent blockage and duodenal obstruction. Stent replacement was required on at least one occasion in 20 patients, ie, 29.5% of those at risk. These patients presented with a recurrence of their jaundice and/or cholangitis. The blocked stents were easily replaced endoscopically in all cases and this required a hospital admission of 2-3 days. Duodenal obstruction requiring bypass surgery occurred in five patients, 6% of those at risk.

Our results are similar to those obtained by Huibregtse at the University of Amsterdam in a larger series of patients with carcinoma of the pancreas palliated with endoscopic stents (Table 11-3).[36] The incidence of duodenal stenosis in both series is lower than expected. A review of a series of patients undergoing biliary bypass surgery without prophylactic gastroenterostomy found reoperation for duodenal stenosis in a mean of 16% (range 6-50%) of patients.[37] The lower incidence in endoscopic series is due to patient selection. Duodenal compression or invasion makes endoscopic stenting technically difficult. We usually do not attempt stenting in these patients as they are best treated by surgical bypass.

The quality of palliation is often difficult to judge. However, we consider that endoscopic stents provide good palliation. After successful stent insertion, pruritis is rapidly relieved, usually within 2-3 days. Jaundice resolves over several weeks. Nutrition is improved by returning bile to the duodenum and many patients without extensive metastatic disease gain weight. Renal impairment due to biliary obstruction resolves after stenting and renal function returns to normal. In the small group of patients who had a biliary fistula, successful stenting resulted in resolution of the fistula within 24-48 hours.

This review of our series and others in the literature shows that endoscopic stents provide effective palliation in patients who are high risks for surgery.

Unresectable Disease in Patients Fit for Surgery

Surgical bypass has traditionally been the standard treatment for patients with unresectable disease. A laparotomy provides the opportunity to biopsy the lesion, obtain proof the tumor is not resectable by surgical exploration, and then a prophylactic gastroenterostomy may be performed. Unfortunately, this surgery has a substantial mortality. In an extensive review of the series in the English literature, Sarr found that the mean 30-day mortality for surgical bypass in carcinoma of the pancreas was 18%.[37] Modern imaging techniques (ultrasound, computed tomography, endoscopic ultrasound) make it easier to select patients with unresectable disease without resorting to a laparotomy. Confirmation of malignancy can be obtained by percutaneous aspiration cytology or trucut biopsy guided by ultrasound or computed tomography.[35] Endoscopic stenting may be an alternative to bypass surgery. Stenting has the advantage of being less traumatic than surgery with a shorter initial hospital stay and possibly a lower 30-day mortality. The disadvantages are readmissions for stent blockages and possibly late duodenal obstruction. In the endoscopic stent series to date, the incidence of late duodenal obstruction is low in patients with an endoscopically normal duodenum on presentation. Whether this low incidence will continue in younger, fitter patients needs to be assessed in further studies.

The results of the current series of endoscopic stents for carcinoma of the pancreas should not be compared with surgical series. The endoscopic patients have been selected because they are not fit for bypass surgery and are older with more extensive disease than surgical patients. Both these factors adversely influence 30-day mortality and overall survival. The two techniques are best compared in a prospective randomized trial and the results of the first such study have been presented.[38] A total of 52 patients with unresectable carcinoma of the pancreas were randomized between endoscopic stents and bypass surgery. The techniques were equally successful in relieving jaundice. The 30-day mortality for endoscopic stents (9%) was less than that for surgery (20%). However, this was not statistically significant due to the small numbers in the trial. The length of the initial hospital admission was significantly less for stents (5 days) compared with surgery (13 days). The number of days spent in hospitals throughout the patient's lifetime was also significantly less for stents. Further studies are required to confirm this result and one such trial is currently being conducted at the Middlesex and London Hospitals. Analysis of the results of these trials may allow identification of patient groups that are best managed by each technique. Probably, surgery will be shown to provide the best palliation for reasonably fit younger patients and stenting to be best in elderly frail patients.

Resectable Tumors

There is a small group of patients with early cancers in the head of the pancreas who are potentially curable.[39] All patients should be thoroughly investigated to identify this group. The morbidity and mortality of surgery in these patients is increased by the presence of obstructive jaundice. Prolonged biliary obstruction causes disturbances in many physiologic processes, including coagulation, renal function, wound healing, and myocardial function.[30,40-42] It has been postulated that preoperative biliary drainage will correct these abnormalities and reduce the incidence of complications following surgery. Preoperative percutaneous transhepatic drainage has been extensively studied. Nakayama, using preoperative drainage, found that operative mortality was reduced compared with historical controls.[14] Two other studies using historical controls and three studies using concurrent but nonrandomized controls have also suggested benefit from percutaneous preoperative drainage.[43-47] However, three prospective randomized trials showed no benefit and emphasized the complications of percutaneous drainage, which appear to outweigh any benefit.[48-50]

Endoscopic stenting is an alternative to percutaneous drainage and avoids the complications of puncturing the liver and external drainage. Patients with endoscopic stents could spend 4–6 weeks at home while their hepatocellular function recovers and nutritional states return to normal. The potential disadvantages of the approach are the possibility that surgery will be more difficult if the bile duct is no longer dilated and that the stent procedure may introduce infection. The role of endoscopic preoperative drainage can only be assessed in a prospective randomized trial and such a study is currently being conducted at the Middlesex and London Hospitals. However, the accrual rate is slow since so few patients have lesions which are resectable.

Hilar Strictures

Malignant hilar strictures pose many technical problems. The strictures are often very irregular and tortuous, and are difficult to cannulate. We reviewed the results of endoscopic stenting in hilar biliary obstruction due to malignancy at the Middlesex Hospital between May 1983 and December 1985. A total of 64 patients were considered for stenting, their lesions were not resectable, and the

Table 11-4 Results of Endoscopic Stenting for Hilar Strictures Subdivided According to Type of Stricture

	Type 1 ($N = 14$)	Type 2 ($N = 9$)	Type 3 ($N = 41$)	Total ($N = 41$)
Successful stent insertion	14 (100%)	8 (89%)	30 (73%)	52 (81%)
Successful relief of jaundice	13 (93%)	8 (89%)	23 (56%)**	44 (69%)
30-day mortality	1 (7%)	2 (25%)	4 (13%)	7 (13%)
Median survival (weeks)	32	20	12	16

* See text for classification of types of stricture.
** Relief of jaundice was significantly more successful in type 1 and 2 strictures compared with type 3 ($p < 0.01 \chi^2$).

patients were considered unsuitable for bypass surgery because of their age, the extent of the disease, or unrelated medical illness. The patients were elderly (median age 68 years), deeply jaundiced, mean bilirubin 405 μmol/liter, and 30% had renal impairment due to prolonged biliary obstruction. Previous bypass surgery had been unsuccessful in 11 (17%). Histologic confirmation of malignancy was obtained in 38 (59%) at fine-needle aspiration biopsy or postmortem examination. The tumors included cholangiocarcinoma ($N = 42$), carcinoma of the gallbladder ($N = 10$), and metastases ($N = 12$). Stents were successfully inserted in 52 (81%) and this relieved the jaundice in 44 (69%). Complications occurred within 2 weeks of the procedures in 10 patients (16%); these were mainly cholangitis (7 patients, or 11%). The stents inserted were 10 FG in diameter ($N = 53$) with some 11.5 FG ($N = 9$), and 8-FG stents were inserted on two occasions when it was not possible to dilate the stricture with the 10-FG dilator. Seven patients (13%) with successfully inserted stents died within 30 days of the procedure. In three of these patients the bilirubin was falling and the causes of death were a pneumothorax following a lung biopsy, bronchopneumonia, and malignancy. In the other four patients there was no fall in bilirubin and the cause of death was progressive liver failure in two, cholangitis and hemorrhage following insertion of a percutaneous drain in the third. The median survival of patients with successfully inserted stents was 16 weeks (mean 22 weeks).

The technical difficulty in stenting depends on the extent of the stricture. We have classified hilar strictures as follows: a stricture involving both right and left hepatic ducts plus intrahepatic ducts, type 3; involving right and left ducts, type 2; and involving the common hepatic duct within 2 cm of the bifurcation but not left or right duct, type 1. Type 3 strictures are usually associated with more extensive malignant disease.

Our results have been subdivided according to the type of hilar stricture as shown in Table 11-4. Stent insertion was more successful in type 1 and 2 strictures compared with type 3 ($p < 0.01 \chi^2$), and once the stent was inserted jaundice was more often relieved. Postmortem examination of two patients with type 3 strictures and successfully inserted stents but no fall in bilirubin showed that the stents were draining segments of liver that were extensively invaded by tumor. Survival was longer in type 1 strictures, although this was not statistically significant with the small numbers involved.

Thirteen patients required stent replacement on at least one occasion, ie, 25% of those at risk. This was easily accomplished endoscopically. Cholangitis developed in undrained segments in two patients (4%) in association with blocked stents. This was managed by percutaneously inserted external drains.

Insertion of a single stent will only drain part of the liver in type 2 and 3 strictures. Some authors—particularly Cremer[51]—advocate the placement of two or more stents in this situation. However, this is technically difficult and succeeds in only about 30% of attempts by endoscopy alone.[52] Other stents must be placed percutaneously or by a combined endoscopic-radiologic procedure. Our results do not suggest that it is imperative to drain all segments unless or until sepsis develops. The majority of our patients had multiple intrahepatic strictures and of course would require multiple stents to obtain complete drainage of the liver. We have used two stents in only two patients in this series. Follow-up of the patients with a single stent in situ has shown that jaundice and the symptoms of biliary obstruction are relieved when as little as 20% of the liver is drained.

Huibregtse obtained similar results in a large series of 275 patients with malignant hilar stricture treated with endoscopic stents.[52] Jaundice was relieved in 72% of these patients, the 30-day mortality was 20%, and the mean survival was 6 months.

Our results suggest that a single endoscopic stent can provide palliation of malignant hilar strictures in patients at high risk for bypass surgery. However, in patients with extensive malignancy and multiple intrahepatic strictures, stenting is technically more difficult, the insertion of a stent does not always relieve jaundice, and the survival of these patients is often short even if jaundice is relieved. Further studies are required to select those patients who will benefit from stenting from those in whom further intervention is meddlesome.

Stent Design

The technique of stent insertion has been modified and improved with increasing experience and expertise since its introduction over 8 years ago. The design of guidewires, catheters, and dilators used for cannulating, negotiating, and dilating the stricture are now well established. However, the optimal diameter and shape of the stent remains controversial. The shape of the stent must conform with the bile duct and provide anchorage to prevent distal and proximal migration. Initially, pigtails were used to provide anchorage. These were straightened out over a guidewire for insertion and the curve reformed when the stent was in position in the bile duct and the guidewire was removed. Huibregtse noted that there was often not enough room for the pigtail to form above obstructions. He cut flaps at the upper and lower ends of the stent to provide anchorage.[53] This proved simple and effective, and is now widely used for lesions at all levels.

The maximum outside diameter of the stent is limited by the diameter of the instrument channel in the endoscope. Initially 7- and 8-FG stents were inserted through a standard endoscope. Large-diameter endoscopes have been developed specifically for biliary stenting. These allow the insertion of 10-FG and, more recently, 11.5-FG stents. However, the larger diameter makes the endoscope less flexible and more cumbersome to use. Some authors claim that small-diameter stents provide good palliation,[54] while others insist that bigger is better.[20,55,56]

We started using flaps for anchorage at the time the large endoscopes became available. Thus we changed from 8-FG stents with pigtails to 10-FG straight stents with flaps. The performance of 8- and 10-FG stents has been reviewed retrospectively.[57]

The two groups of patients were similar. They were elderly; 60% had low strictures due to carcinoma of the pancreas, and the rest had strictures at the hilum or mid-duct. Both groups received antibiotics prophylactically before stenting. A total of 28 patients had 8-FG stents inserted on 38 occasions and 51 patients had 10-FG stents inserted on 61 occasions. The incidence of successful stent insertion and relief of jaundice was similar in both groups. However, the incidence of early cholangitis was significantly higher in patients with 8-FG stents (13, or 34%) than in those with 10-FG stents (3, or 5%); $p < 0.001$ χ^2. The incidence of complications other than cholangitis was similar in the two groups. The higher incidence of early cholangitis with small-diameter stents has been found by other investigators. Deviere *et al* report early cholangitis in 40% with 7-FG stents (internal diameter 1.4 mm) compared with 7% with 10-FG stents.[55] Two other series describe a reduction in cholangitis when changing from small- to large-diameter stents although the precise details are not given.[19,20]

The increased incidence of early cholangitis with 8-FG stents is due to their lower flow capacity. Slow drainage leads to stasis and bacterial overgrowth in the bile resulting in clinical cholangitis. The flow capacity of a tube can be calculated from fluid mechanics. Flow capacity is proportional to the internal diameter raised to the fourth power,[58] thus a small increase in diameter results in a large increase in flow capacity. An increase in diameter from 8 to 10 FG results in a 170% increase in flow capacity.[57] 10-FG stents have a flow capacity well above the physiologic requirement. There is a wide safety margin for unpredictable variables such as clot and debris in the bile, or increased bile viscosity due to infection.

In our comparison of the two groups the 10-FG stents remained patent longer than the 8-FG stents. Stent replacement was required in 12 patients (43%) with 8-FG stents compared with 13 (25%) with 10-FG stents. The time to blockage of the stents was calculated by actuarial life table analysis. The median patency of 10-FG stents—32 weeks—was significantly longer than that of 8-FG stents—12 weeks; $p < 0.001$ log rank analysis. Assuming a constant rate of sludge deposition, we calculated that an increase in diameter from 10 to 11.5 FG would increase median stent survival from 32 to 37.6 weeks.[57] In a recent randomized trial there was no significant difference in stent survival or the rate of stent change between 10- and 12-FG stents. The 12-FG stents were more difficult to insert.[69]

Biliary stents are blocked by a material that resembles biliary sludge. Analysis has shown that it consists mainly of calcium bilirubinate with some calcium palmitate and an organic matrix.[59] We performed light and electron microscopy studies of blocked stents and showed that this material is a matrix of bacterial biofilm containing crystals of calcium bilirubinate, calcium palmitate, and cholesterol.[60] Bacterial biofilm is a general phenonemon occurring regularly in nature[61] and industrial acquatic systems.[62] Bacteria adhere to solid surfaces and then produce a polysaccharide which cements the bacterial cell to the surface and mediates adhesion to sister cells.[63] Further bacterial multiplication leads to the formation of adherent microcolonies which eventually coalesce to form the biofilm. In bile, bacterial enzyme activity, β-glucuronidase, and phosphilipase lead to the formation of calcium bilirubinate, calcium palmitate, and cholesterol within the biofilm. Bacterial biofilms have also been found on the surfaces of other biomedical devices such as urinary catheters,[64] peritoneal dialysis catheters,[65] and intrauterine contraceptive devices.[66] Bacteria adhere to all the materials currently used to manufacture stents—polyethylene, polyurethane, and Teflon. However, a polymer with an intrinsic antibacterial action could prevent bacterial adhesion. It may be possible to incorporate biocides or antibiotics into polymers so that they leach out slowly over a period of time. Further work in this area may result in stents resistant to blockage.

We currently prefer stents of at least 10-FG diameter, manufactured from polyethylene. Flaps at each end prevent migration of the stent out of the stricture. The lower section of the stent is 4 cm long corresponding to the retropancreatic portion of the common bile duct,[67] and there is a gentle curve of approximately 120° corresponding to the shape of the bile duct. The upper portion of the stent is of variable length according to the position of the stricture in the bile duct. We do not put multiple side holes on our stents as the rough-cut edges of these provide anchorage for bacterial biofilm. There is a gentle taper at the upper end to aid insertion. Sharp curves and tapers should be avoided as these cause substantial reductions in flow capacity.[68] The wall thickness of the stent is a compromise between two opposing factors. A thicker wall gives better stiffness and elastic properties required for insertion and greater strength to resist stress fracture in the long term. However, with a fixed outside diameter a thinner wall results in a bigger internal diameter and better flow capacity.

Conclusions

There is a broad spectrum of patients with biliary obstruction due to malignancy (Figure 11-8). Surgery is the established method of managing these patients; however, the probability of surviving an operation decreases with age and with extensive metastatic disease. The patients with the lowest operative mortality are young, fit patients with small tumors. Those at highest risk are elderly frail patients with extensive tumor loads.

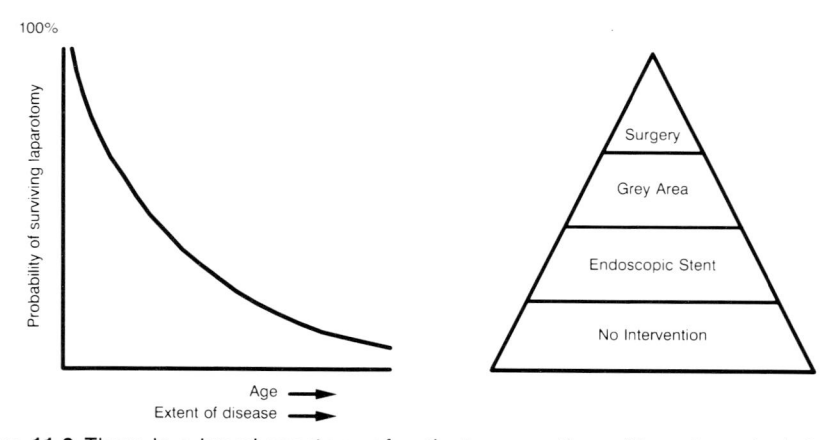

Figure 11-8 There is a broad spectrum of patients presenting with malignant obstructive jaundice. The risk of surgery depends on many factors, particularly increasing age and the extent of the disease. The management chosen for each patient depends on a careful clinical assessment of his or her overall condition.

Perhaps the most difficult decision to make is when *not* to intervene. For many elderly patients with extensive metastatic disease, attempts at intervention may cause more distress than palliation. Multiple intrahepatic strictures usually indicate the presence of extensive metastases. In these patients effective palliation of biliary obstruction is difficult with endoscopic stenting or any other technique.

On the other hand, young patients with localized tumors surely deserve the benefit of surgery with the possibility of a resection and cure. Endoscopic stents may have a role in preoperative drainage of these patients, but this needs to be assessed in prospective randomized trials. Unresectable tumors in patients fit for surgery are currently a "grey" area. The roles of bypass surgery and endoscopic stenting need to be defined in prospective randomized trials. The results of the first such study suggest that stenting is at least as effective as surgery.

The introduction of endoscopic stenting has had its greatest impact on the group with unresectable tumors in patients who are high risks for surgery. Our results and other published series have shown that endoscopic stents provide good palliation for these difficult patients.

References

1. Fraumeni JF, Jr: Cancers of the pancreas and biliary tract. Epidemiological considerations. *Cancer Res* 1975;35:3437–3446.
2. Department of Health and Social Security; Office of Population Censuses and Surveys. Cancer statistics, registrations and mortality. 1962–1982, London, HMSO.
3. Herman RE, and Cooperman AM: Current concepts in cancer. Cancer of the pancreas. *N Engl J Med* 1979;301:482–485.
4. Bismuth H, and Malt RA. Carcinoma of the biliary tract. *N Engl J Med* 1979;301:704–706.
5. Okuda K, Kubo Y, Okazaki N, *et al*: Clinical aspects of intrahepatic bile duct carcinoma including hilar carcinoma; a study of 57 autopsy-proven cases. *Cancer* 1977;39:232–246.
6. Pitt HA, Cameron JL, Postier RG, and Gadacz TR: Factors affecting mortality in biliary tract surgery. *Am J Surg* 1981;141:66–72.
7. Ransohoff DF, Gracie WA, Wolfenson LB, and Neuhauser D: Prophylactic cholecystectomy or expectant management for silent gallstones. *Ann Intern Med* 1983;99:199–204.
8. Lerut JP, Gianello PR, Otte JB, and Kestens PJ: Pancreaticoduodenal resection. Surgical experience and evaluation of risk factors in 103 patients. *Ann Surg* 1984;199:432–437.
9. Andren-Sandberg A, and Ihse I: Factors influencing survival after total pancreatectomy in patients with pancreatic cancer. *Ann Surg* 1983;198:605–610.
10. Blievernicht SE, Neifeld JP, Terz JJ, and Lawrence J, Jr: The role of prophylactic gastroenterostomy for unresectable periampullary carcinoma. *Surg Gynec Obstet* 1980;151:794–796.
11. Ubhi CS, and Doran J: Palliation for carcinoma of head of pancreas. *Ann Royal Coll Surg of Engl* 1986;68:159–162.
12. Feduska NJ, Dent TL, and Lindenaeur SM: Results of palliative operations for carcinoma of the pancreas. *Arch Surg* 1971;103:330–333.
13. Kaude JV, Weidermer L, and Agee CF: Decompression of the bile ducts with the percutaneous technique. *Radiology* 1969;93:69–71.
14. Nakayama T, Ikeda A, and Okada K: Percutaneous transhepatic drainage of the biliary tract. *Gastroenterology* 1978;74:554–559.

15. Hoevels J, and Lunderquist A: Results of percutaneous internal-external drainage. In: Classen M, Geenan J, Kawai K, eds. *Nonsurgical Biliary Drainage*. Berlin, Springer-Verlag, 1984, pp. 43–46.
16. Burcharth F: A new endoprosthesis for non-operative intubation of the biliary tract in malignant obstructive jaundice. *Surg Gynecol Obstet* 1978;146:76–78.
17. Soehendra N, and Reynders-Frederix V: Palliative bile duct drainage. A new endoscopic method of introducing a transpapillary drain. *Endoscopy* 1980;12:8–11.
18. Speer AG, Cotton PB, Russell RCG, et al: Randomized trial of endoscopic versus percutaneous stent insertion in malignant obstructive jaundice. *Lancet* 1987;2:57–62.
19. Hagenmuller F: Results of endoscopic bilioduodenal drainage in malignant bile duct stenoses. In: Classen M, Geenan J, Kawai K, eds. *Nonsurgical Biliary Drainage*. Berlin, Springer-Verlag, 1984, pp. 93–104.
20. Huibregtse K, and Tytgat GNJ: Endoscopic placement of biliary prostheses. In: Salmon PR, ed. *Gastrointestinal Endoscopy: Advances in Diagnosis and Therapy*, London, Chapman and Hall, 1984, pp. 219–231.
21. Leung JWC, Emery R, Cotton PB, Russell RCG, Vallon AG, and Mason RR: Management of malignant obstructive jaundice at the Middlesex Hospital. *Br J Surg* 1983;70:584–586.
22. Mueller PR, Ferrucci JT, Teplick SK, *et al*: Biliary stent endoprosthesis: Analysis of complications in 113 patients. *Radiology* 1985;156:637–639.
23. Dooley JS, Dick R, George P, Kirk RM, Hobbs KEF, and Sherlock S: Percutaneous transhepatic endoprosthesis for bile duct obstruction. *Gastroenterology* 1984;86:905–909.
24. Hoevels J, and Ihse I: Percutaneous transhepatic insertion of a permanent endoprosthesis in obstructive lesions of the extrahepatic bile ducts. *Gastroinstest Radiol* 1979;4:367–377.
25. Burcharth F, Eisen F, Christiansen LA, *et al*: Nonsurgical internal biliary drainage by endoprosthesis. *Surg Gynecol Obstet* 1981;153:857–860.
26. Coons HG, and Carey PH: Large-bore, long biliary endoprostheses (biliary stents) for improved drainage. *Radiology* 1983;148:89–94.
27. Burcharth F: Results of the percutaneous implantation of endoprostheses. In: Classen M, Geenan J, Kawai K, eds. *Nonsurgical Biliary Drainage*. Berlin, Springer-Verlag, 1984, pp. 47–55.
28. Pereiras RV, Jr, Rheingold OJ, Hutson D, *et al*: Relief of malignant obstructive jaundice by percutaneous insertion of a permanent prosthesis in the biliary tree. *Ann Intern Med* 1978;89:589–593.
29. Dooley JS, Hamilton-Miller JMT, Brumfitt W, and Sherlock S: Antibiotics in the treatment of biliary infection. *Gut* 1984;25:988–998.
30. Green J, Beyar R, Sideman S, Mordechovitz D, and Better OS. The "jaundiced heart," a possible explanation for postoperative shock in obstructive jaundice. *Surgery* 1986;100:14–20.
31. Cunningham JT, Cotton PB, and Speer AG: A biliary cannulation sleeve. *Gastroint Endosc* 1986;32:407–408.
32. Classen M, and Phillip J: Endoscopic retrograde cholangiography (ERCP) and endoscopic therapy in pancreatic disease. *Clin Gastroenterol* 1984;13:3819–3842.
33. Axon ATR, and Cotton PB: Endoscopy and infection. *Gut* 1983;24:1064–1066.
34. Van Gansbeke D, Van Gossum A, Schils J, Engelholm L, Cremer M, and Struyven J: Sonographic monitoring of biliary endoprostheses. *Gastrointest Radiol* 1984;9:335–339.
35. Lees WR, Hall-Craggs MA, and Manhire A: Five years experience of fine-needle aspiration biopsy: 454 consecutive cases. *Clin Radiol* 1985;36:517–520.
36. Huibregtse K, Katon RM, Coene PP, and Tytgat GNJ: Endoscopic palliative treatment in pancreatic cancer. *Gastroint Endosc* 1986;32:334–338.

37. Sarr MG, and Cameron JL: Surgical palliation of unresectable carcinoma of the pancreas. *World J Surg* 1984;8:906–918.
38. Shepherd HA, Royle G, Ross APR, et al: Endoscopic biliary endoprosthesis in the palliation of malignant obstruction of the distal common bile duct; a randomized trial. *Br J Surg* 1988;75:1166–1168.
39. Moosa AR, Scott MH, and Lavelle-Jones M: The place of total and extended total pancreatectomy in pancreatic cancer. *World J Surg* 1984;8:895–899.
40. Jedrychowski A, Hillenbrand P, Ajdukiewicz AB, Parbhoo SP, and Sherlock S: Fibrinolysis in cholestatic jaundice. *Br Med J (Clin Res)* 1973;1:640–642.
41. Better OS: Bile duct ligation: An experimental model of renal dysfunction secondary to liver disease. In: *The Kidney in Liver Disease.* Ed Epstein M, New York, Elsevier, 1983.
42. Irvin TT, Vassilakis JS, Chattopadhyay DK, and Greaney MG: Abdominal wound healing in jaundiced patients. *Br J Surg* 1978;65:521–522.
43. Takada T, Hanyu F, Kibayashi S, and Uchida Y: Percutaneous transhepatic cholangial drainage; direct approach under fluoroscopic control. *J Surg Oncol* 1976;8:83–97.
44. Golicz RP, Stanley JH, Soncale CD, et al: Routine pre-operative biliary drainage; effect on management of obstructive jaundice. *Radiology* 1984;152:352–356.
45. Denning DA, Ellison EC, and Carey LC: Pre-operative percutaneous transhepatic biliary decompression lowers operative mortality in patients with obstructive jaundice. *Am J Surg* 1981;141:61–65.
46. Norlander A, Kalin B, and Sundblad R: Effect of percutaneous transhepatic drainage upon liver function and postoperative mortality. *Surg Gynecol Obstet* 1982;155:161–166.
47. Gundry SR, Strodel WE, Knol JA, et al: Efficacy of preoperative biliary tract decompression in patients with obstructive jaundice. *Arch Surg* 1984;119:703–706.
48. Hatfield ARW, Tobas R, Terblanche J, et al: Pre-operative external biliary drainage in obstructive jaundice: A prospective controlled clinical trial. *Lancet* 1982;2:896–900.
49. McPherson GAD, Benjamin IS, Hodgson HJF, et al: Pre-operative percutaneous transhepatic biliary drainage: The results of a controlled trial. *Br J Surg* 1984;71:371–375.
50. Pitt AP, Gomes AS, Lois JF, et al: Does pre-operative percutaneous biliary drainage reduce operative risk or increase hospital cost? *Ann Surg* 1985;201:545–553.
51. Deviere J, Baize M, de Toeuf J, and Cremer M: Long-term follow-up of patients with hilar malignant stricture treated by endoscopic internal biliary drainage. *Gastroint Endosc* 1988;34:95–101.
52. Tytgat GNJ, Huibregtse K, Bartelsman JFW, and Den Hartog Jager: Endoscopic palliative therapy in gastrointestinal and biliary tumors with prostheses. In: Classen M, ed. *Clin Gastroenterol*: Endoscopy, London, W. B. Saunders, 1986, pp. 249–273.
53. Huibregtse K, and Tytgat GN: Palliative treatment of obstructive jaundice by transpapillary introduction of large bore bile duct endoprosthesis. *Gut* 1982;23:371–375.
54. Zimmon DS, and Clemett AR: Experience with 5 French biliary pancreatic endoscopic stents. *Gastroint Endosc* 1985;30:168.
55. Deviere J, Baize M, Buset M, et al: Complications of internal endoscopic biliary drainage. *Acta Endosc* 1986;16:19–29.
56. Siegel JH, Pullano W, Kodsi B, Cooperman A, Ramsey W: Optimal palliation of malignant bile duct obstruction: Experience with endoscopic 12 French prostheses. *Endoscopy* 1988;20:137–141.
57. Speer AG, Cotton PB, and MacRae KD: Endoscopic management of malignant biliary obstruction: Stents of 10 French gauge are preferable to stents of 8 French gauge. *Gastroint Endosc* 1988;34:412–417.
58. Rodkiewicz CM, Otto WJ, and Scott GW: Empirical relationships for the flow of bile. *J Biomech* 1979;12:411–413.

59. Wosiewitz V, Schrameyer B, and Safrany L: Biliary sludge: Its role during bile duct drainage with an endoprosthesis. *Gastroenterology* 1985;88:1706.
60. Speer AG, Cotton PB, Rode J, Seddon AM, Neal CR, and Costerton JW: Bacterial biofilm blocks biliary stents. A light and electron microscopic study. *Ann Intern Med* 1988;108:546–553.
61. Geesey GG, Mutch RJ, Costerton JW, and Green RB: Sessile bacteria: An important component of the microbial population in small mountain streams. *Limnol Oceanogr* 1978;23:1214–1223.
62. McCoy WF, and Costerton JW: Fouling biofilm development in tubular flow systems. *Dev Industr Microbiol* 1982;23:551–558.
63. Costerton JW, Marrie TJ, and Cheng K-J: Phenomena of bacterial adhesion. In: Savage DC, Fletcher M, eds. *Bacterical Adhesion Mechanisms of Physiological Significance*. New York, Plenum Press, 1985, pp. 3–43.
64. Nickel JC, Grant SK, and Costerton JW: Catheter associated bacteriuria. *Urology* 1985;24:369–375.
65. Marrie TJ, Nobel MA, and Costerton JW: Examination of the morphology of bacteria adhering to peritoneal dialysis catheters by scanning and transmission electron microscopy. *J Clin Microbiol* 1983;18:1388–1398.
66. Marrie TJ, and Costerton JW: A scanning and transmission electron microscopic study of the surfaces of intrauterine contraceptive devices. *Am J Obstet Gynecol* 1983;146:384–394.
67. Dawson PM, and Allen-Mersch TG: The anatomical relationship between the retropancreatic part of the duct and the main pancreatic duct. *Ann Royal Coll Surg Engl* 1983;65:188–190.
68. Leung JWC, Favero GD, and Cotton PB: Endoscopic biliary prostheses: A comparison of materials. *Gastroint Endosc* 1985;31:93–95.
69. Dowsett JF, Williams SJ, Hatfield ARW, et al: Does stent diameter matter in the endoscopic palliation of malignant biliary obstruction? A randomized trial of 10 FG versus 12 FG endoprostheses. *Gastroenterology* 1989;96:A128.

Chapter **12**

Preoperative Biliary Decompression

Robert C. Kurtz, M.D.

Over the years, there have been substantial improvements in anesthesia and surgical techniques and in the pre- and postoperative care of the patient, yet major surgical procedures are still associated with high morbidity and mortality in the presence of malignant biliary obstruction and jaundice.

In an attempt to reduce this morbidity and mortality, A. O. Whipple[1] described his two-stage approach to the surgical management of carcinoma of the ampulla in 1935. The first stage was a surgical decompression of the obstructed biliary system. The second stage, performed some time later, was the cancer resection itself. The two-stage procedure was in part necessary to help reverse the abnormal coagulation state of many of the jaundiced patients due to hypoprothrombinemia. This approach was used almost exclusively until 1941, when vitamin K therapy was first introduced.

The single-stage procedure had become the current practice at the Lahey Clinic in 1962, when Warren and colleagues published their results of radical pancreaticoduodenectomy.[2] They recommended reserving the two-stage approach for the older, markedly jaundiced patient with renal insufficiency and a borderline prothrombin time. Mongé and colleagues published their 22-year experience with radical pancreaticoduodenectomy at the Mayo Clinic in 1964.[3] Their series consisted of 239 patients with carcinoma of the head of the pancreas, ampulla, duodenum, and common bile duct. The two-stage procedure was again reserved only for the higher risk patient, yet it is noteworthy that they reported that the hospital mortality of this selected group was lower (11.6%) than that of their entire group of patients (19.2%).

In a retrospective study, Maki and associates at Tohoku University in Sendai, Japan[4] compared the operative mortality of periampullary lesions resected from 1950 through 1959, using a one-stage procedure, with similar lesions treated surgically thereafter utilizing a two-stage approach. They demonstrated an impressive surgical mortality of only 8% with the two-stage technique versus 50% in those patients resected without previous biliary bypass surgery. They felt that there was a direct relationship between the level of jaundice and the surgical mortality, and advocated surgical cholecystostomy 3–4 weeks prior to the definitive cancer resection. They refed the externally drained bile back to the patient during the waiting period.

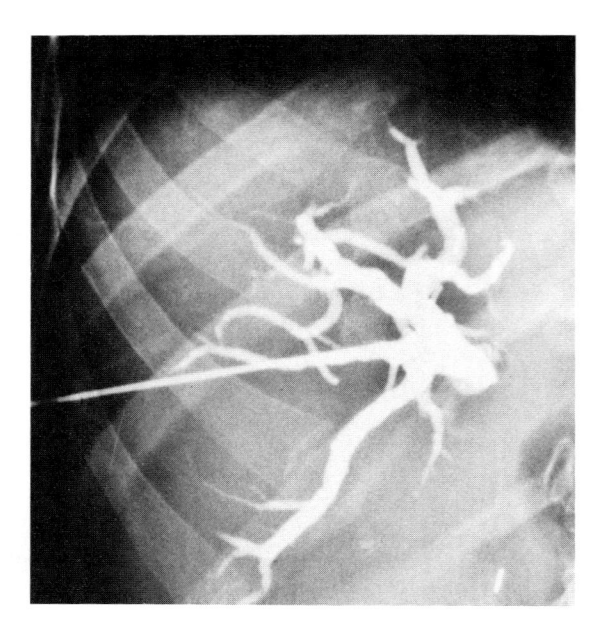

Figure 12-1 Percutaneous transhepatic drainage of a complete hilar obstruction due to cholangiocarcinoma.

Many surgeons believed that jaundiced patients undergoing pancreaticoduodenectomy for cancer had an increased morbidity and mortality which was in some way related to their level of jaundice, but they hesitated at the routine recommendation of the two-stage surgical procedure for all jaundiced patients. The possibility of draining the obstructed biliary tree nonsurgically at the same time a preoperative percutaneous transhepatic cholangiogram was done had obvious appeal (Figure 12-1).

Retrospective Trials

In 1978, Nakayama, Ikeda, and Okuda from the Chiba University in Japan[5] described their retrospective experience of percutaneous transhepatic biliary drainage (PTD) in patients with obstructive jaundice (Table 12-1). PTD was attempted in 105 patients and was successful in 104 of them. A malignancy was the cause of the biliary obstruction in 84 patients. Jaundice had been present

Table 12-1. Retrospective Studies on the Effect of PTD on Postoperative Mortality

Ref.	With PTD	Without PTD
Nakayama[5]	8% (4/49)	28% (36/148)
Dooley[6]	24% (5/21)	—
Denning[7]	16% (4/25)	25% (8/32)
Norlander*[8]	18% (8/44)	33% (14/42)
Gundry[9]	4% (1/25)	20% (5/25)
Total	13.4% (22/164)	25.5% (63/247)

* Patients with malignant obstruction.

for an average of 35 days in the patients with malignant obstruction, and serum bilirubin fell from a mean of 20.4 mg/dl to 10.8 mg/dl after 1 week and 4.1 mg/dl after 1 month of drainage. The decompression effect on serum bilirubin with PTD was similar in scope to 20 other patients who had undergone surgical cholecystostomy for external biliary drainage. A definitive surgical procedure was performed on 69 of the 104 patients with PTD after their serum bilirubin levels had fallen to less than 5 mg/dl. This group included 49 of the original 84 patients with malignant obstruction. The operative or 30-day mortality was 5.8% when all 69 patients were included, and 8.2% when looking at only those 49 patients with a malignant cause for obstruction. The authors compared these results retrospectively with those seen in 148 patients on whom an operation was performed without PTD. The mortality in this group was 28.3%. The difference in postoperative mortality, when compared to the 8.2% in the PTD group, was significant ($p < 0.05$).

Dooley and associates[6] at the Royal Free Hospital in London, England, reported their results with PTD in 41 patients. They were successful in placing the drainage catheter in 40 of 41 patients. Malignant biliary obstruction was present in 30 patients. Seven patients had palliative endoprostheses placed and 33 had external drainage established, with 21 of the 33 patients going on, at a later date, to surgery. The operative mortality in this latter group was 24%.

Denning et al at Ohio State[7] reviewed the records of 57 patients over a 4-year period (1975-1979) who had obstructive jaundice with admission bilirubin levels greater than 5 mg/dl. PTD was performed preoperatively in 25 of these patients. The remaining 32 patients went to surgery without preoperative biliary drainage. Three patients in the PTD group had benign biliary strictures. The remaining 22 patients had malignant biliary obstruction. However, only three patients were considered to have resectable tumors. Of the remaining 19 patients, 14 had a surgical biliary bypass performed and 5 had exploration and biopsy only. Six of the 32 patients who underwent surgery without PTD had a benign cause for their biliary obstruction. In the remaining 26 patients, a malignancy caused the obstruction, and only 6 of these patients were thought to be resectable. The remainder either had a palliative surgical bypass (15) or exploration and biopsy alone (5).

The morbidity rate of the PTD group was 28% (7 of 25) compared to 56% (18 of 32) in those without preoperative biliary decompression. This was statistically significant ($p < 0.05$). There was no difference in operative mortality between the two groups (16% versus 25%). The major postoperative complication was sepsis.

Norlander et al, at the Karolinska Hospital, Stockholm, Sweden,[8] reported on two groups of patients treated at their institution from 1968 to 1980. One group of 109 patients had PTD, and the other group of 65 patients, seen mainly during the earlier years of the study, went to surgery immediately after a diagnostic cholangiogram. In the group of 109 patients with PTD, 58 had at least 1 week of drainage before surgery. There were 44 patients in this group who had malignant biliary obstruction, and there were 42 patients with cancer in the group of 65 without PTD. There was no difference seen in 30-day operative mortality between these two groups. The authors state that if they excluded those patients in the PTD group with an inefficient drainage result from their statistical analysis, then a mortality advantage would be seen favoring the PTD group. Additionally, looking at just those patients with malignant obstruction, the mortality rate was 18% with and 33% without PTD.

The last retrospective series was from the University of Michigan by Gundry and associates.[9] During the 3-year period from 1979 to 1982, they studied 50 consecutive matched patients with either a benign or malignant cause for their biliary obstruction. Twenty-five patients had PTD preoperatively, and 25 patients went to surgery within 3 days following a diagnostic percutaneous cholangiogram. Malignant obstruction was seen in 18 patients in the PTD group and 21 patients in the non-PTD group. Twenty patients in each group had "dense jaundice" (serum bilirubin level greater than 10 mg/dl). Complications related to PTD occurred in nine patients (36%) and were mainly infectious. Postoperative complications occurred in only two patients (8%) in the PTD group compared with 13 patients (52%) in the non-PTD group. Only one postoperative death occurred in the PTD group (4%), whereas there were five postoperative deaths in the non-PTD group (20%). The authors also found that the mean hospital stay was actually shorter in the PTD group and that the postsurgical hyperbilirubinemia resolved more rapidly in this group as well.

It would appear from a review of these retrospective trials that PTD is a safe method of preoperative biliary decompression, with a low procedure-related morbidity and mortality. Most importantly, from these studies it would seem that decreasing the level of jaundice by PTD in patients with malignant biliary obstruction preoperatively should improve the 30-day surgical mortality in this patient population. Thus, many institutions began the routine use of PTD preoperatively. However, in 1982, McPherson *et al*,[10] from the hepatobiliary unit of the Hammersmith Hospital in London, published a prospective evaluation of 37 patients referred to their unit for PTD. All of the patients were jaundiced, and 10 patients had, in addition, severe renal insufficiency with creatinine clearance of 50 ml/min or less. A malignant cause for the obstruction was present in 35 patients (24 hilar lesions and 11 distal bile duct lesions) and two had sclerosing cholangitis. All were treated with prophylactic antibiotics.

The most dramatic findings of this study was the morbidity of PTD itself (Table 12-2). Infection was the most serious complication. Where 10 of the 37 patients had positive bile cultures initially, 25 patients had positive bile cultures, and 10 patients had positive blood cultures during the course of their PTD. Surgery was performed on 33 patients, and 8 died during the hospitalization (24.2%). Two of these deaths were associated with infection acquired during the period of PTD. Multiple liver abscesses were found at postmortem examination. The authors concluded that PTD is associated with a significant complication rate and that controlled trials would be needed to assess the

Table 12-2. Percutaneous Drainage Related Morbidity

Ref.	Mortality
McPherson [10]	54% (20/37)
Hatfield [11]	80% (20/25)
McPherson [12]	36% (13/36)
Total	54% (53/98)

role of preoperative PTD in the management of patients with malignant biliary obstruction.

Prospective Randomized Trials

The first prospective randomized evaluation of preoperative PTD was done by Hatfield and colleagues in Cape Town, South Africa[11] (Table 12-3). They randomly assigned 57 patients to either PTD followed by surgery (29 patients) or surgery alone (28 patients). The PTD patients all received prophylactic antibiotics and the continuous external biliary drainage was into a "sealed bag" system to help avoid infection. Drainage was carried out for at least 7–10 days. PTD was associated with a host of complications including reversible renal failure, pain, bile leak, bleeding, and multiple pulmonary difficulties. Postoperative complications were similar in both the drainage and nondrainage groups. Most importantly, surgical mortality rates were essentially the same for the PTD (14%) and non-PTD (15%) groups. The authors concluded that there was no advantage to the routine preoperative use of PTD and that the significant morbidity of the procedure weighed heavily against using it.

McPherson and colleagues[12] followed up their earlier study with a prospective randomized trial of preoperative drainage. Seventy patients were entered into the trial, 36 in the PTD group and 34 in the non-PTD group. Only patients with malignant biliary tract obstruction were included. Five patients withdrew from the study, leaving 34 patients in the PTD group and 31 in the non-PTD group. PTD lowered the serum bilirubin as expected, but again there were numerous complications of PTD. Five patients required early surgery for bile peritonitis and two of these died of renal failure. Five patients died during the drainage period, two of heart disease, two of pneumonia, and one with cholangitis. The mortality for surgery with PTD was 11 of 34 (32%), which was compared with the mortality of surgery alone which was 6 of 31 (19%). The authors stopped the trial, concluding that there was clearly no benefit from preoperative PTD other than bilirubin reduction and that there may in fact be an increase in mortality in the PTD group. As an aside, the authors were unable to determine an optimal preoperative period for PTD but did note that the PTD group had prolongation of their hospital stay when compared to those patients who went straight to surgery (40 days versus 23 days).

A third prospective randomized trial of preoperative PTD came from the Sepulveda VA Medical Center in California, by Pitt and colleagues.[13] Patients entered into the study could not have end-stage malignancies, had to have a

Table 12-3. Prospective Studies on the Effect of PTD on Postoperative Mortality

Ref.	With PTD	Without PTD
Hatfield[11]	14% (4/29)	15% (4/28)
McPherson[12]	32% (11/34)	19% (6/31)
Pitt[13]	8.1% (3/37)	5.3% (2/38)
Total	17% (17/100)	12.4% (12/97)

serum bilirubin of 10 mg/dl or more, and had five or more of the risk factors affecting biliary tract surgery described by Pitt in an earlier paper.[14] A total of 79 patients were entered into the study. Forty patients were in the preoperative PTD group and 39 in the non-PTD group. Surgery was performed on 37 patients in the PTD group and 38 in the non-PTD group. Percutaneous transhepatic drainage was successfully performed in 32 patients (87%). Drainage was continued for a mean of 10.9 days. Bilirubin and other liver functions were significantly improved. Five patients had a complication of PTD itself (13.6%). Postoperative complications occurred in 16 of 37 PTD patients (43.2%). When the presurgical and postsurgical complications in the PTD group were combined, 21 of 37 patients (56.8%) had complications. This was compared to 20 of 38 patients (52.6%) in the non-PTD group. Three patients in the PTD group (8.1%) and two patients in the non-PTD group (5.3%) died. There was no statistically significant difference in the complication or mortality rate between the two groups. Length of stay postoperatively and in intensive care units was also similar, but the preoperative length of hospitalization and, hence, the overall cost of the hospitalization was significantly higher in the PTD group. As a result, the authors recommended that preoperative PTD should not be routinely performed.

Endoscopic Biliary Drainage

The results of the prospective trials of PTD contrast markedly with those of the retrospective PTD trials. It seems clear that the high rate of infective complications of PTD may very well obscure any potential postoperative mortality benefit. In a recent retrospective review,[15] the failure rate of PTD in 81 consecutive patients was 10%. Emergency surgery was required in 4 patients (4.9%), 10 patients (12.3%) required blood transfusions, the overall sepsis rate was 34.6%, and 38 (47%) patients required 68 catheter manipulations.

The percutaneous method of biliary drainage involves manipulation of catheters through the peritoneal cavity and hepatic parenchyma, risking bile peritonitis and injury to intrapleural and vascular structures. Endoscopically placed biliary drainage catheters (EBD) have been in use in Europe and the United States for several years. Endoscopic placement of biliary stents avoids these problems by providing antegrade drainage through a catheter passed into the bile duct via the ampulla of Vater (Figures 12-2 and 12-3).

Classen and Hagenmuller[16] describe their endoscopic techniques for placement of both nasobiliary and bilioduodenal endoprosthesis. An endoscopic endoprosthesis was placed successfully through a malignant obstruction in 86.4% of the patients attempted at the University Hospitals at Hamburg and Frankfurt, West Germany. Morbidity and mortality of endoscopic biliary drainage was retrospectively compiled by these two authors[17] in 584 patients. There were 22 (3.8%) drainage-related complications (mainly cholangitis) and four deaths (0.7%). An additional eight patients (1.4%) had a nondrainage-related complication, and seven (1.2%) died.

Huibregste and Tytgat[18] described their experience with large-bore (3.2-mm) biliary endoprosthesis successfully used to palliate patients with malignant biliary obstruction. The short-term complications in their series included cholangitis and fever in 11 patients (24.4%). Seven patients had long-term complications of recurrent jaundice, stent migration, and clogging.

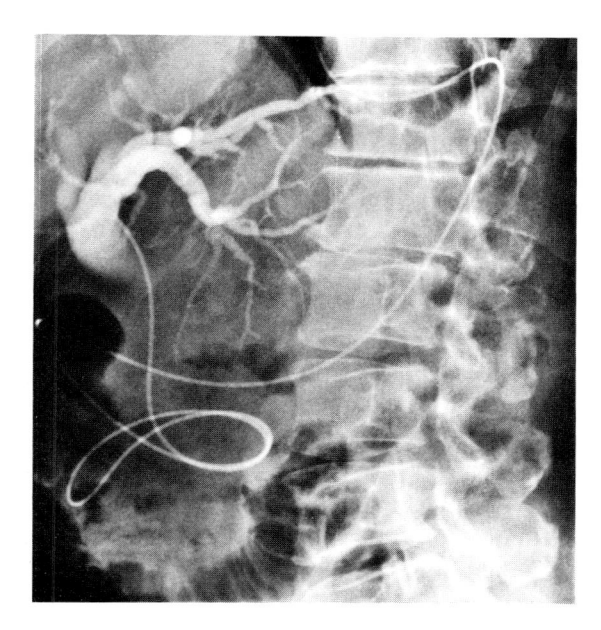

Figure 12-2 Preoperative endoscopically placed nasobiliary drain in a patient with ampullary cancer.

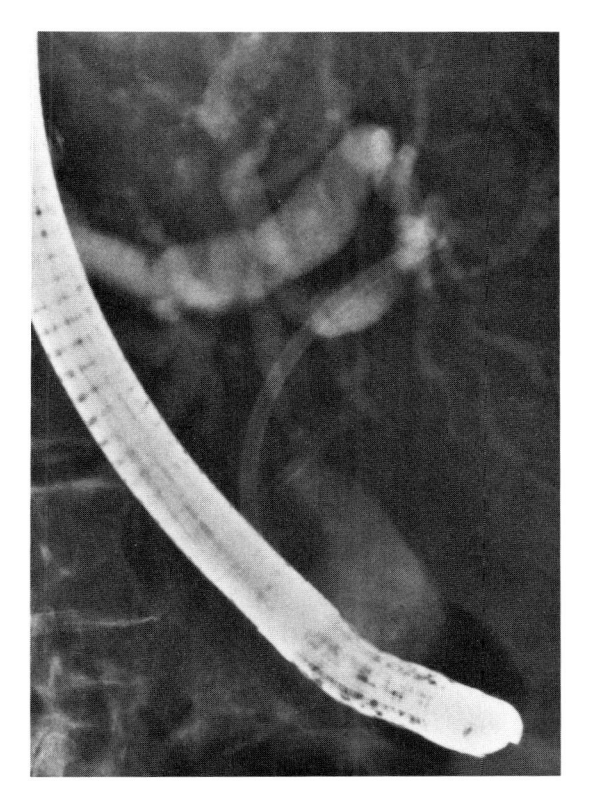

Figure 12-3 Large-bore endoscopically placed internal stent in malignant biliary obstruction due to pancreatic cancer.

The same authors[19] updated their experience by presenting their results of palliating a group of 221 patients with jaundice and pancreatic cancer. The endoscopic stents were placed immediately after the diagnostic endoscopic cholangiogram in 147 patients (66%). A second attempt was required in 45 patients, and 8 patients required a third procedure. The incidence of procedure-related cholangitis was much higher when the biliary stent could not be inserted on the first attempt. Cholangitis occurred in 12 of 53 patients (22.6%) who required a second or third attempt at stent placement, but only in 4 of 147 (2.7%) patients in whom the stent was placed on the first attempt. This was statistically significant ($p = 0.0001$). Serum bilirubin levels were reduced in 194 of 200 patients (97%) and fell into the normal range in 171 of the 181 patients who survived 30 days. In the 21 patients in whom a stent could not be placed, failure in 11 patients was attributable to an inability to perform a papillotomy. In 5 patients, the guidewire could not be passed above the malignant stricture, and in the remaining 5 patients, duodenal obstruction secondary to the tumor prohibited passage of the duodenoscope.

The 30-day hospital mortality in these pancreatic cancer patients was 10% (22 patients), and 4 patients (2%) died as a direct result of the endoscopic procedure. The mean survival for the group was 182 days. The median survival was 149 days, with a range of 1–839 days. Recurrent jaundice occurred in 75 of the stented patients (37.5%). This was felt to be secondary to clogging of the endoprosthesis, and in 42 patients the endoprosthesis was changed. The remaining 33 patients were deemed too ill, and no further studies were performed in them.

Our own Memorial Sloan-Kettering Cancer Center experience with endoscopically placed stents is similar to other reported series. The first attempt success rate in our initial series of 44 patients was 70.5% (31 of 44). Cholangitis with or without sepsis occurred in 14%. It is of interest that, when we compared the fall in mean serum bilirubin at 1 week of those patients who had preoperative endoscopic biliary drainage with the fall in bilirubin in those with inoperable advanced pancreatic cancer or metastatic cancer, the decrease in mean bilirubin in the preoperative group was much more impressive (Figure 12-4), reconfirming the advanced stage of disease of the palliated patients and the decrease in stent benefit in this group.

Stanley and associates[20] retrospectively compared EBD with PTD, both with and without subsequent surgery. The success rate of PTD was 98% compared with EBD (92%). Seven major complications occurred in the group of 35 EBD patients (20%). There were 14 drainage-related complications in the 59 patients who underwent PTD (23.7%). Too few patients were in the study to statistically compare the groups' survival rates. They concluded that EBD should be viewed as a good alternate to PTD and that fewer bleeding complications and better patient acceptance were important factors in favor of EBD.

Speer and colleagues[21] recently reported the results of a prospective randomized study comparing PTD and EBD in 75 high-risk patients with malignant biliary obstruction treated at the London or Middlesex Hospital. The patients had a mean age of 73 years, were deeply jaundiced, and 20% had renal insufficiency. Twenty-nine patients had hilar bile duct strictures due to bile duct or gallbladder cancer, while 46 patients had distal bile duct strictures due to pancreatic cancer. The endoscopic stents were significantly ($p = 0.017$) more successful in relieving the jaundice (81% versus 61%) and had a significantly lower

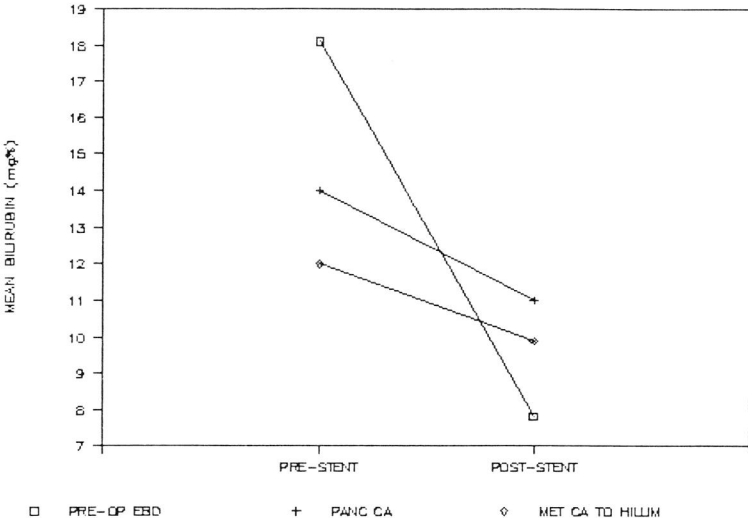

Figure 12-4 Comparison of fall in serum bilirubin at 1 week in patients with endoscopic stents either placed preoperatively or palliatively.

30-day mortality rate (15% versus 33%). Complications occurring within 30 days were seen in 7 of the 37 patients with the endoscopic stents (19%) and 22 of 33 patients (67%) with percutaneously placed stents. Cholangitis occurred in 7 patients with EBD and 5 patients with PTD. Renal insufficiency was more common in the PTD group (4 patients versus 1 patient). The large number of remaining complications occurred in the PTD group and consisted mainly of hemorrhage (5 patients) and bile peritonitis (7 patients). The authors conclude that the higher mortality after percutaneous stents was related to the higher morbidity of this procedure and that the endoscopic method should be used first, especially in elderly or frail patients, with the percutaneous approach used if the endoscopic method fails.

As EBD has less morbidity associated with it than PTD, a prospective randomized trial comparing patients with malignant bile duct obstruction who have EBD preoperatively with those who go directly to surgery should help to answer the question of the usefulness of preoperative biliary drainage. Such a trial has been initiated at Memorial Sloan-Kettering Cancer Center but, unfortunately, to date too few patients have been entered to yield any meaningful results.

There are several other confounding variables which may have impact on the surgical morbidity and mortality in jaundiced patients. These variables include the length of time or duration of preoperative biliary decompression and whether the biliary drainage is internal, into the duodenum, or external, into a bag.

Duration of Preoperative Biliary Drainage

Koyama and associates[22] induced obstructive jaundice in mongrel male dogs and then relieved the jaundice with a cholecystogastrostomy after 4, 6, and 12 weeks. Hepatic mitochondrial respiratory function, ketogenesis, and collagen metabolism were studied. Even though serum bilirubin levels rapidly returned to normal after biliary bypass surgery in the dogs, parameters of mitochondrial respiratory function and ketogenesis improved slowly. Even in the dogs with the shortest duration of biliary obstruction, over 3 weeks of biliary decompression was needed to see improvement. Similar studies were done in patients who had undergone surgery for pancreaticoduodenal cancers. Severe liver mitochondrial respiratory dysfunction was also seen in patients who had had long-term biliary obstruction. Only slight improvement was seen in 5-6 weeks after relief of the obstruction. It is interesting to speculate that with this prolonged recovery period of subcellular injury, the goal of normalization of serum bilirubin by 1 or 2 weeks of preoperative drainage may be a naive one, and that a much longer period, perhaps a month or more, will be needed to really improve hepatic function. Failure of preoperative PTD to improve surgical mortality may then be in part due to too short a period of biliary drainage.

Internal Versus External Drainage

Gouma and colleagues[23] studied the effect of internal and external biliary drainage on the mortality of jaundiced Sprague-Dawley rats. The animals were placed in four groups. Group 1 consisted of 15 animals who underwent bile duct ligation, followed 2 weeks later by cecal ligation and puncture. Group 2 had 16 animals with bile duct ligation with a subsequent internal biliary drainage procedure, followed in 2 weeks by cecal ligation and puncture. Group 3 consisted of 11 animals that had the same procedures as those in group 2, except that the biliary drainage procedure was external rather than internal. Group 4 consisted of 18 animals that had a sham operation, followed in 2 weeks by cecal ligation and puncture. Body weight was initially the same for the animals in all four groups. However, those animals with external biliary drainage weighed less at the time of cecal ligation and perforation despite daily replacement of bile loss with subcutaneous saline injections. Serum albumin concentrations were the same for all groups initially, then fell after bile duct ligation. There was no difference in serum albumin levels between the internal and external drainage groups. The albumin values for both drainage groups were significantly lower than for the sham group ($p < 0.001$). No differences in serum creatinine levels were noted in any group throughout the study.

Serum bilirubin levels increased similarly in the three groups with bile duct ligation and fell to normal levels without difference in both the external and internal drainage groups. Alkaline phosphatase levels remained elevated in both drainage groups, and aspartate aminotransferase and alanine aminotransferase levels returned to normal after either the internal or external drainage procedures.

The major result of this study was seen in the animal mortality rates. Biliary ligation followed by cecal ligation and puncture caused a significantly higher mortality rate in the animals from day 3 to day 7. When the jaundice was relieved by internal drainage, the animal mortality decreased to levels similar to that seen in the sham group. However, there was no mortality reduction seen in the animals with external biliary drainage This lack of decrease in mortality with external biliary drainage was not related to infectious complications of the ex-

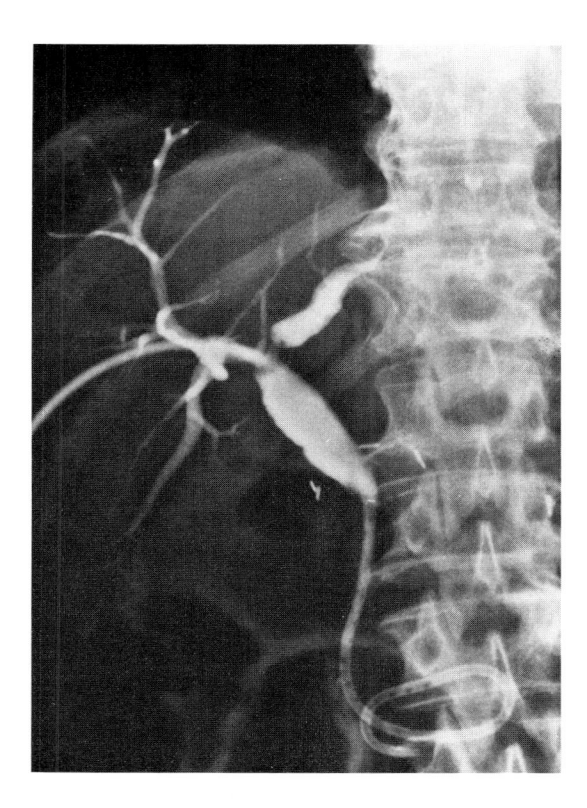

Figure 12-5 Percutaneously placed large-bore internal stent palliatively draining a hilar cholangiocarcinoma.

ternal drainage system, as these animals had no overt signs of sepsis. The authors theorized that the reduced mortality seen in the internal drainage animals was due to reestablishment of the enterohepatic circulation of bile salts, which helped to modify the endotoxemia, that potentially could occur more readily when bile salts were absent from the intestinal tract.

Bailey[24] in 1976 had suggested after studying both humans and rats that endotoxemia in the jaundiced human subjects accounted for decreased renal function postoperatively, as measured by creatinine clearance. In the animal studies done subsequently, he demonstrated that the lack of normal concentrations of bile salts in the intestine allowed the absorption of endotoxin, which theoretically could be prevented by feeding patients bile salts. Furthermore, Kupffer cells, their function hindered by hyperbilirubinemia, allow spillage of endotoxin into the peripheral circulation.

The method of stent placement, whether endoscopic or percutaneous, may have less to do with postoperative mortality than whether the bile is drained externally or internally. The prospective randomized trials of preoperative percutaneous biliary drainage did not stratify for external or internal drainage when comparing morbidity and mortality data. In a recent prospective randomized study from Australia,[25] an attempt was made to internalize all of the percutaneous stents (Figure 12-5). Those patients who were drained internally had fewer complications than those who went directly to surgery ($p < 0.02$). This advantage was reduced when the morbidity of the percutaneous procedure was included in the analysis. The major cause of morbidity in those patients who went directly to surgery without preoperative PTD was renal insufficiency in 4 of 15 patients (27%). Only 1 patient out of 15 in the PTD group developed renal insufficiency. Overall, there were 10 complications in the immediate surgery group (67%) and 3 deaths (20%). One patient died postoperatively in the PTD group (6.7%) and nine had complications (60%) (two postoperatively and seven related to the PTD).

Conclusion

It is clear that preoperative percutaneous biliary drainage should not be used routinely in patients with malignant biliary obstruction. If there is a potential advantage to relieving the hyperbilirubinemia before surgery, it is masked by the significant procedure-related morbidity that has been demonstrated by the randomized prospective trials. Endoscopic placement of internal biliary stents would appear to have a lower associated early and later complication rate. The stents placed in this fashion are generally internal and, therefore, the biliary decompression is more "physiologic," with a return of bile salts to the intestinal tract. In addition, the patient can be discharged from the hospital and the biliary decompression followed as an outpatient, reducing hospitalization costs and allowing for a longer drainage period, which may lead to improved subcellular hepatic function and potentially further reduce the operative morbidity and mortality rates. Of course, this is all speculative. Whether the endoscopic approach to preoperative biliary drainage will actually prove to be better than the percutaneous technique awaits completion of the present ongoing clinical trials.

References

1. Whipple AO, Parsons WB, and Mullino CR: Treatment of carcinoma of the Ampulla of Vater. *Ann Surg* 1935;102:763–779.
2. Warren KW, Cattell RB, Blackburn JP, and Nora PF: A long-term appraisal of pancreaticoduodenal resection for periampullary carcinoma. *Ann Surg* 1962;155:653–662.
3. Mongé JJ, Judd ES, and Gage RP: Radical pancreaticoduodenectomy: A 22-year experience with the complications, mortality rate, and survival rate. *Ann Surg* 1964;160:711–722.
4. Maki T, Sato T, and Kakizaki G: Pancreaticoduodenectomy for periampullary carcinomas: Appraisal of two-stage procedure. *Arch Surg* 1966;92:825–833.
5. Nakayama T, Ikeda A, and Okuda K: Percutaneous transhepatic drainage of the biliary tract. Technique and results in 104 cases. *Gastroenterology* 1978;74:554–559.
6. Dooley JS, Dick R, Olney J, and Sherlock S: Nonsurgical treatment of biliary obstruction. *Lancet* 1979;ii:1040–1043.
7. Denning DA, Ellison EC, and Carey LC: Preoperative percutaneous transhepatic biliary decompression lowers operative morbidity in patients with obstructive jaundice. *Am J Surg* 1981;141:61–65.
8. Norlander A, Kalin B, and Sundblad R: Effect of percutaneous transhepatic drainage upon liver function and postoperative mortality. *Surg Gynecol Obstet* 1982;144:161–166.
9. Gundry SR, Strodel WE, Knol JA, Eckhauser FE, and Thompson NW: Efficacy of preoperative biliary tract decompression in patients with obstructive jaundice. *Arch Surg* 1984;119:703–708.

10. McPherson GAD, Benjamin IS, Habib NA, Bowley NB, and Blumgart LH: Percutaneous transhepatic drainage in obstructive jaundice: Advantages and problems. *Br J Surg* 1982;62:261–624.
11. Hatfield ARW, Tobias R, Terblanche J, Girdwood AH, Fataar S, Harries-Jones R, Kernoff L, and Marks IN: Preoperative external biliary drainage in obstructive jaundice: A prospective controlled clinical trial. *Lancet* 1982;2:896–899.
12. McPherson GAD, Benjamin IS, Hodgson HJF, Bowley NB, Allison DJ, and Blumgart LH: Preoperative percutaneous biliary drainage: The results of a controlled trial. *Br J Surg* 1984;71:371–375.
13. Pitt HA, Gomes AS, Lois JF, Monn LL, Deutsch LS, and Longmire WP: Does preoperative percutaneous biliary drainage reduce operative risk or increase hospital cost? *Ann Surg* 1985;201:545–553.
14. Pitt HA, Cameron JL, Postier RG, and Gadacz TR: Factors affecting mortality in biliary tract surgery. *Am J Surg* 1981;141:66–72.
15. Joseph PK, Bizer LS, Sprayregen SS, and Gliedman ML: Percutaneous transhepatic biliary drainage: results and complications in 81 patients. *J Am Med Assoc* 1986;255:2763–2767.
16. Classen M, and Hagenmuller F: Biliary drainage. *Endoscopy* 1983;15:221–229.
17. Hagenmuller F, and Classen M: Therapeutic endoscopic and percutaneous procedures. In: Popper H and Schaffner F, eds. *Progress in Liver Diseases*, Vol 2. New York, Grune and Stratton, 1982, pp. 299–317.
18. Huibregste K, and Tytgat GNJ: Palliative treatment of obstructive jaundice by transpapillary introduction of large bore bile duct endoprosthesis: Experience in 45 patients. *Gut* 1982;23:371–375.
19. Huibregste K, Katou RM, Coene PP, and Tytgat GNJ: Endoscopic palliative treatment in pancreatic cancer. *Gastroint Endosc* 1986;32:334–338.
20. Stanley J, Gobien RP, Cunningham J, and Andriole J: Biliary decompression: An institutional comparison of percutaneous and endoscopic methods. *Radiology* 1986;158:195–197.
21. Speer AG, Cotton PB, Russell RCG, Mason RR, Hatfield ARW, Leung JWC, MacRae KD, Houghton J, and Lennon CA: Randomized trial of endoscopic versus percutaneous stent insertion in malignant obstructive jaundice. *Lancet* 1987;2:57–62.
22. Koyama K, Takagi Y, Ito K, and Sato T: Experimental and clinical studies on the effect of biliary drainage in obstructive jaundice. *Am J Surg* 1981;142:293–299.
23. Gouma DH, Coelho JCU, Schlegel JF, Li YF, and Moody FG: The effect of preoperative internal and external biliary drainage on mortality of jaundiced rats. *Arch Surg* 1987;122:731–734.
24. Bailey ME: Endotoxin, bile salts, and renal function in obstructive jaundice. *Br J Surg* 1976;63:774–778.
25. Smith RC, Pooley M, George CRP, and Faithful GR: Preoperative percutaneous transhepatic internal drainage in obstructive jaundice: A randomized, controlled trial examining renal function. *Surgery* 1985;97:641–646.

Chapter **13**

Iridium-192 Irradiation of Biliary Tract Malignancy

B. H. Laurence, M.B., B.S., B.Med. Sci (Hons), F.R.A.C.P.

In spite of developments in nonsurgical biliary drainage, the need for improved palliation in biliary tract malignancy continues. The endoscopic insertion of a stent can provide rapid relief of jaundice and in elderly or poor-risk patients is an acceptable alternative to surgery.[1,2] This approach does, however, have serious limitations. There is a high morbidity—early cholangitis (10%), inadequate drainage (10–20%), and late stent blockage (25–30%)[3–5]—and the technique is significantly less successful in hilar malignancy than in pancreatic carcinoma.[6–8] Survival remains short—6 months on average—and intractable pain is a frequent terminal problem.

In malignant biliary obstruction, radiation-induced tumor regression can improve biliary drainage, relieve pain, and prolong survival.[9,10] Experience with external radiotherapy is limited and the reports are difficult to compare because of inadequate clinical data (e.g., site of obstruction, extent of disease), varying dose schedules (2,000–8,000 cGy), or different treatment regimens (e.g., surgical or nonsurgical drainage, adjuvant chemotherapy). External irradiation (5,000–7,000 cGy) has been used successfully in the palliation of both pain and jaundice from pancreatic carcinoma[9,11]; combined with surgery or chemotherapy (5-fluorouracil), it can significantly increase survival time.[12–14] Similar results have been obtained in cholangiocarcinoma. A dose of 4,000–6,000 cGy can reduce pain and relieve jaundice[15,17–19]; when combined with surgery, tube drainage (transhepatic, T tube, U tube), or chemotherapy it can significantly improve survival compared with that following biliary drainage alone.[15,16,20,21]

This form of radiotherapy has the disadvantage, however, of including radiosensitive, normal tissue in the treatment field. Damage to the intestine or liver can occur with significant morbidity and death.[15,20] A number of methods have been devised to increase the local tumor dose with minimization of the risk to adjacent organs—intraluminal irradiation, interstitial therapy with radioactive implants (radium, ^{125}I), and intraoperative radiotherapy.[9,10] In the elderly, poor-risk patient, the most appropriate of these is intraluminal irradiation, alone or combined with external radiotherapy.

Experience with intraluminal radiotherapy in biliary tract malignancy is again limited (Table 13-1). The radiation source—radium needles, iridium-192 seeds or iridium-192 wire—has been inserted with an afterloading technique

Table 13-1 Intraluminal Radiotherapy in Malignant Bile Duct Obstruction

				Radiotherapy Intraluminal		Radiotherapy External		
	No.	Tumor	Drainage	Source	Dose (cGy)	No.	Dose (cGy)	Survival (months)
Conroy et al[22]	6	2° (4) Panc (2)	Percutn.	Radium	20,000+	1	3,000	1–6
Jones et al[24]	10	Chol	Percutn.	Ir 192	4,400	7	4,400	11.5 (3–26)
Prempree et al[25]	1	Chol	Surg	Ir 192	12,000			36
Mornex et al[26]	7	Chol	Surg Percutn.	Ir 192	7,600	4	2,550	3–23
Johnson et al[27]	11	Chol (7) Panc (1) 2° (3)	Surg Percutn.	Ir 192	5,655	11	4,820	8.5 (0.5–22.5)
Karani et al[28]	30	Chol	Surg Percutn.	Ir 192	4,470			16.8 (1–66)
Molt et al[29]	15	Chol (7) Panc (1) 2° (7)	Surg Percutn.	Ir 192	2,150	11	3,275	4.5 (0.5–11.0)

following either surgical or percutaneous insertion of a catheter through the tumor. The aim of most studies has been to deliver 4,000–6,000 cGy at 0.5 cm from the source but there has been a wide range of both dose (1,250–20,000 cGy) and treatment times (21–177 hours). Additional external radiotherapy, with a mean dose of 3,600 cGy (2,550–4,820 cGy), was administered to 42% of the patients.[22,24,26,27,29] Almost 80% of the patients treated had cholangiocarcinoma and the remainder pancreatic carcinoma or hilar metastases. The specific effect of intraluminal radiation alone on the palliation of symptoms is difficult to assess. Jones reported cholangiographic evidence of tumor regression from between 3 and 24 months in half of patients with cholangiocarcinoma treated with combined radiotherapy.[23,24] This response has not been observed by others.[29] Good biliary drainage without an indwelling catheter was achieved in three of six patients (four with hilar metastases, two with pancreatic carcinoma) treated by Conroy and colleagues.[22] A patient of Prempree et al with cholangiocarcinoma had no evidence of malignancy at laparotomy 2 months after treatment and was alive with normal liver function 3 years later.[25]

Survival times range between 1 and 66 months with a reported median survival of 4.5 months and mean survivals between 8.5 and 16.8 months. Without suitable control groups it is not possible to determine the influence of the various therapeutic maneuveres (drainage, intraluminal and external radiotherapy) on these survival figures. The results of the largest study are encouraging.[28] Thirty patients with hilar cholangiocarcinoma had either surgical (15) and/or percutaneous biliary drainage (23) followed by intraluminal irradiation with iridium-192 wire (4,000–5,000 cGy). The overall mean survival was 16.8 months (1–66), almost twice as long as the mean survival of an unmatched group of patients treated with biliary drainage alone (8.5 months).

Immediate complications attributable directly to intraluminal irradiation

Table 13-2 Physical Properties of Iridium-192 Wire

External diameter	0.3 mm
Platinum filtration	0.1 mm
Radial dose constant	3.48×10^{-17} Gy m² Bq⁻¹ S⁻¹
Half-life	74.02 days
HVL in lead	3 mm
Principal γ-energy range	0.3–0.6 MeV

were uncommon and included nausea, vomiting, weight loss, and duodenitis.[27,29] There were no major late complications; minor gastrointestinal bleeding from duodenal ulceration and hemobilia were recorded in two patients treated with combined internal and external radiotherapy.[29] Drainage-related complications were, however, an important cause of morbidity, with cholangitis occurring in 40% of patients (contributing to the death of two) in one study.[28] Percutaneous biliary drainage can certainly provide effective palliation in malignant obstructive jaundice,[30–32] but has a significant incidence of early complications (6–38%)[33]; the most frequent of these, hemorrhage (13.8%)[34] and bile leakage (16%),[35] are directly related to hepatic puncture. A study comparing endoscopic and percutaneous bypass in high-risk patients with malignant bile duct obstruction has demonstrated significantly fewer early complications (6% versus 33%) and a lower 30-day mortality (15% versus 34%) with the endoscopic techniques.[36] Similar advantages could be expected from using the endoscopic (transpapillary) route for placement of both the intraluminal radiation source and subsequent stent.

We developed a technique of intraluminal irradiation which utilizes an endoscopically placed nasobiliary catheter. Iridium-192 wire—a γ-ray emitter with a half-life of 74 days—was chosen as the radiation source (Table 13-2). The wire is an active platinum-iridium alloy encased in an 0.1-mm-thick platinum sheath for filtering out β emissions; the small diameter and flexibility allows its insertion into a standard guidewire and facilitates passage through the curves of a nasobiliary catheter.

Technique

Placement of the radioactive source using an afterloading technique requires an indwelling nasobiliary catheter. This is inserted along with a large-diameter biliary stent which enables bile to drain both through and around the catheter during irradiation. On completion of treatment, the catheter can be removed leaving the stent draining into the duodenum.

Insertion of Nasobiliary Catheter and Stent

Using a standard technique, a guidewire (Cook, 0.035) is inserted through the malignant stricture. A Teflon guide catheter (400 cm, 6.5 FG) with a distal pigtail is then passed over the wire until its tip is at least 5 cm above the stricture. The stricture is dilated and a large-diameter (10–11.5 FG), straight polyethylene

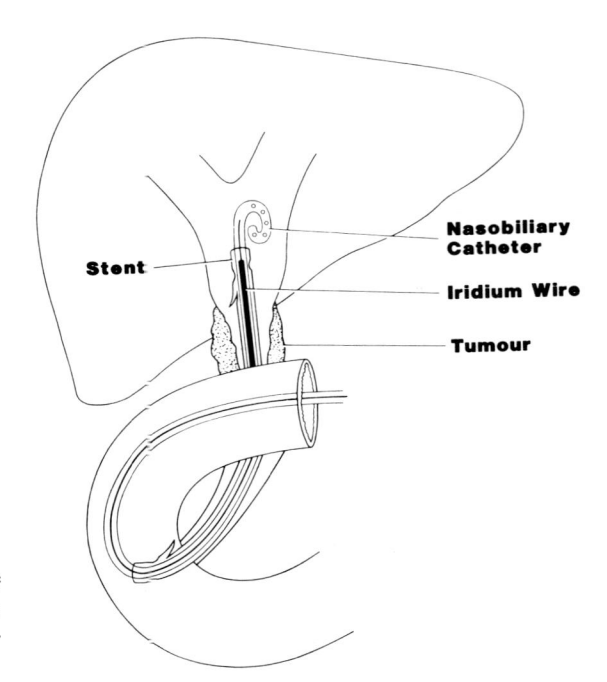

Figure 13-1 Combined insertion of nasobiliary catheter and stent with iridium-192 wire within the catheter.

stent is pushed through the obstruction over the guide catheter; the pushing catheter and guidewire are removed allowing the pigtail on the guide catheter to form above the stricture (Figure 13-1). If placement of a large-diameter stent is not possible (e.g., a hilar stricture), a nasobiliary catheter alone is inserted; this is replaced by a stent on completion of treatment. The duodenoscope is removed over the catheter and the catheter rerouted through the nose. The total length of the catheter is reduced to 120 cm to accommodate the radiation source (145 cm); a Y connector (Cook PSFLL-PCF-MLL-30) is then attached to the proximal end and external drainage of bile is established through one of the limbs (Figure 13-2).

The patient can eat and move about freely without the catheter being displaced; vigorous vomiting, however, can dislodge the catheter and if nausea develops, an antiemetic should be given immediately. The bile is cultured daily and prophylactic antibiotics are administered while the catheter is in place. If the diagnosis of malignancy has not been confirmed by biliary cytology or endoscopic biopsy, the nasobiliary tube (following a nasobiliary cholangiogram) provides a ready target for percutaneous fine-needle aspiration or biopsy of the stricture.

Preparation of the Radiation Source

The radiation source is prepared by incorporating a length of iridium-192 wire into a standard guidewire. The length of wire used is equal to one and a half times the length of the malignant stricture, corrected for radiologic magnification against the known diameter of the duodenoscope. This provides a 25% overlap of wire at either end of the stricture; when the stricture is at the lower

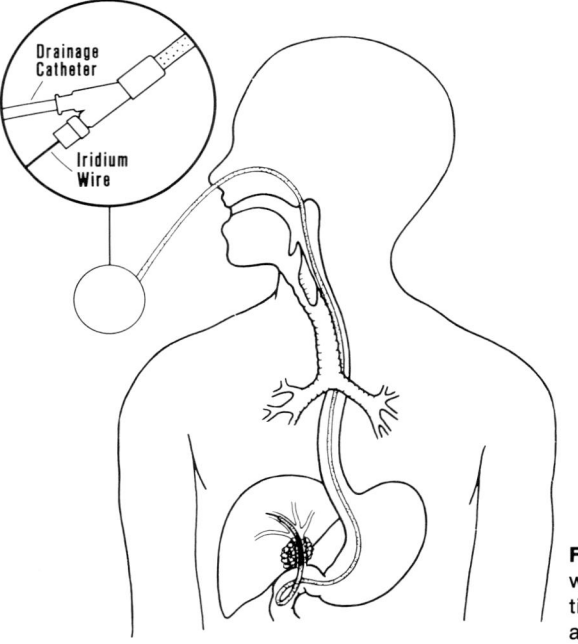

Figure 13-2 Nasobiliary catheter with proximal Y connector for fixation of iridium wire and bile drainage.

end of the common bile duct, the overlap is shortened to prevent duodenal irradiation.

The central stilette of a straight, moveable-core, Teflon-coated wire (0.035, 145 cm, Medrad TM351451) is removed. A nylon thread, 1–2 cm long, is then inserted into the outer sheath followed by the appropriate length of iridium-192 wire (usually 3–10 cm long). The stilette is replaced, pushing the nylon spacer and iridium-192 wire to the sealed distal end of the sheath (Figure 13-3). Long forceps are used to manipulate the wire which limits the dose of irradiation to the hands of the operator to 200 μSV per loading; lead windows and L-shaped shields reduce body exposure to less than 100 μSV, well within the accepted safety limits. The loaded guidewire is heat-sterilized in an autoclavable transport container.[37]

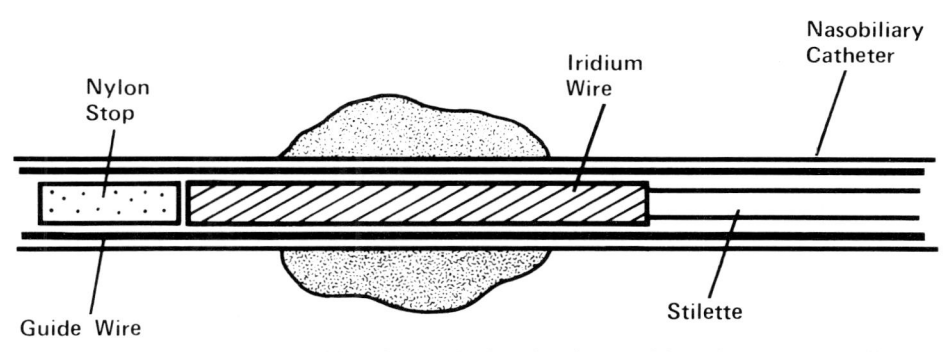

Figure 13-3 Iridium-192 wire within the guidewire showing position of spacer and stilette.

Loading of the Source

Immediately before inserting the radiation source, a nasobiliary cholangiogram is carried out to delineate the upper margins of the malignant stricture. The active end of the guidewire is then advanced from the transport container and directed with long, sterile forceps through the rubber seal of the Y connector. The iridium-192 wire is positioned across the stricture under fluoroscopic control, its localization being facilitated by a higher radiodensity than the guidewire. The wire is fixed by tightening the rubber seal of the Y connector and taping. The stilette can be removed from the guidewire without altering the position of the iridium wire and this may reduce the risk of displacement due to excessive bowing of the catheter within the duodenum.

Treatment is planned to administer 6000 cGy with 100% of the dose delivered at a distance of 0.5 cm from the iridium-192 wire (Figure 13-4). The duration of therapy is determined by the length and radioactivity of the wire and the dose rate (estimated from a locally calculated "Escargot", similar to the Paris system).[38] The wire is usually in position for 3–4 days, the length of time increasing as the radioactivity of the source diminishes. The position of the wire is checked daily by fluoroscopy and repositioned as necessary. Standard radiation therapy procedures are followed, with radiation monitoring of all personnel in contact with the patient. The maximum activity of the iridium-192 wire results in an exposure rate of only 400 μSV/hr at 50 cm in air and 200 μSV/hr when in the patient. The nursing attendants may safely spend 1 hr/week at 50 cm from the patient undergoing treatment.

When additional external radiotherapy is given, it is an advantage to plan the fields while the nasobiliary tube is in position and cholangiographic delineation of the stricture is possible. Treatment is carried out 1–4 weeks after completion of intraluminal irradiation. A total of 3,000 cGy can be administered by a 4-Mev linear accelerator in 10 fractions over 2 weeks with minimal morbidity; AP/PA fields to a volume not exceeding 10 × 10 cm are used, with no more than 50% of the right kidney included in the treatment volume.

On completion of intraluminal irradiation, the pigtail is straightened with a guidewire and the catheter carefully removed under fluoroscopic control. Three months after therapy, the stent is removed and retrograde cholangiography repeated to determine the need for continued stent drainage.

Results

Experience with transpapillary irradiation of biliary tract malignant is limited.

Philip and colleagues[39] treated three patients—cholangiocarcinoma 2, hilar metastases 1—with iridium-192 incorporated in a nasobiliary catheter; a dose of 6,000 cGy was administered. There were no complications and all were alive 4–5 months after treatment; in one patient, adequate biliary drainage was achieved without a stent. Siegel et al[40] used a double-lumen stent preloaded with iridium-192 wire to treat 12 patients—cholangiocarcinoma in 5, pancreatic carcinoma in 4, and ampullary carcinoma in 3. A mean dose of 5,000 cGy was delivered and large-diameter stents (10–12 FG) were inserted after therapy. There were no complications and both improved drainage and tumor mass regression were observed. Combined external beam (4,500 cGy) and transpapillary irradiation with iridium-192 seeds (2,100 cGy) have been used to treat a

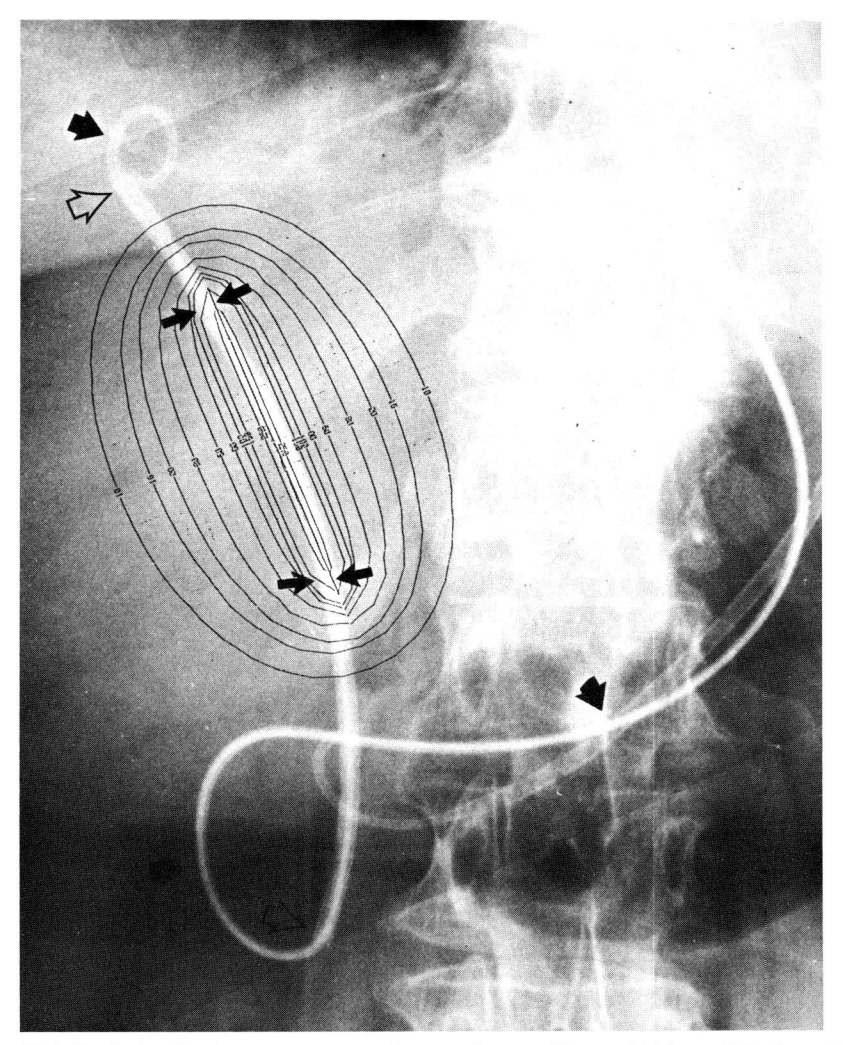

Figure 13-4 Radiation isodose curves superimposed on an X ray of iridium-192 wire within a malignant stricture. Small arrows: limits of iridium wire; open arrows: stent; large closed arrows: nasobiliary catheter.

patient with cholangiocarcinoma; there was a 50% increase in the internal diameter of the stricture and liver function tests were normal 1 year after therapy.[41]

We have treated 25 patients using the afterloading technique described— 7 with cholangiocarcinoma, 12 with pancreatic carcinoma, 3 with hilar metastases,[42] 2 with carcinoma of the gallbladder, and 1 with carcinoma of the papilla. All were elderly (median age 69 years) and were considered unsuitable for surgical palliation; none of the patients with pancreatic or cholangiocarcinoma had evidence of metastatic disease at the time of treatment. The diagnosis was confirmed histologically in 20 (80%); the clinical course of the other five patients was consistent with the radiologic diagnosis of a malignant stricture.

Iridium-192 therapy was administered through a nasobiliary catheter in 24 patients; this approach was unsuccessful in one patient and intraluminal irradiation was subsequently carried out through a transhepatic catheter. Biliary drainage was established immediately after treatment in all but one patient with carcinoma of the ampulla; 21 had endoscopic stents (10 or 11.5 FG), one a percutaneous stent, and two a surgical biliary bypass.

Treatment was designed to deliver 6,000 cGy; two patients had only 4,500 cGy because of displacement of the catheter. The mean duration of therapy was 90 hr (70–109). Two patients with cholangiocarcinoma were given a second course of intraluminal irradiation for local extension of the disease, 15 and 35 months after the initial treatment; five patients with pancreatic carcinoma received additional external radiotherapy (3,000 cGy) 1–4 weeks after intraluminal therapy.

There were no immediate side effects (e.g., nausea, vomiting) or long-term complications (e.g., fistula) directly attributable to radiotherapy. One patient died 10 days after treatment from a cerebrovascular accident (a 30-day mortality of 4%). This is similar to the 3.3% mortality reported with intraluminal therapy by the percutaneous route.[28] It compares favorably with the mortality following surgical biliary bypass (pancreatic carcinoma, 6–19%[43-45]; cholangiocarcinoma, 11–35%[46-48]) or biliary drainage alone by the endoscopic approach (8–19%[1,6,7]).

Early cholangitis occurred in 29%, an incidence considerably higher than after endoscopic drainage alone (19%).[36] In almost all cases it developed within 48 hr of inserting the radiation source and responded rapidly to antibiotics. Karani *et al* also reported a high incidence of cholangitis (40%) in patients undergoing intraluminal irradiation.[28] The increased risk of cholangitis is probably due to partial obstruction of the drainage catheter by the loaded guidewire, with repeated manipulation within an obstructed and infected biliary tree a contributing factor. The simultaneous insertion of a large-diameter stent with the nasobiliary catheter allows rapid drainage of bile both through and around the catheter, confirmed radiographically. It is anticipated that this technique will reduce the incidence of cholangitis but there is insufficient experience so far. The simultaneous use of two lengths of iridium-192 wire within a stent could also be of value, by reducing the treatment time by up to 48 hr.

Blockage of the stent was the most common late complication and stent replacement was required in 25%. The median survival of the first stent was 4.4 months, and in 12 patients (57%) biliary drainage with the initial stent was still adequate at the time of death. In three patients—one with pancreatic and two with cholangiocarcinoma—blocked stents were removed but were not replaced because of a significant increase in the diameter of the stricture (Figure 13-5); liver function tests in these patients remained normal at 2, 4, and 6 months. Duodenal obstruction necessitating surgical bypass developed in two patients with pancreatic carcinoma 16 and 34 weeks after radiotherapy.

Twenty patients died of their malignancy from 60 to 532 days after treatment; five are still alive after 150, 240, 285, 317, and 1,340 days. The overall median survival for patients with pancreatic carcinoma was 250 days (approximately 8.3 months) and for cholangiocarcinoma, 300 days (10 months). These results compare favorably with our earlier experience of transpapillary drainage alone—a survival in pancreatic carcinoma of 147 days (5.2 months) and in cholangiocarcinoma 84 days (3 months). The mean survival of patients with cholangiocarcinoma treated with iridium-192 by Karani *et al*[28] was almost double that of historical controls treated by biliary decompression alone (16.8

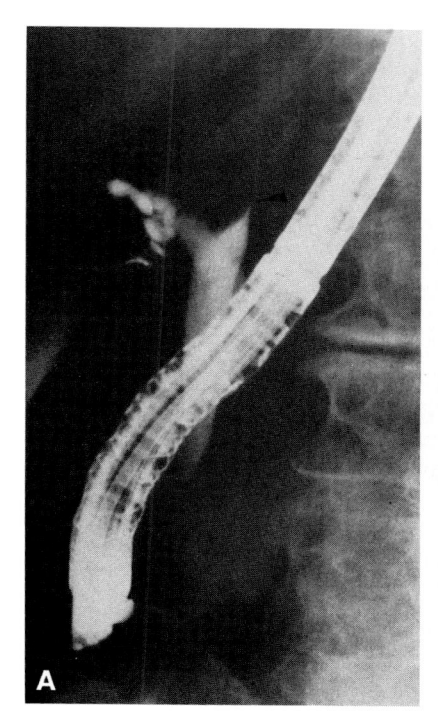

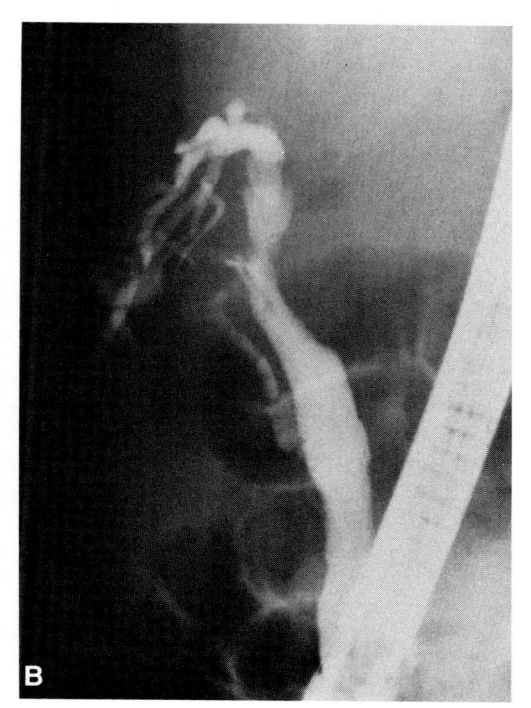

Figure 13-5 Hilar obstruction due to cholangiocarcinoma before **(A)** and 3 months after intraluminal irradiation **(B)**.

months versus 8.5 months); the mean survival of our equivalent treatment group was 12 months. In the absence of a controlled study, the relevance of these survival figures is uncertain; they do not differ greatly from those after palliative drainage or bypass alone (pancreatic carcinoma, 6–7 months[6,43,45]; cholangiocarcinoma, 8–19 months[28–49]).

There are fundamental problems to treating biliary tract malignancy by intraluminal irradiation. Intrinsic to all γ-ray emitters such as iridium-192 is the rapid decline in radiation intensity with increasing distance from the source. The therapeutic effect with intraluminal irradiation is influenced by both tumor size and the relationship of the source to the tumor center. In cholangiocarcinoma, annular involvement of the duct and the relatively small size of many tumors at presentation favor effective treatment. In pancreatic carcinoma, the peripheral position of the obstructed bile duct in a large tumor will result in eccentric and incomplete tumor irradiation; although this may relieve the duct obstruction, a significant effect on pain or long-term survival is unlikely. Intraluminal "boost" therapy to the primary tumor followed by external radiotherapy is probably preferable to intraluminal irradiation alone. Our experience with combined therapy is confined to five patients with pancreatic carcinoma; by limiting the external dose to 3,000 cGy it was possible to administer a total dose of 9,000 cGy with minimal morbidity. Survival in these patients ranges from 44 to 501 days without any obvious additional benefit in terms of improved palliation.

The transpapillary approach to intraluminal irradiation in malignant bile duct involvement is certainly technically feasible and relatively safe. It can provide prolonged improvement in biliary drainage and relief of cholestatic symptoms without a stent. In view of the high morbidity association with a stent, this alone is likely to be a significant contribution to better palliation. The risk of early cholangitis, however, must be justified by demonstrating additional benefits in quality of life, pain control, or longevity. This information will only be obtained by a controlled trial of combined internal and external radiotherapy against surgical or stent drainage alone.

References

1. Tytgat GW, Bartelsman JF, Den Hartog-Jager FC, Huibregtse K, and Mathusvliegen EM: Upper intestinal and biliary tract endoprosthesis. *Dig Dis Sci* 1986;31(Suppl):57S–76S.
2. Shepherd HAD, Diba A, Ross AF, Arthur M, Royle G, and Colin-Jones D: Endoscopic biliary prosthesis in the palliation of malignant biliary obstruction: A randomized trial. *Gut* 1986;27:A1284.
3. Haber GB, and Kortan PP: Complications of endobiliary prosthesis. *Gastroint Endosc* 1985;31:168.
4. Safrany L, Schott B, Krause S, Balint T, and Portocarero G: Endoskopische transpapillare Gallengangs drainage bei tumorbedingten Verschlussikterus. *Dtsch Med Wschr* 1982;107:1867–1871.
5. Riemann JF, Lux G, Rosch W, and Beickert-Sterba A: Non surgical biliary drainage: Technique, indications and results. *Endoscopy* 1981;13:157–161.
6. Huibregtse K, Katon RM, Coene PP, and Tytgat GNJ: Endoscopic palliative treatment in pancreatic cancer. *Gastroint Endosc* 1986;32:334–338.
7. Speer AG, and Cotton PB: Endoscopic biliary prosthesis in 102 poor risk patients with carcinoma of the pancreas. *Gut* 1986;27:A1278.
8. Speer AG, Cotton PB, and Dineen LP: Endoscopic palliation of malignant hilar strictures. *Gut* 1986;27:A601.
9. Dobelbower RR, and Milligan AJ: Treatment of pancreatic cancer by radiation therapy. *World J Surg* 1984;8:919–928.
10. Kopelson G, Gunderson LL: Primary adjuvant radiation therapy in gallbladder and extrahepatic biliary tract carcinoma. *J Clin Gastroenterol* 1983;5:43–50.
11. Miller TR, and Fuller LM: Radiation therapy of carcinoma of the pancreas. *Am J Roentgenol* 1958;80:787–790.
12. Kalser MH, and Ellenberg SS: Pancreatic cancer. Adjuvant combined radiation and chemotherapy following curative resection. *Arch Surg* 1985;120:899–903.
13. Moertel CG, Frytak S, Hahn RG, O'Connell MJ, Reitemeier RJ, Rubin J, Schutt AJ, et al: Therapy of locally unresectable pancreatic carcinoma. A randomized comparison of high dose (6000 Rads) radiation alone, moderate dose radiation (4000 Rads) and 5-fluorouracil and high dose radiation plus 5-fluorouracil. *Cancer* 1981;48:1705–1710.
14. Whittington R, Dobelbower RR, Mohiuddin M, Rosato FE, and Weiss SM: Radiotherapy of unresectable pancreatic carcinoma: A 6 year experience with 104 patients. *Int J Rad Oncol Biol Phys* 1981;7:1639–1644.
15. Hanna SS, and Rider WD. Carcinoma of the gallbladder or extrahepatic bile ducts: The role of radiotherapy. *Can Med Assoc J* 1978;118:59–61.
16. Hishikawa Y, Shimada T, Miura T, and Imajyo Y: Radiation therapy of carcinoma of the extrahepatic bile ducts. *Radiology* 1983;146:787–789.
17. Pilepich MV, and Lambert PM: Radiotherapy of carcinoma of the extrahepatic biliary system. *Radiology* 1978;127:767–770.
18. Smoron GL: Radiation therapy of carcinoma of the gallbladder and biliary tract. *Cancer* 1977;40:1422–1424.

19. Green W, Mikkelsen MD, and Kernen JA: Cancer of the common hepatic bile duct: Palliative radiotherapy. *Radiology* 1973;109:687–689.
20. Buskirk SJ, Gunderson LL, Adson MA, Martinez A, May GR, McIlrath DC, Nagorney DM, Edmundson GK, Bender CE, and Kirkmartin J: Analysis of failure following curative irradiation of gallbladder and extrahepatic bile duct cancer. *Int J Rad Oncol Biol Phys* 1984;10:2013–2023.
21. Langer JC, Langer B, Taylor BR, Zeldin R, and Cummings B: Carcinoma of the extrahepatic bile ducts: Results of an aggressive surgical approach. *Surgery* 1985;98:752–759.
22. Conroy RM, Shahbazin AA, Edwards K, Moran E, Swingle KF, Lewis GJ, and Pribram HFW. A new method for treating carcinomatous biliary obstruction with intracatheter radium. *Cancer* 1982;49:1321–1327.
23. Chitwood WR, Meyers WC, Heaston DK, Herskovic AM, McLeod ME, Scott Jones R. Diagnosis and treatment of primary extrahepatic bile duct tumours. *Am J Surg* 1982;143:99–106.
24. Jones RS, Chitwood WR, Heaston DK, and Herskovic AM: The combined use of percutaneous transhepatic drainage and irradiation for carcinoma of the extrahepatic bile ducts. *Contemp Surg* 1983;22:59–69.
25. Prempree T, Cox EF, Sewchand W, and Tang CK. Cholangiocarcinoma: A place for brachytherapy. *Acta Radiol Oncol* 1983;22:353–359.
26. Mornex F, Ardiet JM, Bret P, and Gerard JP: Radiotherapy of high bile duct carcinoma using intracatheter Iridium-192 wire. *Cancer* 1984;54:2069–2073.
27. Johnson DW, Safai C, and Goffinet DR: Malignant obstructive jaundice: Treatment with external beam and intracavitary radiation therapy. *Int J Radiat Oncol Biol Phys* 1985;11:411–416.
28. Karani J, Fletcher M, Brinkley D, Dawson JL, Williams R, and Nunnerly H. Internal biliary drainage and local radiotherapy with iridium-192 wire in the treatment of hilar cholangiocarcinoma. *Clin Radiol* 1985;36:603–606.
29. Molt P, Hopfan S, Watson RC, Botet JF, and Brennan MF: Intraluminal radiation therapy in the management of malignant biliary obstruction. *Cancer* 1986;57:536–544.
30. Nakayama T, Ikeda A, and Okuda K: Percutaneous transhepatic drainage of the biliary tract: Techniques and results of 104 cases. *Gastroenterology* 1978;73:554–559.
31. Hoevels J, and Lunderquist A: Results of percutaneous internal-external drainage. In: Classen M, Geenen J, Kawai K (Eds) *Nonsurgical Biliary Drainage.* Berlin, Springer-Verlag, 1984, pp. 43–46.
32. May GR, Bender CE, Williams HJ, and Macarty RL. Percutaneous biliary decompression. *Sem Intervent Radiol* 1985;2:21–30.
33. Wittich GR, Van Sonnenberg E, and Simeone JF. Results and complications of percutaneous biliary drainage. *Sem Intervent Radiol* 1985;2:39–49.
34. Monden M, Okamura J, Kobayashi N, Shibita N, Horikawa S, Fujimoto T, Kosaki G, Kuroda C, and Uchida H: Haemobilia after percutaneous transhepatic biliary drainage. *Arch Surg* 1980;115:161–164.
35. Carrasco CH, Zornoza J, and Betchel WJ: Malignant biliary obstruction: Complications of percutaneous biliary drainage. *Radiology* 1984;152:343–346.
36. Speer AG, Cotton PB, Russell RC, Mason WR, Hatfield AR, Leung JW, Macrae KD, Houghton J, and Lennon CA: Randomized trial of endoscopic versus percutaneous stent insertion in malignant obstructive jaundice. *Lancet* 1987;2:57–62.
37. Deans T, and Rafferty MW: An autoclavable transport container for guidewires containing iridium-192. *Br J Radiol* 1986;59:1223–1224.
38. Pierquin B, Dutreix A, Paine CH, Chassagne D, Marinell G, and Ash D: The Paris system in interstitial radiotherapy. *Acta Radiol Oncol* 1978;17:33–48.
39. Philip J, Hagenmuller F, Manegold J, Szepesi S, and Classen M. Endoscopic intraductal radiotherapy of high bile duct carcinoma. *Dtsch Med Wschr* 1984;109:422–426.
40. Siegel JH, Pullano W, Ramsey WH, Rosenbaum A, Halpern G, Nonkin R, Jacob H, and

Lichenstein J: Endotherapy: Iridium implantation and drainage. One step therapy for malignant biliary obstruction. *Gastroint Endosc* 1987;33:177–178.
41. Venu RP, Geenen JE, Hogan WJ, Johnson GK, Klein K, and Stone J. Intraluminal radiation therapy for biliary tract malignancy: An endoscopic approach. *Gastroint Endosc* 1987;33:236–238.
42. Levitt MD, Laurence BH, Cameron F, and Klemp PF. Transpapillary iridium-192 wire in the treatment of malignant bile duct obstruction. *Gut* 1988;29:149–152.
43. Van Heerd NJ, Heath P, and Alden C. Biliary bypass for ductal adenocarcinoma of the pancreas. Mayo Clinic Experience, 1970–1975. *Mayo Clin Proc* 1980;55:537–540.
44. Morrow M, Hilaris B, and Brennan MF: Comparison of conventional surgical resection, radioactive implantation, and bypass procedures for exocrine carcinoma of the pancreas 1975–1980. *Ann Surg* 1984;199:1–5.
45. Brooks BC, et al: Evaluation of palliative procedures of pancreatic cancer. *M J Surg* 1981;141:430–433.
46. Tompkins RK, Thomas D, Wile A, and Longmire WP: Prognostic factors in bile duct carcinoma. *Ann Surg* 1981;194:447–457.
47. Evander A, Fredlund P, Hoevels J, Ihse I, and Bengmark S: Evaluation of aggressive surgery for carcinoma of the extrahepatic bile ducts. *Ann Surg* 1980;191:23–29.
48. Blumgart LH, Benjamin IS, Hadjis NS, and Beazley R: Surgical approaches to cholangiocarcinoma at confluence of hepatic ducts. *Lancet* 1984;1:66–70.
49. Broe PJ, and Cameron JL: The management of proximal biliary tract tumours. In: McLean LD, Ed. *Advances in Surgery,* Vol 15. Chicago, Year Book, 1984:172–174.

Chapter **14**

Direct Cholangiopancreatoscopy

Richard A. Kozarek, M.D.

Direct, nonoperative cholangiopancreatoscopy has been a goal of endoscopists for many years. The development of small-caliber endoscopes which could be passed through prototype side-viewing duodenoscopes to visualize the pancreatic and biliary ducts was first reported in Japan in 1975.[1] Over the next several years there was a flurry of activity in both Europe and Japan utilizing such mini- (daughter, fileal, baby) scopes at the time of diagnostic and therapeutic ERCP.[2,3] Most reported series were small and documented the feasibility of the procedure, the largest noting an 84% technical success rate in the 50 patients in whom it was employed.

Despite the initial enthusiasm for this procedure, miniscopes never enjoyed widespread application and have remained technical curiosities to most practicing endoscopists. Several factors have been associated with this. First and foremost was the improvement in CT and ultrasound imaging which precluded the need for more invasive diagnostic procedures. These studies, coupled with skinny-needle aspiration of imaged lesions, have proved variably cost-effective and reasonably sensitive and specific, particularly in diagnosing neoplasms of the liver and pancreas. Two other factors were associated with the decline in enthusiasm for miniscopes. Early small-caliber instruments proved quite fragile and could be totally fractured over the parent scope's elevator tip or at the level of the proximal biopsy channel at the time of introduction. This fragility might have been acceptable if the instruments had either been designed with disposable shafts or priced inexpensively. However, original instruments approximated $10,000, a price in excess of most conventional endoscopes.

Several factors have evolved in the past 13 years suggesting that a reevaluation of this technology is in order. First, diagnostic studies including ERCP, CT, ultrasound, MRI, and angiography remain imperfect diagnostic tools of the pancreatobiliary tree. Thus, intramural or small luminal lesions can be missed or misinterpreted. Retained common bile duct stones, evaluationn of a pancreatic duct stricture, and differentiation between some instances of cholangiocarcinoma and sclerosing cholangitis are cases in point. Miniscopes, particularly with the miniaturization of accessory tools such as cytology brushes and biopsy forceps, have the potential for improving our diagnostic capabilities.

In addition to improved diagnoses, the potential of applying directed pancreatobiliary therapy must now be viewed as possible. For instance, tunable dye and q-switched Nd-YAG lasers were recently developed that can effect gallstone fracture.[4-7] These high-power lasers deliver their energy in milli- and nanosecond pulses, respectively, that can be applied directly to the stone using a 250-μm quartz fiber. Such a fiber can be passed through a variety of miniscopes to allow large, impacted common bile duct stones to be fractured under direct endoscopic evaluation. Use of similar quartz fibers could also allow application of Nd-YAG and other laser modalities to unresectable and obstructing pancreatobiliary neoplasms and even pancreatic duct calculi. Finally, use of directional miniscopes may allow placement of guidewires through difficult-to-cannulate biliary stenoses in preparation for balloon dilation or stent placement.

Because of the potential for both improved diagnostic and therapeutic capabilities in the pancreatobiliary tree,[8,9] I have evaluated a number of miniscopes during the past 3 years.[10-12] Instruments evaluated included those manufactured by Schott Fiberoptics (formerly Reichert): 5- and 7-Fr, 180-cm, 3- and 1.8-Fr working channels; Microvasive Inc.: 3-Fr, 70-cm, no channel, and 6-Fr, 180-cm, 2.8-Fr channel; American-Edwards: 1- and 3-Fr, 200-cm, no channel and 7-Fr, 200-cm, 3-Fr channel; and Olympus Inc.: 184-cm, 11.1-Fr, 3.6-Fr channel, 188-cm, 14.1-Fr, 5.1-Fr channel, 121-cm, 8.6-Fr, and containing 2, 1.2-Fr and 1.3-Fr working channels (see Figure 14-1). Only the larger Olympus scopes had directionality utilizing two-way tip deflection. The largest Olympus instrument was also the only one to include automatic suction capabilities as well as air-water insufflation. Instruments were either passed directly through a T (or percutaneous biliary) tube or at time of ERCP using diagnostic or therapeutic duodenoscopes (4.2-mm working channel). Instruments above 7 Fr required the

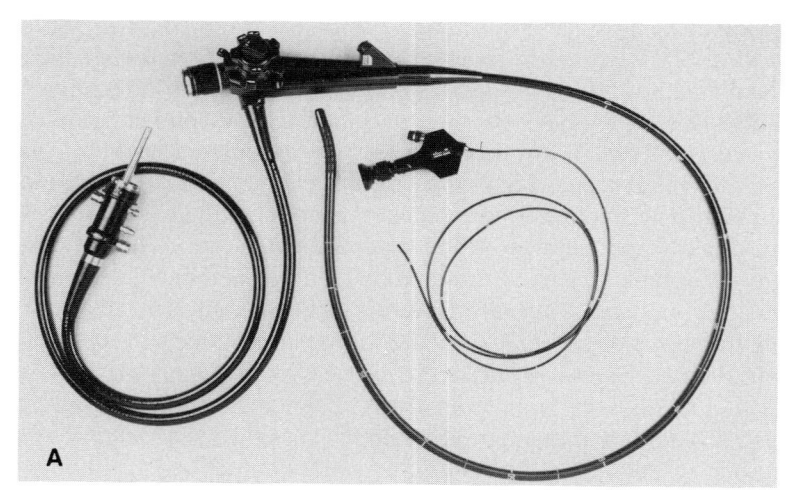

Figure 14-1 (A) 7 Fr Schott miniscope shown with therapeutic Olympus duodenoscope (4.2 mm channel). **(B)** Microvasive miniscope. Head is reusable, variable diameter/length scope shafts are interchangeable and ultimately disposable. **(C)** 14.1 Fr Olympus "ultra-thin" passed through prototype 5.5 mm channel mother scope. Note automatic air-water, two-way tip deflection. **(D)** 5 (left) and 7 (right) Fr miniscopes protruding from diagnostic and therapeutic duodenoscopes respectively. **(E)** 7 (11 o'clock), 6, 3, and 1 Fr miniscopes arranged clockwise around pediatric endoscope for comparison.

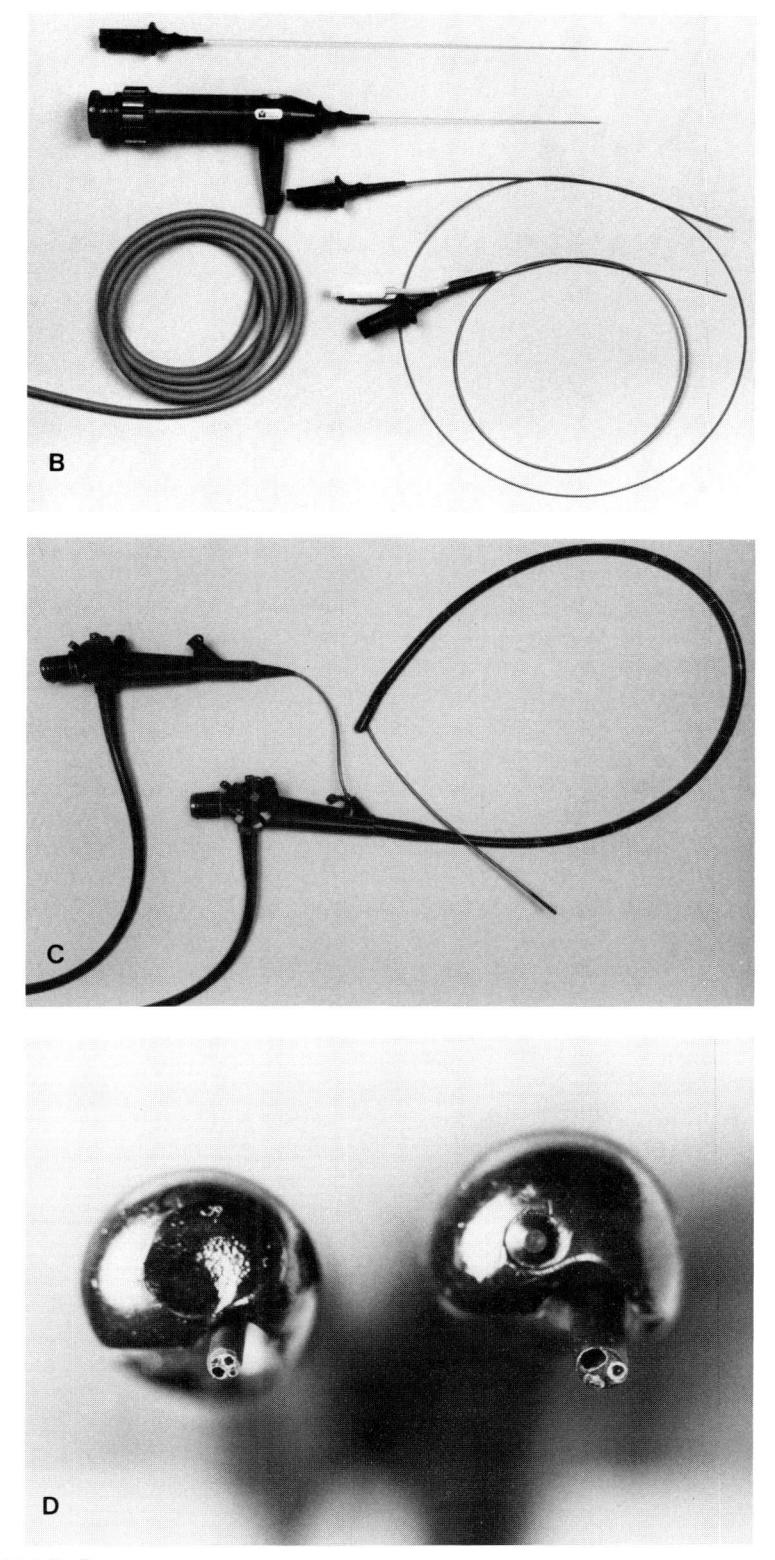

Figure 14-1 B–D

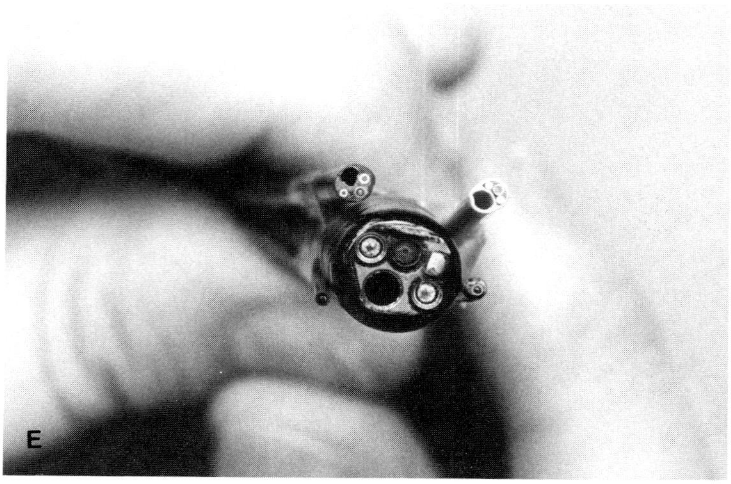

Figure 14-1 E

latter, and the largest Olympus instrument was passed through a prototype duodenoscope with a 5.5-mm channel. For the most part, miniscopes were passed over guidewires, although 3-Fr instruments were passed directly and the 1-Fr instrument was designed to pass through a toposcopic balloon. All procedures were utilized in conjunction with fluoroscopy.

In the 42 patients in whom I have attempted direct cholangiopancreatoscopy (9 T-tube, 33 at time of ERCP), I have been technically successful in 35 of 42 instances. These results include all 9 patients in whom miniscopes were used through percutaneous tracts and 26 of the 33 patients studied post-ERCP. Diagnoses were often multiple and included common bile duct (CBD) stones, 20, pancreatic carcinoma, 4, chronic pancreatitis, 5, cholangiocarcinoma, 5, papillary stenosis/ampullary spasm, 5, sclerosing cholangitis, 4, and postoperative or stone-induced biliary stricture, 4. Of the 35 successful patients, visualization was judged to be good to excellent in two-thirds and fair-to-poor in the remaining one-third. Several of the latter cases were related to bundle fracture after the miniscope was in the desired duct. Scopes 7 Fr or larger were used in conjunction with sphincterotomy in all but two cases. Additional diagnoses or clarification of stenotic biliary lesions were noted in 12 patients and included a firm diagnosis of cholangiocarcinoma, 5, missed CBD stone or intrahepatic, 3, inflammatory common hepatic duct (CHD) stricture, 3, and papillary stenosis (see retrograde through a choledochoduodenostomy and originally felt to be a distal CBD neoplasm), 1 (Figures 14-2 to 14-8, **Plate 6**). An improved diagnostic yield was also confirmed by Ponchen et al in a recent report, utilizing the larger of the Olympus miniscopes for directed biopsy of biliary stenoses.[13,14]

In addition to improved diagnostic capabilities in the pancreatobiliary tree, miniscopes have also been utilized therapeutically.[11,12,15,16] In a combined series with Peter Cotton of Duke, we utilized tunable dye laser lithotripsy through the directable Olympus miniscope to fracture large or impacted CBD stones unremovable by conventional therapy. Successful and without complication in all seven patients in whom it was utilized, complete stone evacuation was effected in only four cases (unpublished data).

255

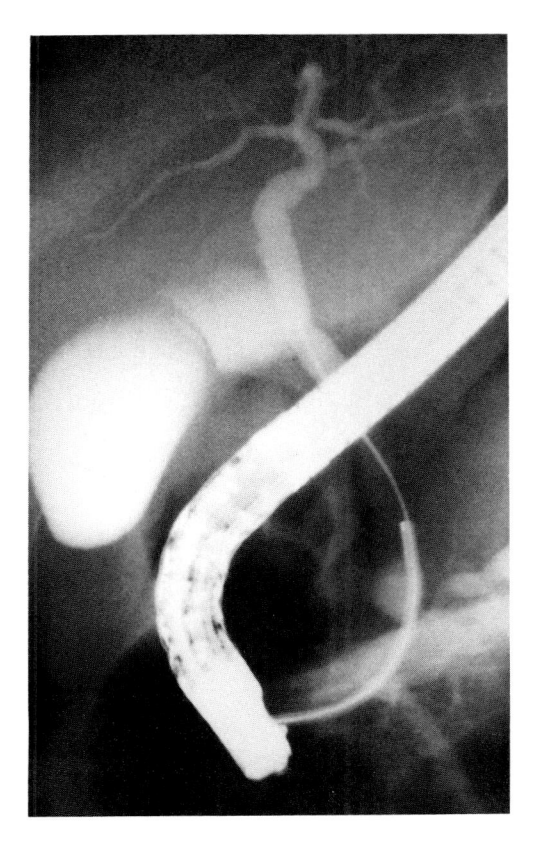

Figure 14-2 7 Fr miniscope passed over guidewire and into mid-CBD without endoscopic sphincterotomy.

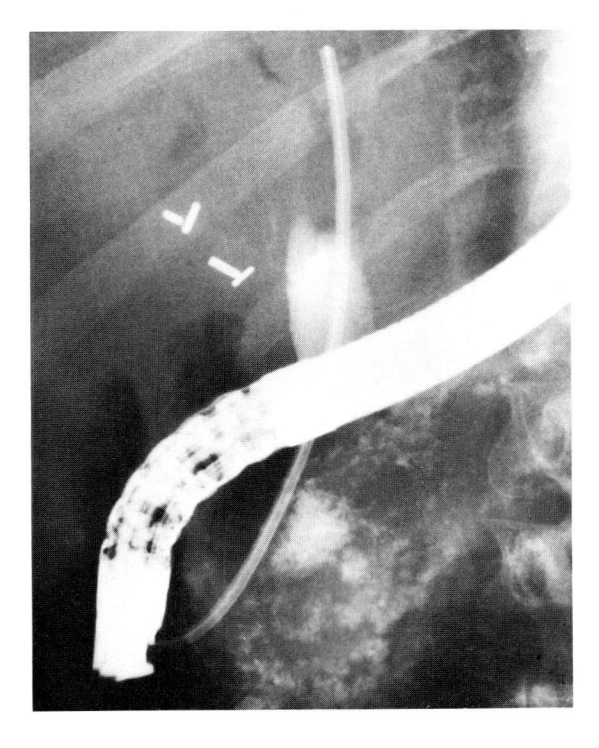

Figure 14-3 7 Fr miniscope at level of bifurcation. Note air in CBD.

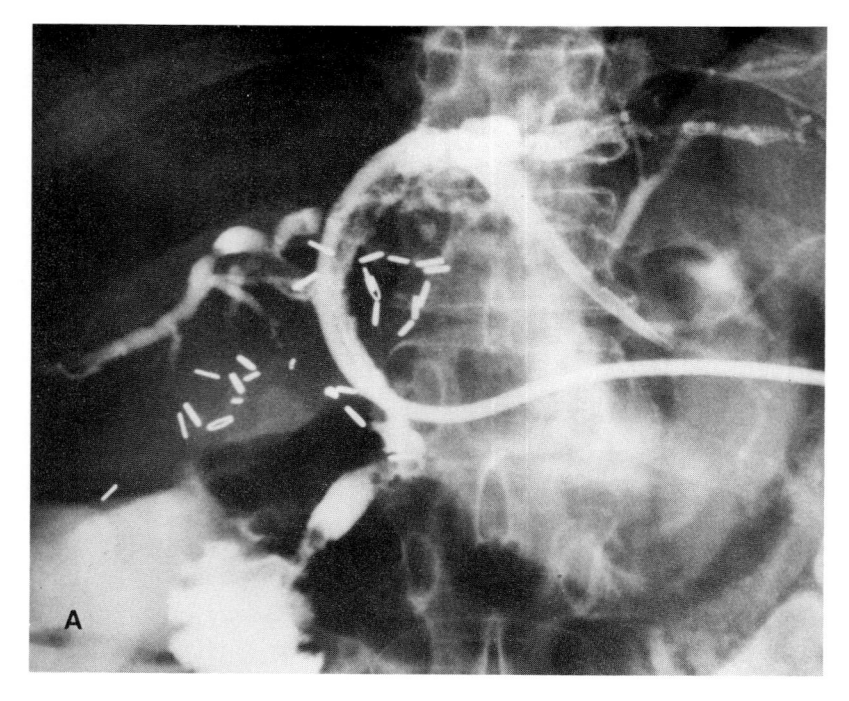

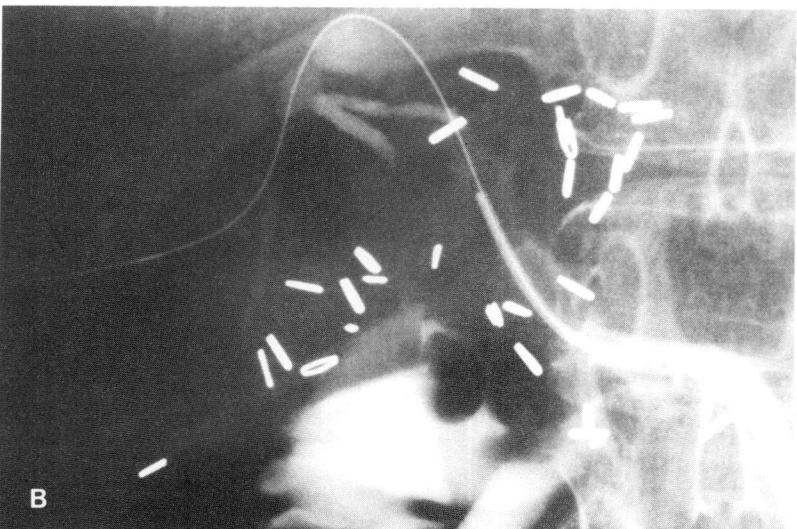

Figure 14-4 (A) Percutaneous cholangiogram in patient with cholangiocarcinoma. **(B)** 5 Fr miniscope passed through biliary drainage catheter in patient depicted in Figure 4A.

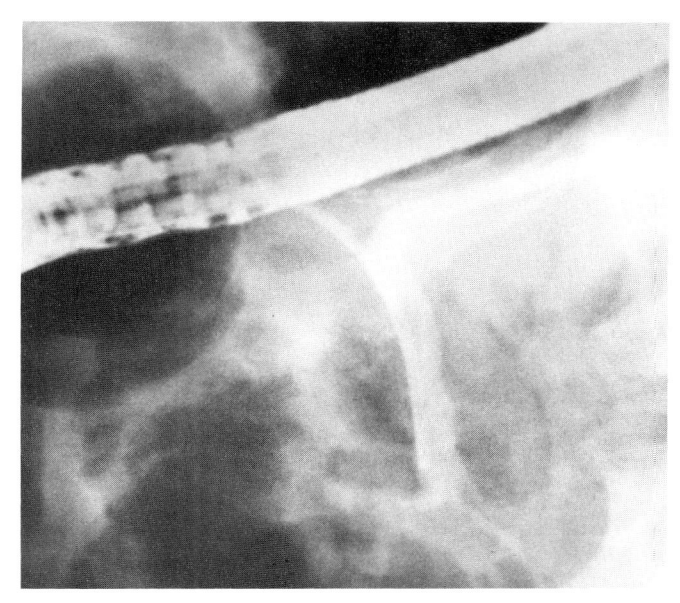

Figure 14-5 Retrograde cholangioscopy through choledochoduodenotomy in patient originally felt to have distal cholangiocarcinoma. Endoscopic diagnosis: Papillary stenosis.

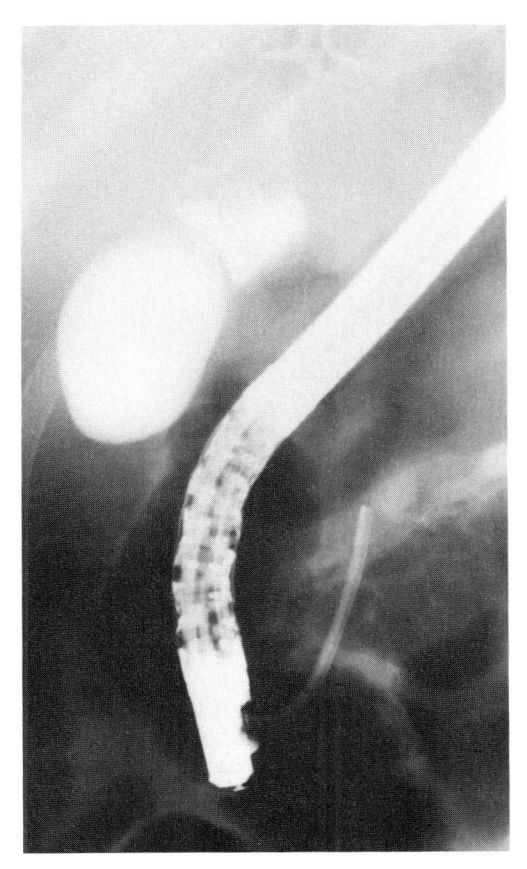

Figure 14-6 Direct pancreatoscopy utilizing a 7 Fr scope in patient with carcinoma of head of the pancreas.

258

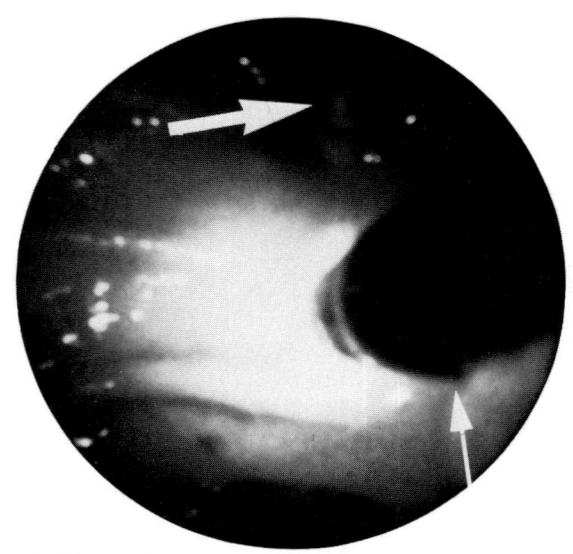

Figure 14-7 (Plate 6) 6 Fr miniscope (small arrow) at time of insertion into papilla (large arrow).

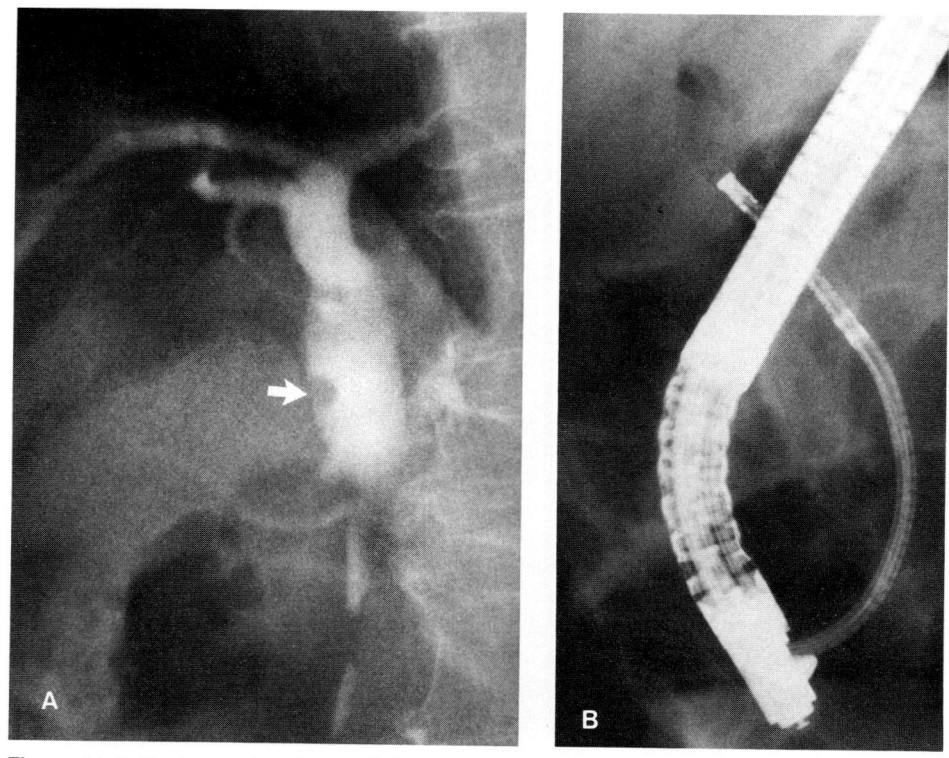

Figure 14-8 (A) Arrow depicts small filling defect in CBD in elderly patient with recurrent cholangitis. **(B)** 11 Fr miniscope evaluating filling defect depicted in 8A. Lesion was submucosal nodule at cystic duct entrance. Patient had previous cholecystectomy.

Multiple limitations were noted with most of the instruments tested. Most important was scope fragility. This was a particular problem with miniscopes that utilized a fused as opposed to an individual fiber bundle system. Fused bundle systems, while much cheaper to produce than acid-leached fiber bundles, will fracture altogether, leading to a total loss of vision and system blackout. This occurred frequently in early production models of some Microvasive and American-Edwards instruments and has been the target of extensive study by these companies. The use of finer fibers, more durable sheath material, and passage over guidewires or through protective sheaths are all mechanisms of protection that have been recently addressed. Moreover, the development of a "disposable" shaft system in conjunction with a permanent head is a unique approach that will allow the endoscopist to vary fiber diameter and length to fit the technical situation. Most instruments sustained damage at the level of the mother scopes' elevator or proximally at the biopsy channel. Olympus addressed the latter problem by using an introducer system which helps to feed the miniscope through the biopsy channel and prevent kinking at the insertion point. It has also contained its larger "ultrathin" scope in metal and Teflon sheathing, assuring greater durability but at a much higher cost than the other miniscopes evaluated.

A number of other limitations were shared by most of the miniscopes used. For instance, all but the largest Olympus instruments lacked tip deflection and an automatic suction device. In addition, only the largest Olympus instrument had a port for automatic air or water installation. In the former case, lack of tip deflection was partially compensated for by use of the miniscope over a guidewire and position or elevator change with the parent scope. Nevertheless, this led to only piecemeal ductal visualization if the miniscope tip was against the ductal wall. Lack of automatic suction and air/water installation was a problem in the setting of previously injected contrast solution or with viscous bile or pancreatic juice. Accordingly, use of a syringe on the biopsy port to aspirate fluid or inject air or water to ensure a clear visual medium was often necessary. In most cases this required guidewire removal, making further scope passage tenuous.

Additional problems included the clumsiness associated with two eye pieces (those of the conventional endoscope plus miniscope). This can be obviated with a second endoscopist in the room or using a minicam and monitor system for the parent instrument. Ultimately, with chip miniaturization and refinement, both the mini and conventional endoscopes could be video systems with images projected on a split-screen monitor system. Finally, photographic capabilities were limited with most instruments (Figure 14-9A–E, **Plates 7–11**). A high-speed film (400 or greater) and 300 W light source were necessary to obtain photographs, even with larger instruments. The long exposure time required to ensure adequate light with 7-Fr or smaller miniscopes was often associated with motion artifact. Even when clear and adequately illuminated, however, the image can appear minute on a 35-mm slide.

Despite the litany of concerns and technical limitations elaborated above, the 13 years that have transpired since the introduction and "rediscovery" of miniscopes has assured their continued evolution. With additional technologic refinements to include improved light bundles and sheath material, directionability, accessory equipment miniaturization, and the testing of ancillary therapeutic modalities, very small caliber cholangiopancreatoscopes should ultimately play a limited but definite role in the future of GI endoscopy.

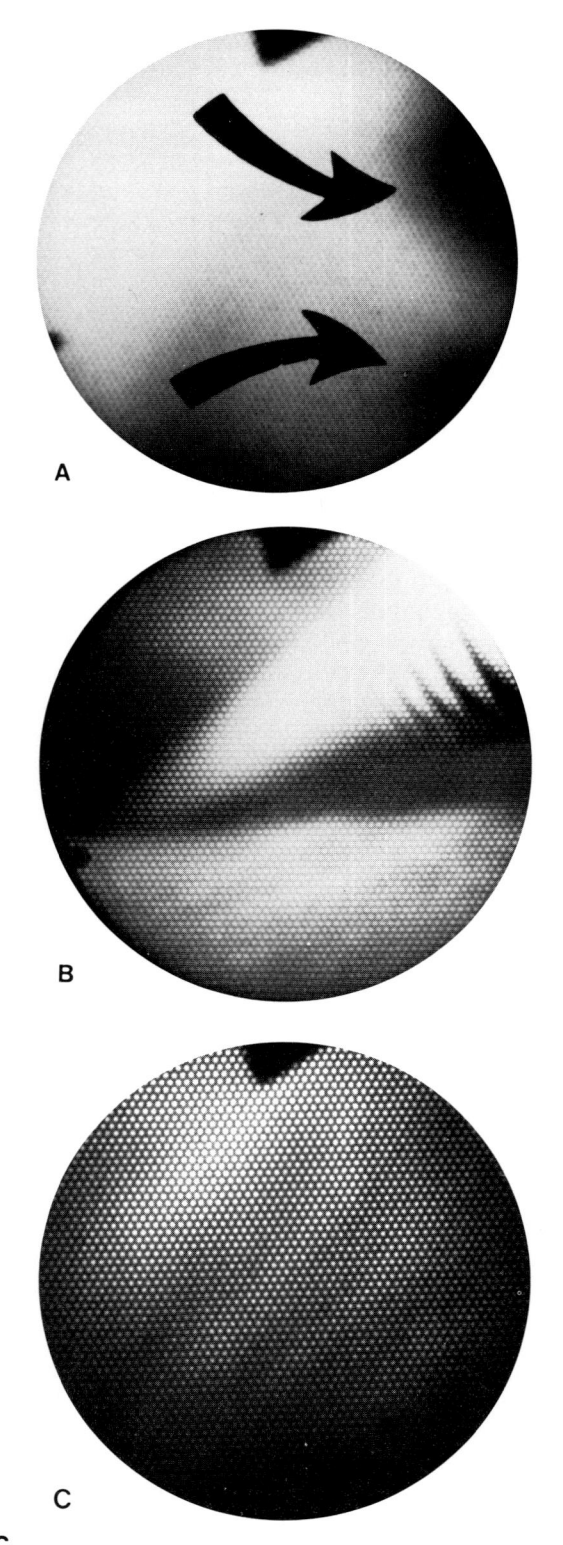

Figure 14-9 A, B, C

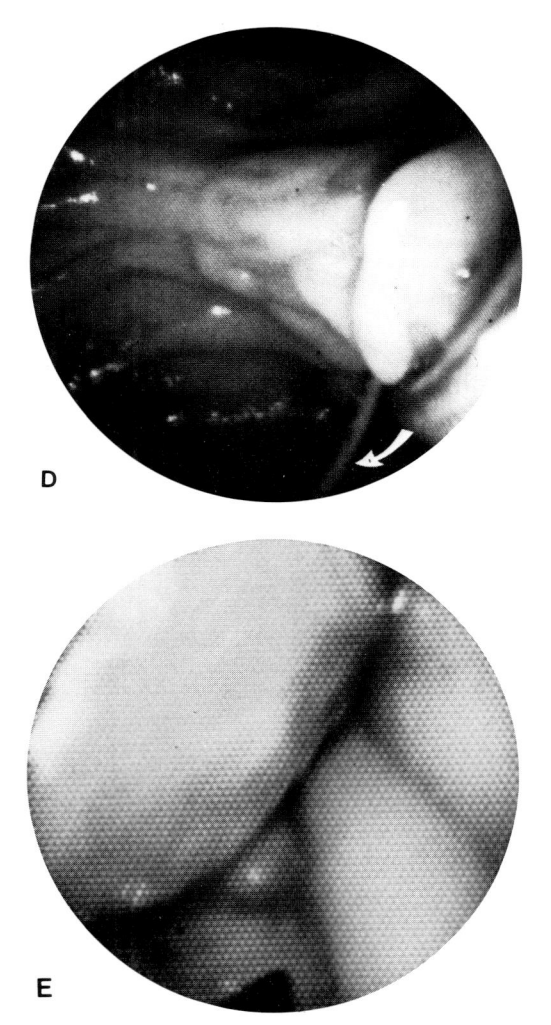

Figure 14-9 (A) (Plate 7) Bifurcation of common hepatic duct (arrows) seen with miniscope. **(B) (Plate 8)** Common bile duct seen through 8.7 Fr miniscope. Note guidewire. **(C) (Plate 9)** Pancreatic duct wall in patient with chronic pancreatitis. Note ductal irregularity. **(D) (Plate 10)** 14 Fr miniscope in patient who underwent laser lithotripsy for large CBD stone. Arrow shows nasobiliary drain. **(E) (Plate 11)** CBD stone in patient depicted in Figure 9D. Note nasobiliary drain.

References

1. Takekoshi, Mariyama M, Sugiyama N, et al: Retrograde cholangiopancreatoscopy. *Gastroent Endosc (Japan)* 1975;17:678–683.
2. Rösch W, Koch H, and Demling L: Peroral cholangioscopy. *Endoscopy* 1976;8:172–173.
3. Nakajima M, Akasaka Y, and Yamaguchi K: Direct endoscopic visualization of the bile and pancreatic duct systems by peroral cholangiopancreatoscopy (PCPS). *Gastrointest Endosc* 1978;24:141–145.

4. Nishioka NS, Teng P, Deutsch TF, and Anderson RR: Mechanism of laser-induced fragmentation of urinary and biliary calculi. *Las Life Sci* 1987;1:231–245.
5. Nishioka NS, Levins PC, Murray SC, et al: Fragmentation of biliary calculi with tunable dye lasers. *Gastroenterology* 1987;93:250–255.
6. Ell CH, Hochberger V, Müller D, et al: Laser lithotripsy of gallstones by means of a pulsed Neodymium-YAG laser: In vitro and animal experiments. *Endoscopy* 1986;18:92–94.
7. Ell CH, Lax G, Hochberger J, et al: Laser lithotripsy of common bile duct stones. *Gut* 1988;29:746–751.
8. Bar-Meir S, and Rotmensch S: A comparison between peroral choledochoscopy and endoscopic retrograde cholangiopancreatography. *Gastrointest Endosc* 1987;33:13–14.
9. Bar-Meir S, and Rotmensch S: Investigation of obstructive jaundice by an ultra-thin caliper endoscope: A new technique for potential use in pregnancy. *Ann J Obstet Gynecol* 1984;150:1003–1004.
10. Kozarek, RA. Direct cholangioscopy and pancratoscopy at time of endoscopic retrograde cholangiopancreatography. *Am J Gastroenterol* 1988;83:55–57.
11. Kozarek RA, Ball TJ, and Low DE: Therapeutic uses of miniscopes. *Gastrointest Endosc* 1988;34:205 (Abstract).
12. Kozarek RA: Miniscopes: A technology in search of an application. *J Clin Gastroenterol,* to be published.
13. Ponchon T, Chavallion A, Ayela P, Lambert R, et al: Retrograde biliary endoscopy for biopsy of stenoses and for lithotripsy. *Gastrointest Endosc* 1988;34:191 (Abstract).
14. Riemann JF, Kohler B, Harloff M, and Weber J: Peroral cholangioscopy—An improved method in the diagnosis of common bile duct diseases. *Gastroenterology* 1988;94:37 (Abstract).
15. Kozarek RA, Low DE, and Ball TJ: Tunable dye laser lithotripsy: In vitro studies and in vivo treatment of choledocholithiasis. *Gastrointest Endosc* 1988;34:418–420.
16. Faulkner DJ, Kozarek RA: Effect of tunable dye laser fragmentation on subsequent gallstone dissolution with methyltert-butylether in vitro. *Radiology,* to be published.

Index

A

Acalculous cholecystitis, association with sphincter of Oddi dysfunction, 153
Accessory papilla, 30
Accessory papillary stenosis
 association with pancreas divisum, 31–32
 problems of assessment, 33
Acute cholangitis. *See* Cholangitis, acute
Acute recurrent pancreatitis. *See* Pancreatitis, acute recurrent
Alcohol, etiological factor in acute pancreatitis, 103
Alcoholic pancreatitis, 75–76
Alkaline phosphatase, serum, elevation in sphincter of Oddi dysfunction, 153
Ampulla of Vater
 reasons for enlargement, 11
 tumors, 11
Ampullary carcinoma
 associated with acute cholangitis, 93
 choice of approach in jaundiced patient, **17**
 endoscopic view of, *12*
 results, in transluminal radiotherapy, 244–245
Ampullary tumors
 associated with Gardner's familial polyposis, 13
 treatment of, 11
Angiography, diagnosis of pancreatic carcinoma, 19
Antibiotics
 indication with ERCP, 10
 use of for poststent management, 213
Atropine, effect of on sphincter of Oddi, 148

B

Bacterial biofilm, mechanism, in stent blockage, 219
Bactobilia, after ES, 128
Balloon
 removal of large common bile duct stones, 80
 treatment, of common bile duct stones, 79
 use during sphincterotomy, stone removal, 52–53
Balloon catheter, method, in treatment of benign biliary duct stricture, 173–175, *173*

Balloon dilation, 157
 need for stent after, 178
 treatment
  pancreatic sphincter dysfunction, 163
  sclerosing cholangitis, 182
Basal sphincter pressure, 140
 in pancreatic and common duct, 142
Basket extraction, as alternative to balloon stone removal, 53
Baskets, in removal of large common bile duct stones, 80
Benzylpenicillin, in treatment of acute cholangitis, 94
Bile
 cholesterol saturation, 128
 contaminated after ES, 128
Bile duct
 common, usual course of, *45*
 correlation of US and ERCP measurements, 14
 free cannulation
  technical options, **45**
  technique, 44–48
 identification of mechanical obstruction with ultrasound, 13–14
 options for stone removal, **56**
Bile duct stones, management after sphincterotomy, 75–89
Biliary colic, clinical sign of bile duct stones, 75
Biliary decompression, preoperative, 225–237
Biliary disease, diagnosis with ERCP, 9–39
Biliary drainage
 external vs. internal, 234–236
 endoscopic, 230–233
 preoperative, endoscopic, 3
 preoperative. *See* Preoperative biliary drainage, duration
Biliary drainage, percutaneous transhepatic. *See* Percutaneous transhepatic biliary drainage (PTBD)
Biliary duct stricture
 appearance, *24*
 benign
  distribution, **176**
  treatment, 173–178
 cause of, 171
 cholangiogram, *172*
 distribution, **176**

263

Biliary duct stricture [cont.]
  endoscopic management, 171–188
  patient profile, **176**
  repair, 171
  results of treatment, **177**
  secondary to chronic pancreatitis, 28
  success of treatment, 175–178
  treatment, complications of, 175–178
Biliary fistulae, 178–181
  treatment, 179
  treatment modalities, **180**
Biliary obstruction
  diagnosis with computerized body tomography, 14
  etiology, **14**
  malignant
    percutaneous transhepatic insertion of catheter in, 204–207
    stents for, 203–224
    surgical bypass, 203–204
Biliary pain, sphincter of Oddi dysfunction, 152
Biliary sphincter ablation, effectiveness against pancreatitis, 162
Biliary sphincter disease
  benign, success of ES following, 159–160
  complications of ES treatment, 158–159
Biliary sphincter dysfunction, 139
  effect of Neocholex in, *146*
Biliary stricture
  benign, treatment of, 3
  choice of approach in jaundiced patient, **17**
Biliary tract fistulae, treatment of with stents, 171
Biliary tract malignancy, iridium-192 irradiation in, 239–250
Biliary-cutaneous fistulae, 178
Biliary-pancreatic sphincter dysfunction
  gastrointestinal smooth muscle disorders associated with, 164
  treatment, 157–158
Biliary-peritoneal fistulae, 178
Bilirubin
  levels in choledocholithiasis, 76
  serum, levels after biliary drainage, 232, 234
Billroth II anastomsosis
  indication for percutaneous transhepatic retrograde endoscopy, 57
  and success with ERCP, 10
Billroth II gastrojejunostomy, and ERCP, 16
Bleeding. *See* Hemorrhage
Bubbles, air, distinguishing from common bile duct stones, 77
Bypass surgery, carcinoma of pancreas, 215–216

C

CA 19-9, serologic assay, pancreatic carcinoma, 19
Calcium bilirubinate stones, characteristics of RPC, 101
Calcium channel blockers, effect on sphincter of Oddi, 148–149
Cannulation
  free, technique with ERCP, 44–48
  selective, use of in endoscopic stenting, 210–211
Carcinoma
  ampulla, preoperative biliary decompression, 225–237
  gallbladder, 203
  pancreas, 203, 213–220
  surgical bypass, mortality of, 204
Catheter, percutaneous
  mortality of, 205
  treatment, in biliary obstruction, 204–207
Catheters, types of, *197*
CBD. *See* Bile duct, common, usual course
CBT. *See* Computerized body tomography
CCK. *See* Cholecystokinin
Cephalosporin, treatment
  acute cholangitis, 94
  acute pancreatitis, 105
Charcot's triad, clinical sign, bile duct stones, 75
Chiba thin-needle technique, 1
Cholangiocarcinoma. *See also* Carcinoma, gallbladder
  associated with sclerosing cholangitis, 185
  choice of approach in jaundiced patient, **17**
  radiotherapy, 239
  results, transluminal radiotherapy, 244–245
  use of PTC, 16
Cholangiogram, multiple calculi, *78*
Cholangiography, choice in jaundiced patient, **17**
Cholangiopancreatoscopy, direct, 251–263
Cholangitis,
  acute
    associated with acute pancreatitis, 115–118
    association of ampullary carcinoma with, 93
    bacteria involved, **94**
    biochemical features, **115**
    causes, **93**
    clinical features, 91–92, **92**
    comparison of complications, **98**
    comparison of risk factors, **97**, **99**
    empyema of gallbladder as complication, 99
    etiology, 92–93
    management, 93–94
    medical treatment, 94–95
    outcome of various treatments, **96**
    parasitic infestation as cause, 117–118
    pathogenesis, 93
    surgical decompression, 95
    treatment
      endoscopic sphincterotomy, 96–101
      PTBD, 95
  after biliary drainage, 232
  clinical sign of bile duct stones, 75
  complication, endoscopic sphincterotomy, 65–68
  as late complication, endoscopic sphincterotomy, 70–71
  recurrent pyogenic, 101–102, 115
    stones characteristic of, 101
    treatment, 102
  sclerosing, treatment, 172

Cholecystectomy
  effect of sphincter pressure and response to hormones, 151
  following acute pancreatitis attack, 114
  following ES, 131
  role of ES before, 134–136
Cholecystitis
  acalculous, association with sphincter of Oddi dysfunction, 153
  acute
    as late complication, endoscopic sphincterotomy, 70
    complication, endoscopic sphincterotomy, 70
  following ES, 130–131
  nonvisualization of gallbladder is predictive, 131, 134
  risk of after endoscopic sphincterotomy, 128
  symptoms similar to sphincter of Oddi dysfunction, 151
Cholecystokinin
  challenge test with to evaluaton adequacy of ES, 158
  effect on sphincter of Oddi, 144
  paradoxical response of sphincter of Oddi and pancreatic sphincter, 145–147
Cholecystostomy, treatment, acute cholangitis, 95
Choledochal cysts, detection following acute pancreatitis, 114
Choledochocele, as cause of acute recurrent pancreatitis, **191**
Choledochoduodenal fistulotomy. *See* Cannulation, free, technique with ERCP
Choledochoduodenostomy, treatment, acute cholangitis, 95
Choledocholithiasis. *See also* Bile duct stones
  appearance, *52*
  assessment for surgery, 15
  diagnosis with ultrasound, 13
  laboratory findings, 76
  minimally dilated duct, *56*
  sensitivity of ultrasound in, **13**
  sphincterotomy as treatment of choice, 2
  symptoms similar to sphincter of Oddi dysfunction, 151
Chorangioscopy, retrograde, cholangiocarcinoma, *257*
Chronic pancreatitis, 191–194. *See* Pancreatitis, chronic
Clonorchis sinensis, implication in RPC, 101
Computerized body tomography, 9
  comparison with ERCP, diagnosis of pancreatic carcinoma, 20
  diagnosis of biliary obstruction, 14
Congestive heart failure, differential diagnosis from common bile duct stones, 77
Cystoduodenostomy, treatment, chronic pancreatitis, 193, 194
Cystogastrostomy, endoscopic, treatment, chronic pancreatitis, 193, 194

D

DAT. *See* Duodenal appearance time
Dietary fat, paradoxical response of sphincter of Oddi and pancreatic sphincter, 145–147
Dietary management, treatment, biliary-pancreatic sphincter dysfunction, 157
Dissolution techniques, treatment, common bile duct stones, 84–86
Diverticulum, indication for percutaneous transhepatic retrograde endoscopy, 57
Dormia basket, 1, 95
Double-duct sign, indicator of pancreatic carcinoma, 21
Drains, placement, percutaneous vs. endoscopic, 16–18
Duct of Santorini, 31
Duct stones, common
  choice of approach in jaundiced patient, **17**
  diagnosis, 14
Duct of Wirsung, appearance, *31*
Duodenal appearance time, 156

E

EBD. *See* Endoscopic biliary drainage
Electrohydraulic lithotripsy, 3
Empyema, gallbladder
  complication of acute cholangitis, 99
  following ES, 130
  treatment, 100–101
Endoprostheses. *See* Stents
Endoscopes
  small caliber, 251
  type for stent placement, 207
Endoscopic biliary drainage, 230–233
  cholangitis following, 232
  success rate, 232
  success rate in relieving jaundice, 232–233
  techniques, 230
  treatment
    jaundice, 233
    pancreatic cancer, 232
Endoscopic retrograde cholangiopancreatography (ERCP)
  accuracy in pancreatic carcinoma diagnosis, 21
  acute cholangitis, 91–102
  acute pancreatitis, 102–120
  acute pancreatitis following, 191
  as therapeutic tool, 172
  combined with manometry, complications, 144
  comparison
    with CBT, diagnosis of pancreatic carcinoma, 20
    with percutaneous transhepatic cholangiography, 15–16
  complication rate, 10
  complications, treatment biliary duct stricture, 175–178
  contributions to diagnosis, 11–13
  cost, 10–11
  detection of common bile duct stones, 190
  development, 1
  diagnosis
    of biliary disease, 9–39
    of jaundiced patient, 13–18
    of pancreatic carcinoma, 18–22

Endoscopic retrograde [cont.]
   of pancreatic disease, 9–39
     sclerosing cholangitis, 182
  diagnostic
    free cannulation technique, 44–48
    technique, 43–44
  indications for antibiotic treatment, 10
  initial resistance to procedure, 9–11
  major advantage of, 11
  role in management of acute pancreatitis, 110–114
  routine use in acute pancreatitis, 190
  safety in diagnosis and treatment of acute pancreatitis, 189
  safety of in treatment of acute pancreatitis, 107–109, **108**
  training for, 10
  treatment
    benign biliary duct stricture, 173–176
    biliary fistula, 179
  value in pancreatitis, 22–29
Endoscopic retrograde sphincterotomy
  importance of disinfection, 41–42
  indications for, **42**
  preparation for, 41–43
  technical steps, **42**
  technique, 41–59
  treatment, common bile duct stones, 79
Endoscopic sphincterotomy
  acute cholecystitis as complication, 70
  appearance, *54–55*
  cholangitis as complication, 65–66
  cholecystectomy following, 131
  cholesterol saturation of bile after, 128
  complication rate, 61
  complications, 61–73
  complications for biliary sphincter disease, 158
  complications following, 98, **98**
  early complications, **62**
  evaluation of adequacy, 158
  factors associated with mortality, 96
  follow-up of patients, 128
  gallstone formation following, 128–129
  hemorrhage, 61–63
  history, 1
  impacted basket as complication, 69
  late complications, 70–71
  long-term follow-up of patients with intact gallbladder, **132–133**
  pancreatitis as complication, 63–65
  in patients with intact gallbladder, 127–137
  physiological alterations in biliary tract, 127–128
  as preferred treatment for duct stones, 1–2
  results of treatment of acute pancreatitis with, 107
  retroperitoneal perforation as complication, 66–69
  risk of cholecystitis after, 128
  risk of gallbladder disease following, 129
  role before cholecystectomy, 134–136
  safety of for treatment of acute pancreatitis, 107–109, **108**
  success after benign biliary sphincter disease, 159–161
  success rate, 98
  treatment
    acute cholangitis, 96–101
    biliary fistula, 179
    biliary fistula, success, 181
    biliary sphincter dysfunction, 157
    chronic pancreatitis, 192
    pancreatic sphincter dysfunction, 163–164
    pancreatic sphincter stenosis, 163–164
Endoscopic stents. *See* Stents, endoscopic
Endoscopic techniques, management of benign strictures, 171–188
Endoscopic treatment. *See also* Balloon dilation; Nasobiliary tube, treatment, biliary fistula; Spincterotomy; Stents
  nonmalignant pancreatic disease, 189–201
  sclerosing cholangitis, 181–182
Endoscopic ultrasound, diagnosis of pancreatic carcinoma, 20
Endoscopy. *See also* Miniscopes
  complications, 212
Epigastric pain, sphincter of Oddi dysfunction, 152
Epinephrine, treatment of hemorrhage, post sphincterotomy, 63
ERCP. *See* Endoscopic retrograde cholangiopancreatography
ERS. *See* Endoscopic retrograde sphincterotomy
Escherichia coli, implication in RPC, 101
Esophageal motility disorders, 164
Ethylene diamine teraacetic acid (EDTA), dissolution of common bile duct stones, 85
EUS. *See* Endoscopic ultrasound, diagnosis of pancreatic carcinoma
Extracorporeal shock wave lithotripsy, 3

F

Familial polyposis, Gardner's, association of ampullary tumors with, 13
Fatty meal. *See* Neocholex
Fatty meal ultrasonography, sphincter of Oddi, 147–148
Fever, as complication of ERCP, 10
Fistulae
  biliary. *See* Biliary fistulae
  identification with ERCP, 112

G

Gallbladder
  carcinoma, 203
    results, transluminal radiotherapy, 245–246
  disease
    ES patients compared with general population, 134
    following ES, 130
  empyemia
    as complication of acute cholangitis, 99, 100–101
    following ES, 130
  intact, long-term follow-up of patients following ES, 132–133

Gallbladder-related illness, risk factors, 131–134
Gallstone pancreatitis, 106–109
  advisability of ERCP, 25
Gallstones
  associated with acute pancreatitis, 103
  detection of following acute pancreatitis, 114
  endoscopic sphincterotomy, 127–137
  fate after ES, 129
  formation after ES, 128–129
  fracture with lasers, 253
Gastrointestinal smooth muscle disorders, associated with biliary-pancreatic sphincter dysfunction, 164
Gentamicin, treatment, acute cholangitis, 94
Glucagon
  effect on sphincter of Oddi, 145
  use in manometry, 141
Guidewire
  free cannulation, 44–46
  placement of stent in pancreatic duct, 196, *196*

H
HBS. *See* Hepatobiliary scintigraphy
Hemorrhage
  complication, sphincterotomy, 212
  occurrence with endoscopic sphincterotomy, 61–63
Hemosuccus pancreaticus, diagnosis with ERCP, 113–114
Hepatic abscess. *See* Liver abscess
Hepatobiliary scintigraphy, sphincter of Oddi dysfunction, 156–157
Hepatocellular disease, choice of approach in jaundiced patient, 17
Hilar metastases, result, transluminal radiotherapy, 245–246
Hilar strictures, malignant, 216–218
Hormones, gastrointestinal, effects on sphincter of Oddi, 144–145
Hyperamylasemia, complication, endoscopic sphincterotomy, 63

I
Idiopathic recurrent pancreatitis, monometry to diagnose, 161
Imaging techniques, 9
Impacted basket, complication, endoscopic sphincterotomy, 69
Iridium-192, physical properties, **241**
Iridium-192 irradiation, biliary tract malignancy, 239–250
Iridium-192 radiotherapy, complications, 246
Iridium-192 wire, structure, 243

J
Jaundice
  clinical sign of bile duct stones, 75
  diagnosis of common bile duct stones, methods, 77
  malignant obstructive, management, *220*
  treatment, endoscopic biliary drainage, 232

Jaundiced patient
  choice of cholangiography, **17**
  diagnosis with ERCP, 13–18

L
Laser therapy, 3
Lasers, treatment
  common bile duct stones, 84
  treatment, stones, 254
Lipase, elevated in acute pancreatitis, 103
Lithotripsy, 3
  electrohydraulic, fragmentation of common bile duct stones, 82–83
  extracorporeal, dissolution of stones, 44
  extracorporeal focused shock wave, treatment of duct and gallbladder stones, 83–84
  extracorporeal shock wave, in case of impacted basket, 69
  mechanical, in case of impacted basket, 69
  mechanical or electrohydraulic, removal of bile duct stones, 56
  ultrasonic, treatment, gallbladder and common bile duct stones, 84
Lithotripter
  electrohydraulic, *83*
  mechanical, removal of large common bile duct stones, 81
  mechanical or electrohydraulic, dissolution of stones, 44
Liver abscess
  bile duct stones as complication, 76
  differential diagnosis from common bile duct stones, 76

M
Magnetic resonance imaging, 9
Malignancy, biliary tract, iridium-192 irradiation, 239–250
Malignant hilar strictures, 216–218
Manometry
  endoscopic biliary-pancreatic, complications, 144
  method, sphincter of Oddi, 140–141
  pancreatic sphincter dysfunction, 161
  precautions for pancreas divisum, 141
  use of transducers, 141
Mediastinal pseudocyst, diagnosis with ERCP, 112
Methyl tert-butyl ether
  dissolution, common bile duct stones, 84
  removal of bile duct stones, 56
  treatment, acute cholangitis, 95
Metoclopramide, treatment, gastric retention, 164
Metranidazole, treatment, acute cholangitis, 94
Microtransducers, use during manometry, 141
Migrating motor complex, sphincter of Oddi, 142
Miniscopes, 251, *254. See also* Cholangiopancreatoscopy, direct
  bifurcation of common hepatic duct, *261*
  in common bile duct, *255*
  diagnostic use, 254–255

Miniscopes [*cont.*]
    evaluation, 252, 254
    insertion in common bile duct, recurrent cholangitis, 260f
    insertion into papilla, *258*
    limitations, 257–258
    therapeutic use, 255–256
    types, 254
Monooctanion
    dissolution
        common bile duct stones, 84
        of stones, 44
    removal of bile duct stones, 56
    treatment, acute cholangitis, 95
Morphine
    effect on sphincter of Oddi, 148
    effect on sphincter pressures, *150*
Morphine-prostigmine test
    for biliary-pancreatic sphincter dysfunction, 154–155
    skepticism about utility of, 155
MPT. *See* Morphine-prostigmine test
MTBE. *See* Methyl tert butyl ether
Myocardial infarction, acute, differential diagnosis from common bile duct stones, 76–77

N

Nasobiliary catheter
    intraluminal irradiation, 241–242
    treatment, sclerosing cholangitis, 182
Nasobiliary drainage, importance following endoscopic sphincterotomy, 66
Nasobiliary tube, treatment, biliary fistula, 179
Needle knife, 47–48
Neocholex. *See also* Fatty meal
    utrasonography, sphincter of Oddi
    effect on basal sphincter pressures, *149*
    effect of choledochal sphincter pressure, *146*
Neodynium-YAG laser, treatment, common bile duct stones, 84
Nifedipine
    effect on cholecochal sphincter pressure, *151*
    effect on sphincter of Oddi, 149
Nitrates, treatment, biliary-pancreatic sphincter dysfunction, 157
Nitrites, treatment, biliary-pancreatic sphincter dysfunction, 157
Nitroglycerin, effect on sphincter of Oddi, 148
Nuclear medicine scans, 9
5-Nucleotidase, levels during choledocholithiasis, 76

P

Pain
    abdominal, pancreas divisum as cause, 194
    sphincter of Oddi dysfunction, 152–153
    unexplained, suspected pancreatic or biliary, 29–33
    upper abdominal, biliary and pancreatic sphincter disorder, 164–165
Pancreas, carcinoma, 203, 213–220

Pancreas divisum, 194–196
    appearance, *27*
    as cause of acute pancreatitis, 194
    as cause of acute recurrent pancreatitis, **191**
    association with accessory papillary stenosis, 31–32
    association with sphincter of Oddi dysfunction, 154
    connection with recurrent pancreatic pain, 31
    description, 30
    diagnosis, 31
    incidence, 30
    obstructive pancreatitis, 162
    precautions for during manometry, 141
    treatment, ES, 163
Pancreatic ascites, treatment, 29
Pancreatic cancer
    characteristic ERCP appearance, *22–23*
    choice of approach in jaundiced patient, **17**
    ERCP diagnosis, basis for, 21
    treatment, endoscopic biliary drainage, 232
Pancreatic carcinoma
    diagnostic strategies, 18–22
    diagnostic strategy, 21–22
    double-duct sign, 21
    radiotherapy, 239
    results, transluminal radiotherapy, 244–245
    serologic assays, 18–19
    treatment, surgical bypass, 215–216
Pancreatic disease
    benign, stent placement, **193**
    diagnosis with ERCP, 9–39
    endoscopic therapy, 3
    nonmalignant, endoscopic treatment, 189–201
Pancreatic duct pressures, 143
Pancreatic fistula, treatment, 29
Pancreatic pseudocysts, treatment, 28
Pancreatic sphincter
    dysfunction
        cause, idiopathic pancreatitis, 162–163
        treatment, 163–164
    effect of drugs, 148–150
Pancreatic sphincterotomy, 198–199
Pancreatic-type pain, patients with pancreatic sphincter stenosis or dysfunction, 161–163
Pancreatitis
    acute
        appearance of pseudocysts, 110
        associated with acute cholangitis, 115–118
        biochemical features, **115**
        clinical course, 104–105
        complications, 104
        CT scan, *116*
        definition, 103
        ERCP as treatment, 109–110
        etiology, 103–104
        following ERCP, 191
        management, 105, **105**
        parasitic infestation as cause, 117–118
        pathogenesis, 103–104
        prediction of severity of outcome, **104**, 104–105

results of ES treatment, **107**
role of ERCP in management, 110–114
routine use of ERCP, 190
safety of ERCP diagnosis and treatment, 189
safety of sphincterotomy, 189
surgery as treatment, 109
treatment, 105–106
acute gallstone, safety of ERCP and ES as treatment, **108**, 107–109
acute recurrent, 190–191
etiology, 190
alcoholic, 75–76
and bile duct stones, 75
chronic, 191–194
bile duct strictures secondary to, 28
choice of approach in jaundiced patient, **17**
ductal changes following stent insertion, *195*
ductal morphology determined by ERCP, 25
etiology, **192**
sphincterotomy, 192
treatment approach, 26
treatment with stents, 192
treatment, removal of pancreatic debris, 193
complicated by pseudocyst formation, 193
complication of endoscopic sphincterotomy, 63–65
complication, sphincterotomy, 212
gallstone
advisability of ERCP, 25
diagnosis, 106–109
mortality, 106
treatment, 106–109
hereditary, treatment approach, 25–26
idiopathic
appearance, *26*
basal pancreatic duct sphincter pressures, 162
caused by pancreatic sphincter dysfunction, 162–163
dysfunction of pancreatic sphincter associated with, 154
recurrent, manometry to diagnose, 161
obstructive, pancreas divisum, 162
in patients with pancreatic sphincter stenosis, dysfunction, 161–163
prevention of following endoscopic sphincterotomy, 65
prevention of recurrent attacks, 114
recurrent, pancreas divisum, *27*
sphincterotomy as treatment, 2
and success rate of ERCP, 1
technique for placing stent, 196–199
treatment after ERCP, 64
treatment with somatostatin, 163
value of ERCP, 22–29
Pancreatography, avoidance for ERCP, 44
Pancreatorrhagia, diagnosis with ERCP, 113–114
Pancreatoscopy, carcinoma of head of pancreas, 257

Papillotome, precut, use in free-cannulation technique, 46
Parasitic infestation, cause of acute pancreatitis or cholangitis, 117–118
Precutaneous cholangiogram, cholangiocarcinoma, *256*
Percutaneous fistulae, diagnosis, 178
Percutaneous transhepatic biliary drainage (PTBD)
effect on postoperative mortality, **226**
mortality, **228, 229**
prospective randomized trials, 229–230
retrospective trials, 226–229
success in relieving jaundice, 232–233
success rate, 232
treatment, acute cholangitis, 95
Percutaneous transhepatic cholangiography, development, 1
Percutaneous transhepatic cholangiography
advantage in cholangiocarcinoma, 16
comparison with ERCP, 15–16
Percutaneous transhepatic retrograde endoscopy, indications for, 57
Perforation
complication, sphincterotomy, 212
as result of ERCP, 10
retroperitoneal
complication of endoscopic sphincterotomy, 66–68
predisposing factors, 69
treatment, 67, 69
Peritoneal fistula, diagnosis, 178
Peritoneal lavage, value as treatment, acute pancreatitis, 106
Phasic wave activity, 140
sphincter of Oddi, 142
Postcholecystectomy syndrome, 29
sphincter of Oddi dysfunction associated, 154
PRBD, treatment option in acute cholangitis, 101
Precut papillotomy. *See* Cannulation, free, technique with ERCP
Preoperative biliary decompression, carcinoma of ampulla, 225–237
Preoperative biliary drainage, duration, 233–234
Prostheses. *See* Stents
Pseudocyst
appearance in acute pancreatitis, 110
complication, pancreatitis, 193
pancreatic, treatment, 28
pancreatitis related, 194
treatment, 110
Pseudomomas
complicating factor in ES treatment of acute cholangitis, 99
risk of infection from in ERS, 42
Pseudomonas aeruginosa
infection with following ES, 129
role in post-ERCP cholangitis, 66
PTBD. *See* Percutaneous transhepatic biliary drainage
PTC. *See* Percutaneous transhepatic cholangiography, development

PTD. *See* Percutaneous transhepatic biliary drainage
PTHC, treatment option in acute cholangitis, 101
Puestow procedure, 27
 success rate, 30

Q

Quantitative biliary scintigraphy, sphincter of Oddi, 147–148

R

Radiotherapeutic agents, implantation through endoscopes, 3
Radiotherapy
 intraluminal
  complications, 241
  malignancy, bile duct, **240**
  technique, 241–244
 iridium-192, 239–250
 survival times, 240
 transluminal
  complications, 246
  preparation of radiation source, 242–244
  results, 244–248
  survival rates, 246–247
Recurrent pyogenic cholangitis, 101–102, 115
Retroduodenal artery
 detection with Doppler ultrasound, 62
 source of hemorrhage after sphincterotomy, 62
Retroduodenal phlegmon, duodenal perforation, *69*
Roux-en-Y anastomosis, and ERCP, 16
RPC. *See* Recurrent pyogenic cholangitis

S

Sclerosant, treatment of hemorrhage post sphincterotomy, 63
Sclerosing cholangitis
 associated with cholangiocarcinoma, 185
 with biliary duct stricture, cholangiogram, *184*
 choice of approach in jaundiced patient, *17*
 cholangiogram, *183*
 course of treatment, 185
 therapy, **181**
 treatment, 3, 172
 results, **185**
Secretin, effect on sphincter of Oddi, 144–145
Secretin-ultrasound provocation test, sphincter of Oddi stenosis, 156
Selective cannulation, bile duct, endoscopic stenting, 210–211
Serum alkaline phosphatase, levels in choledocholithiasis, 76
Serum amylase
 elevation in acute pancreatitis, 103
 elevation in sphincter of Oddi dysfunction, 153
Serum glutamicoxaloacetic transaminase, levels during choledocholithiasis, 76

Skinny needle, 95
SO. *See* Sphincter of Oddi
Somatostatin
 effect on sphincter of Oddi, 145
 treatment, pancreatitis, 163
Sphincter dysfunction, biliary-pancreatic, morphine-prostigmine provocative test, 154–155
Sphincter of Oddi
 clinical manifestations of dysfunction, 151–153
 detection of stenosis, test for, 156
 determination of motility, 140–142
 diagnosis of dysfunction, 140
 dysfunction
  as cause of acute recurrent pancreatitis, **191**
  association with biliary-pancreatic disorders, 153–154
  biliary pain, 152
  epigastric pain, 152
  episodes of pain, 152–153
  hepatobiliary scintigraphy, 156–157
  laboratory abnormalities, 153
 effect of
  drugs, 148–150
  gastrointestinal hormones, 144
  glucagon, 145
  secretin, 144–145
  somatostatin, 145
 fatty meal ultrasonography, 147–148
 function and dysfunction, 139–170
 historical perspective, 139–140
 manometric studies, 140–141
 manometry, 3
 normal values, 142–144
 quantitative biliary scintigraphy, 147–148
 response to CCK, 145–147
 tachyarrhythmia, 142
Sphincteroplasty, testing patients who would benefit, 154–155
Sphincterotome, *46*
 preferred design, 48
 two-channel, use in free-cannulation technique, 45–46
 types, *47*
 use in selective cannulation, 210–211
 wire-guided, 57
Sphincterotomy
 complication rate, 2
 endoscopic. *See* Endoscopic sphincterotomy
 indication for, 48
 management of bile duct stones retained after, 75–89
 other techniques, 57–58
 pancreatic, 198–199
 standard, technique, 48–57
 wire position during, *51*
Sphincters. *See* Biliary sphincter; Pancreatic sphincter; Sphincter of Oddi; specific entries
 basal pressures, 142
Stents
 advisability in treatment of acute cholangitis, 101
 biliary, blockage, 219–220

biliary obstruction, malignant, 203–224
blockage, diagnosis, 213
causes of occlusion, 176–177
choice of material for, 177
chonic pancreatitis, 191–192
design, 218–220
endoscopic
  as alternative to bypass surgery for carcinoma of pancreas, 215–216
  hilar strictures, 217, **217**
  mortality and complication data vs. percutaneous stents, **206**
  mortality, 205
  placement, 2–3
  results, treatment carcinoma of pancreas, **214**, 214
  selective cannulation, 210–211
  technique, 207–210
  treatment, carcinoma of pancreas, 213–215
failure in pancreatic diseases, **194**
intraluminal irradiation, 241–242
management after placement, 213
maximum outside diameter, 218
method of placement and postoperative mortality, 235–236
percutaneous, mortality and complications data vs. endoscopic stents, **206**
pigtail, removal of bile duct stones, 56
position, pancreas, **198, 199**
placement in benign pancreatic disease, **193**
placement, percutaneous vs. endoscopic, 16–18
problems with placement in pancreas divisum patients, **196**
straight-barbed, *197*
structure, 220
technique for placing in pancreatic duct, 196–199
treatment, biliary tract fistulae, 171
treatment, large common bile duct stones, 81–82
treatment, pancreas divisum, 194
use, biliary duct stricture, 176–177
wandering, removal, *199*
Stones. *See also* Choledocholithiasis
  bile duct
    clinical manifestations, 75–76
    management after sphincterotomy, 75–89
    options for removal, **56**
  common bile duct
    as complication of liver abscess, 76
    comparison of surgical and ES treatment, **100**
    detection with ERCP, 190
    diagnosis, 77–78
    differential diagnosis, 76–77
    distinguishing from air bubbles, 77
    ERS treatment, 79

fragmentation techniques, 82–84
laboratory findings, 76
large, management, **80**
occurrence in acute pancreatitis, 103
problems with large stones, 80–82
treatment, 78–79
  dissolution techniques, 84–85
gallbladder, comparison of surgery and ES treatment, **100**
methods for dissolution in ERS, 44
removal, balloon vs. basket, 52–53
Stricture
  bile duct
    appearance, *24*
    secondary to chronic pancreatitis, 28
  biliary duct. *See* Biliary duct stricture
  hilar, complication, endoscopy, 212
  intubation and dilation, 211–212
Surgery, carcinoma of pancreas, resectable, 216
Surgical bypass, mortality, 204
Surgical decompression, treatment, acute cholangitis, 95

T

T tube
  cholangiogram, treatment, common bile duct stones, 79
  complications of placement, 178
Tachyoddia, 142
Trypsin, factor in acute pancreatitis, 103
Tunable dye laser, treatment, common bile duct stones, 84
Two-channel sphincterotome, use in free cannulation technique, 45–46

U

Ultrasound, 9
  after acute pancreatitis attack, 114
  diagnosis of jaundiced patient, 13
  diagnosis of pancreatic carcinoma, 20
  fatty meal, sphincter of Oddi, 147–148
  identification of mechanical obstruction, bile ducts, 13–14
  sensitivity in choledocholithiasis, **13**
  value in management of acute cholangitis, 94
Ursodeosycholic acid, treatment, large common bile duct stones, 82
US. *See* Ultrasound

W

Whipple pancreatoduodenectomy, 28
Whipple procedure, 11
Wire-guided sphincterotome, 57